IMPACT OF PROCESSING ON FOOD SAFETY

ADVANCES IN EXPERIMENTAL MEDICINE AND BIOLOGY

Recent Volumes in this Series

Volume 450
ADVANCES IN MODELING AND CONTROL OF VENTILATION
Edited by Richard L. Hughson, David A. Cunningham, and James Duffin

Volume 451
GENE THERAPY OF CANCER
Edited by Peter Walden, Uwe Trefzer, Wolfram Sterry, and Farzin Farzaneh

Volume 452
MECHANISMS OF LYMPHOCYTE ACTIVATION AND IMMUNE REGULATION VII:
Molecular Determinants of Microbial Immunity
Edited by Sudhir Gupta, Alan Sher, and Rafi Ahmed

Volume 453
MECHANISMS OF WORK PRODUCTION AND WORK ABSORPTION IN MUSCLE
Edited by Haruo Sugi and Gerald H. Pollack

Volume 454
OXYGEN TRANSPORT TO TISSUE XX
Edited by Antal G. Hudetz and Duane F. Bruley

Volume 455
RHEUMADERM: Current Issues in Rheumatology and Dermatology
Edited by Carmel Mallia and Jouni Uitto

Volume 456
RESOLVING THE ANTIBIOTIC PARADOX:
Progress in Understanding Drug Resistance and Development of New Antibiotics
Edited by Barry P. Rosen and Shahriar Mobashery

Volume 457
DRUG RESISTANCE IN LEUKEMIA AND LYMPHOMA III
Edited by G. J. L. Kaspers, R. Pieters, and A. J. P. Veerman

Volume 458
ANTIVIRAL CHEMOTHERAPY 5: New Directions for Clinical Application and Research
Edited by John Mills, Paul A. Volberding, and Lawrence Corey

Volume 459
IMPACT OF PROCESSING ON FOOD SAFETY
Edited by Lauren S. Jackson, Mark G. Knize, and Jeffrey N. Morgan

---

IMPACT OF PROCESSING ON FOOD SAFETY

Edited by

Lauren S. Jackson

U.S. Food and Drug Administration
Summit-Argo, Illinois

Mark G. Knize

Lawrence Livermore National Laboratory
Livermore, California

and

Jeffrey N. Morgan

U.S. Environmental Protection Agency
Cincinnati, Ohio

Kluwer Academic / Plenum Publishers
New York, Boston, Dordrecht, London, Moscow

Library of Congress Cataloging-in-Publication Data

Impact of processing on food safety / edited by Lauren S. Jackson, Mark G. Knize and Jeffrey N. Morgan.
p. cm. -- (Advances in experimental medicine and biology ; v. 459)
Includes bibliographical references and index.
ISBN 0-306-46051-3
1. Food industry and trade--Congresses. 2. Food--Contamination--Congresses. 3. Food--Effects of heat on--Congresses. I. Jackson, Lauren S. II. Knize, Mark G. III. Morgan, Jeffrey N. IV. Series.
TP372.5.I53 1999
664--dc21 99-11924
CIP

Proceedings of the American Chemical Society Symposium on Impact of Processing on Food Safety, held April 14 – 18, 1997, in San Francisco, California

ISBN 0-306-46051-3

233 Spring Street, New York, N.Y. 10013

10 9 8 7 6 5 4 3 2 1

A C.I.P. record for this book is available from the Library of Congress.

Printed in the United States of America

PREFACE

The contents of this book are the proceedings of the ACS symposium, "Impact of Processing on Food Safety," which was held April 16–17, 1997, at the American Chemical Society National Meeting in San Francisco, CA. This symposium brought together researchers from diverse backgrounds in academia, government, and industry. Twenty speakers discussed topics ranging from the regulatory aspects of food processing to the microbiological and chemical changes in food during processing.

The main goal of food processing is to improve the microbial safety of food by destroying pathogenic and spoilage organisms. Food processing can also improve food safety by destroying or eliminating naturally occurring toxins, chemical contaminants, and antinutritive factors. Unfortunately, processing can also cause chemical changes that result in the formation of toxic or antinutritive factors. The purpose of this book is to summarize our knowledge of both the beneficial and deleterious effects of processing. Chapter 1 considers the consumer's perceptions about food contaminants and food processing. Chapter 2 summarizes the effects of traditional and nontraditional processing methods on microorganisms in food. Chapters 3–6 review the effects of processing on lipids (fatty acids and cholesterol) in food. Changes in the nutritive value of vitamins and minerals as a result of processing are discussed in chapter 7. Chapter 8 concentrates on how processing reduces the allergenicity of some foods. The remaining 8 chapters of the book summarize the effects of processing on the formation and destruction of chemical contaminants (glycoalkaloids, lysinoalanine, heterocyclic aromatic amines, pesticides, environmental contaminants, veterinary drug residues, heavy metals, and mycotoxins) in food.

The symposium organizers would like to thank the ACS Division of Agricultural and Food Chemistry for their approval and financial support of this symposium. We also express our gratitude to the following sponsors: International Fragrances and Flavors (IFF), Flavor and Extract Manufacturers Association (IFF), and Quadralux, Inc. Most of all, the organizers gratefully acknowledge the contribution of the speakers. Without their dedication, expertise, and hard work, publication of these proceedings would not be possible.

Lauren S. Jackson
Mark G. Knize
Jeffrey N. Morgan

CONTENTS

1

CONSUMER PERCEPTIONS AND CONCERNS ABOUT FOOD CONTAMINANTS

Christine M. Bruhn

Center for Consumer Research
University of California
Davis, California 95616-8598

1. ABSTRACT

More consumers are concerned about microbiological hazards than any other area. Pesticide residues generate concern, especially among low income consumers with less formal education. Use of antibiotics and hormones in animal production is considered a serious hazard by fewer consumers. Consumer attitudes are influenced by media coverage. An increasing number of consumers expect food producers and retailers to assume a major role in providing safe food. A majority of consumers express interesting in purchasing irradiated food when specific benefits are described and the percentage increases when irradiation is more fully described. In actual market experiences, irradiated produce and poultry have been well received. Similarly, most consumers are positive toward biotechnology, with greatest support for environmental applications. The scientific community should use the media to reach the public with information identifying risks and protective strategies, including the use of new technology.

2. INTRODUCTION

The lay person may view a contaminant as something unwanted and not naturally present in a food. This review will focus on consumer attitudes toward intentional additions or modifications in processing which some may consider contamination. To place concerns in perspective, consumer confidence in the safety of food in the supermarket has increased in the last ten years. In 1989, 81% were mostly or completely confident in the safety of food in the supermarket. By 1992, confidence dipped to 72%. It gradually increased to 84% in 1996 (Abt Associates, 1996; Opinion Research, 1990).

Impact of Processing on Food Safety, edited by Jackson et al.,
Kluwer Academic / Plenum Publishers, New York, 1999.

3. CONSUMER FOOD SAFETY CONCERNS

Microbiological contamination is the consumer's greatest concern, followed by chemical contamination, such as pesticide or animal drug residues. Nationwide surveys by the Food Marketing Institute indicated more people volunteer concerns about microbiological hazards than any other potential food safety issue. From 1992 to 1996 volunteered concern about microbiological safety increased from 36% to 49% (Abt Associates, 1996). When concern about contamination by bacteria or germs was specifically asked, 77% acknowledged it as a serious hazard. More consumers consider this a serious hazard than any other potential food risk.

Pesticide residues continue to generate concern among a major segment of the population, with 66% of consumers ranking it a serious hazard in 1996. Concern about pesticides has decreased from 82% in 1989 to the current level.

Concern about other food safety areas has also decreased. Those expressing serious concern with antibiotics and hormones used in poultry or livestock decreased from 61% in 1989 to 42% in 1996. Those rating the use of nitrites in food as a serious hazard decreased from 44% in 1989 to 24% in 1996, while those rating use of additives and preservatives as a serious hazard decreased from 30% in 1989 to 20% in 1996.

Concern about pesticide residue contamination seems logical since pesticides are used for their toxic effect. Several attitude studies noted that concern about pesticide residues was higher among those with lower income and less formal education (Packer, 1992; Center for Produce Quality, 1992; Eom, 1992). Eom (1992) found that consumers with less than $15,000 income per year were willing to pay a higher price premium to reduce the risk of pesticide residues, $0.83 per unit compared to $0.64 and $0.58 per unit among persons with income of $15,000–45,000 or more than $45,000.

Concern also could impact produce consumption. In anticipation of a report from the National Academy of Science, consumers were asked what they would do if pesticide regulations were considered inadequate to account for children's risks (Center for Produce Quality, 1992). Most consumers (93%) indicated they would wash produce better, while many (63%) would peel the skin off produce. However, 15% said they would reduce the amount of produce served. This response, which is not consistent with recommendations to increase the consumption of fruits and vegetables, was highest among those with the lowest income. Of those with income less than $15,000 per year, 33% said they would reduce the amount of produce served, compared to 8% among those with income above $50,000. Less formal education was also related to the tendency to reduce produce consumption, with 20% of those with a high school education or less reporting this response, compared to 8% for those with post graduate schooling. Response also differed by race with 25% of non-Caucasians indicating they would reduce consumption compared to 12% of Caucasians.

Correspondingly, interest in organic production was highest among those with less formal education, with 31% of those with only some high school education expressing an interest in organic produce compared to 18% of college graduates (Packer, 1992). Those with a lower income also showed greater interest in organic products with 32% of those with an annual income of $12,500 saying organic production was important in produce selection compared to 14% among those with income of $50,000 or more. Preference for organic among lower income consumers was unexpected since organic products generally demand a premium price in the marketplace.

Many consumers perceive organic as a pesticide-free production method (Jolly et al., 1989). This misconception may be corrected when the organic standards board recommendations are accepted. The Organic Foods Production Act of 1990 directed the U.S. Department of Agriculture to implement federal rules covering organic farming. The advisory body, the National Organic Standards Board, has developed a set of recommendations to be used as a basis of USDA regulation. The National Organic Standards Board clearly indicates that organic is a not a pesticide-free claim, but rather a system of managing crops and livestock which emphasized natural feeds, medications, pest control methods and soil inputs (Food Chemical News, 1996). It will be interesting to track efforts made to inform consumers about the true nature of organic production and the affect of this definition on consumer purchase.

Natural toxicants seldom generate high levels of concern. Natural is often equated with safe and wholesome. Except for consumption of toad stools, or red tide affecting seafood, people seldom hear about the dangers of natural toxins. In a California survey, people were surprised when they heard that common foods like peanut butter or organic apple juice may contain natural toxins. That pesticides may prevent the development of hazardous natural toxins was new information and not believed by some consumers (Bruhn et al., 1998). Consumer education is needed in this area.

Similarly some in the food industry were unaware of the potential hazards associated with their product. That *E. coli O157:H7* could survive in a juice product was not recognized by the Odwalla company. A fresh apple juice manufacturer in Northern California claimed their product was safe because the juice was squeezed in small batches and immediately frozen. Freezing isn't effective, against *E. coli O157:H7* but pasteurization by heat or energy are protective. Food safety education should be directed toward the industry as well as consumers.

4. INFLUENCES ON CONSUMER CONCERN

Concerns are shaped by the media, the food industry, and the consumer's own knowledge and perception. Surveys indicate people obtained most of their information about food safety from the media with television first followed by newspapers and magazines (Bruhn et al., 1992; Hoban, 1994; Hoban and Kendall, 1993). Other people were also a significant source of information. Many people were skeptical about stories in the media and evaluated information sources to judge credibility. Consumers consider how frequently they heard a message, the credibility of the source, and if the information was reasonable to them. Consumers considered health authorities, such as the American Medical Association or the American Dietetic Association, as the most credible, followed by university scientists and regulatory groups like FDA. The food industry, activist groups, and retailers were considered least credible (Bruhn et al., 1992; Hoban, 1994). No source was believed by everyone.

5. RESPONSIBILITY FOR SAFE FOOD

An interesting shift has occurred in consumer perception of responsibility for safe food. The national Food Marketing Institute survey recorded on whom consumers rely to ensure the products they bought in the supermarket were safe. In 1986 most consumers (48%) responded "yourself as an individual" (Abt Associates, 1996). The government received the second most frequent response with 33%. Over time consumer reliance has shifted. In 1996, fewer consumers relied on themselves, only 25%, and fewer counted on the government, 21%. An increased number of consumers look to manufacturers and food processors, up from 8% in 1986 to 21% in 1996, and food stores, up from 2% in 1986 to 16% in 1996.

This shift may be related to retailer activities or media coverage of food safety issues. Consumers may feel they have little control over pesticide residues since it is not visible. Some retailers appear to be accepting the responsibility for residue-safe products by offering "certified" produce.

Similarly media reports indicate foodborne illness was caused by "contaminated" or "tainted" food. This suggests that someone else unfairly exposed the consumer to a substandard product. The need for proper cooking or high standards of hygiene were given little attention. That government standards do not permit the presence of salmonella, *E. coli O157:H7* or other microorganisms further supports this perception.

6. NEW TECHNOLOGIES

The demand for higher standards of microbiological quality drives the search for new technologies to reach these goals. Consumers are receptive to new technologies which offer benefits. The process of asking consumers about a technology can increase sensitivity to potential harm. Nevertheless, consumers have responded positively to new technologies used in production or processing.

6.1. Laser Processing

Lasers produce light with properties similar to those in the natural solar radiation light spectrum. This spectrum includes electric and radio waves, infrared and visible rays, and UV and shorter wavelengths. Portions of this spectrum have been recognized as effective in controlling microorganisms. Recent research at the University of California, Davis demonstrated that pulsed, high-peak power narrow band laser light is an effective non-thermal, non-additive process to reduce microbial contamination. Dr. Manuel Lagunas-Solar has shown laser light effectively reduces surface bacteria, mold and viral contamination. Because the effect depends on light penetration, the laser treatment is effective in thick transparent fluids, in thin streams of relatively clear liquid or at surfaces.

Consumer attitudes toward laser processing were explored through focus groups held in California (Bruhn et al., 1996). People responded positively toward the potential laser applications, recalling its use in supermarket scanners, medicine, and entertainment. About half of consumers were willing to purchase laser-treated foods based on minimal information about the process. This increased to two-thirds following a brief discussion. Consumers indicated that when a new process is introduced, they wanted information about process benefits, the safety of the treatment, community, environmental and worker safety, and endorsement by recognized health experts.

6.2. Food Irradiation

Exposing food to high levels of electromagnetic energy has been approved in the United States for several applications, including reduction of salmonella and other pathogens in poultry and improving the sanitary quality of spices (Diehl, 1995). The FDA approved irradiation of a variety of meats in the fresh and frozen state in 1997. USDA approval is pending.

Attitude surveys and marketing experience consistently demonstrate that consumers will purchase irradiated food (Bruhn, 1995). National surveys indicate consumer concern about irradiation was less than other food related concerns. When specifically asked, 29% identified irradiation as a potential serious health hazard contrasted to 77% who identified bacteria as a serious hazard (Abt Associates, 1996). The percentage of consumers concerned about irradiation has decreased significantly over time. In the late 1980's between 42%-43% classified irradiation as a serious concern. Those expressing concern decreased to 29% in 1996. A relative ranking of food processing methods surveyed by the Gallup Organization found that irradiation, food preservatives, and use of chlorination generated a similar concern rating (Gallup Organization, 1993).

In the 1996 Food Marketing Institute survey, 69% of consumers indicated they were very or somewhat likely to purchase products irradiated to kill germs or bacteria (Abt Associates, 1996). Surveys completed in several areas of the country indicate 60%-70% of consumers believe irradiation is necessary and would prefer it (Bruhn, 1995). A Gallup survey found 60% were willing to pay extra for hamburger irradiated to reduce bacteria (Gallup Organization, 1993). After consumers received information about irradiation, interest in purchasing increased to 90% of consumers in one study, and education plus food samples increased purchase intent to 99% (Pohlman et al., 1994). Irradiation is not for everyone, but the advantages appeal to a significant segment of the population.

Consumers have purchased irradiated food in select locations across the United States since 1992 (Bruhn, 1995). A significant amount of tropical fruit from Hawaii was sold at several Midwest markets and in ethnic markets in California in collaboration with a study to determine quarantine treatment. From 1995 through October, 1996, eleven shipments of fruit consisting of papaya (10,020 pounds), atemoya (7,302 pounds), rambutan (1,168 pounds), lychee (3,080 pounds), starfruit (2,264 pounds), banana (380 pounds), Chinese taro (30 pounds), and oranges (200 pounds) were irradiated near Chicago and sold (Wong, 1996). The fruit was well received by consumers, however one retailer withdrew due to threats from an activist organization.

The market response to irradiated poultry was tested in Kansas. In 1995 labeled irradiated poultry captured 60% of the market share when priced 10% less than store brand, 39% when priced equally, and 30% when priced 10% higher (Anonymous, 1995b). In 1996 market share increased to 63% when the irradiated product was priced 10% less than the store brand, 47% when priced equally, and 18% and 17% when priced 10% or 20% higher (Fox, 1996). The irradiated product sold better in the more up-scale store, capturing 73% of the market when priced 10% lower, 58% when priced equally, and 31% and 30% when priced 10% or 20% higher. This is consistent with other attitude surveys and marketplace data that indicate irradiation is more accepted in up-scale markets.

Chicken which has been irradiated to destroy bacterial contamination is being used for employee and patient food service in some Florida health care facilities (Anonymous, 1995a). These marketplace activities indicate that many consumers will purchase irradiated food when they see a safety or quality advantage.

6.3. Biotechnology

Techniques of recombinant DNA and other advanced methods of biotechnology can be used in agricultural production or processing. Although few consumers are knowledgeable about biotechnology, many are aware of the technology and consumer attitudes are generally positive. When people hear about the potential benefits of this technology and the endorsement by the health community, positive attitudes increase.

A 1997 national survey of 1,004 U.S. adults found high awareness of food biotechnology and strong support for its benefits. Nearly eight out of ten (79%) Americans were aware of biotechnology, with more than half (54%) saying biotechnology has already provided benefits to them and three out of four consumers (78%) predicting they will benefit from biotechnology in the next five years (International Food Information Council, 1997). Nearly half of the respondents realized foods produced through biotechnology were already in supermarkets.

The 1996 national Food Marketing Institute survey found 62% indicated they were very or somewhat likely to buy a product modified to taste better or fresher with 17% of these very likely. Additionally 74% were very or somewhat likely to buy a product modified to resist insect damage and require fewer pesticide applications (Abt Associates, 1996). Similar attitudes were found in Canada, Japan, and Australia (Hoban, 1996; Kelley, 1995; Walter, 1994) Concern about personal or environmental safety has led to opposition among some consumer and activist groups.

Positive attitudes are increased when consumers receive additional information about the technology from a credible source. An increased number of consumers from California and Indiana viewed biotechnology positively after participating in a discussion and viewing a 10 minute videotape (Bruhn and Mason, 1996). When asked to consider overall benefits and risks, 72% of the participants initially believed the potential impact of biotechnology on human health and well being would be positive After viewing the video tape and participating in the discussion, this increased to 90%. Similarly, after participating in the program, 83% believed biotechnology would have a positive impact on the environment, up from an initial 66%.

7. CONCLUSION

Consumers are sensitive and aware of food safety hazards, however the health professional, food industry, and regulatory agencies must collaborate to provide on-going consumer education. The message must acknowledge that no technology replaces safe food handling and environmental stewardship, and that food safety does not occur automatically, but must be achieved through care in selection and handling. Technologies, whether they are as traditional as pasteurization or as novel as irradiation, laser light, or biotechnology, have unique benefits. These benefit must be highlighted and accompanied with safety criteria. Understanding is enhanced if a new technology is compared to a process familiar to the public. Worker and environmental safety must be addressed. Consumers need to hear when new technologies are endorsed by recognized health professionals.

REFERENCES

Anonymous. Florida hospitals make irradiated chicken buy. *Food Service Director* 1995a, 8, 1.

Anonymous. *The Irradiation Option*. Food Safety Consortium 1995b, 5, 1–5.

Abt Associates Inc. *Trends in the United States, Consumer Attitude And The Supermarket 1996*. Food Marketing Institute, Washington, D.C. 1996.

Bruhn, C. M. Consumer attitudes and market response to irradiated food. *J. Food Protect.* 1995, 58, 175–181.

Bruhn, C. M.; Diaz-Knauf, K.; Feldman, N.; Harwood, J.; Ho, G.; Ivans, E.; Kubin, L.; Lamp, L.; Marshall, M.; Osaki, S.; Stanford, F.; Steinbring, Y.; Valdez, I.; Williamson, E; Wunderlich, E. Consumer food safety concerns and interest in pesticide-related information. *J. Food Safety* 1992, 253–262.

Bruhn, C. M.; Mason, A. *Science and Society Final Report*. USDA Project 94-EFSQ-1–4141. 1996.

Bruhn, C. M.; Schutz, H. G.; Johns, M. C.; Lamp, C.; Stanford, G.; Steinbring, Y.; Wong, D. Consumer response to the use of lasers in food processing. *Dairy, Food, Environ. Sanitat.* 1996, 16, 810–816.

Bruhn, C. M.; Winter, C. K.; Beall, G. A.; Brown, S.; Harwood, J. O.; Lamp, C. L.; Stanford, G.; Steinbring, Y. J.; Turner, B. Consumer response to pesticide/food safety risk statements; Implications for consumer education. In press, *Dairy, Food, and Environmental Sanitarian.*

Center for Produce Quality. *Fading Scares-Future Concerns: Trends In Consumer Attitudes Toward Food Safety.* Alexandria, VA. 1992.

Diehl, J. F. *Safety Of Irradiated Foods.* Marcel Dekker, Inc., New York, 1995.

Eom, Y. S. Consumers respond to information about pesticide residues. *Food Review* 1992, 15, 6–10.

Food Chemical News. *Organic Standards Backgrounder. Food Labeling and Nutrition News Special Report.* CRC Press. 1996.

Fox, J. A. Personal Communication. Department of Agricultural Economics, Kansas State University, Manhattan, Kansas. 1996.

Gallup Organization. *Irradiation: Consumers' Attitudes.* American Meat Institute. New Jersey, 1993.

Hoban, T. *Consumer Awareness and Acceptance of Bovine Somatotropin.* Grocery Manufacturers of America. 1994.

Hoban, T. How Japanese consumers view biotechnology. *Food Technology* 1996, 50, 85–88.

Hoban, T.; Kendall P. A. *Consumer Attitudes About the Use of Biotechnology in Agriculture and Food Production.* North Carolina State University. 1993.

International Food Information Council (IFIC). *Americans Say Yes To Food Biotechnology.* News release, 1997.

Jolly, D. A. Organic foods: consumer attitudes and use. *Food Technology* 1989, 43, 60,62,64,66.

Kelley, J. *Public Perceptions Of Genetic Engineering: Australia, 1994.* International Social Science Survey/Australia. 1995.

Opinion Research, *Trends 90, Consumer Attitudes And The Supermarket 1990.* Food Marketing Institute, Washington, DC., 1990.

Packer. *Fresh Trends 1992*, Vance publications, Lincolnshire, IL 1992, 76–78.

Pohlman, A. J.; Wood O. B.; Mason A. C. Influence of audiovisuals and food samples on consumer acceptance of food irradiation. *Food Technol.* 1994, 48, 46–49.

Walter, R. *Baseline Study Of Public Attitudes To Biotechnology.* Canadian Institute of Biotechnology, Ottawa, Ontario, Canada. 1994.

Wong, L. Personal Communications. Department of Agriculture, State of Hawaii, Honolulu, Hawaii. 1996.

2

MICROORGANISMS AND MICROBIAL TOXINS

D. S. Reid and L. J. Harris

Department of Food Science and Technology
University of California-Davis
Davis, California 95616

1. ABSTRACT

The primary concern in food safety issues focuses on microorganisms and microbial toxins. Effective food preservation requires that the growth and proliferation of hazardous microorganisms be well controlled, and that the presence of significant quantities of microbial toxins in foods be prevented. The traditional effective preservation methodologies, such as canning, are being supplemented by new technologies which are less destructive of the food qualities. New strategies are therefore needed to prevent the transmission of microbial contamination or to prevent the formation of microbial toxins which remain in food. This paper discusses the role of modern processing methodologies in helping protect consumers from hazards of microbial origin.

2. INTRODUCTION

Food preservation has evolved considerably since the initial developments, somewhere in prehistory, of salting and drying as methods to extend the availability of a food resource beyond the immediate harvest period. Processing techniques such as canning and freezing have been available now for a considerable time, and have become routine. The consumer expects that processed foods will be of high quality, nutritious, and safe to consume. A primary concern in food safety focuses on microorganisms and microbial toxins. Effective food preservation requires that the growth and proliferation of hazardous microorganisms be well controlled, and that the presence of significant quantities of microbial toxins in foods be prevented. The traditional effective preservation methodologies, such as canning and drying, are being supplemented by newer techniques which are less destructive of the food qualities. New strategies are, therefore, needed to prevent the transmission of microbial contamination, or the formation of microbial toxins which may remain in the food.

Impact of Processing on Food Safety, edited by Jackson et al.,
Kluwer Academic / Plenum Publishers, New York, 1999.

A wide range of techniques are now utilized for food preservation. These include the thermal methods of traditional canning processes, and of the newer aseptic processing procedures and also newer non-thermal methods (Barbosa-Canovas et al 1995). Heating for microbial control can be by traditional methods, or may involve novel technologies, such as some of the new electrical methods. In addition to employing electrical heating methods, there are other procedures which may lead directly to reduction of microbial populations. Recently, the use of high pressure technologies for decreasing microbial load has been investigated. Additionally, some investigators have utilized high intensity pulses of light to obtain microbial inactivation. Irradiation, using gamma radiation for inactivation of microorganisms, is also a potentially effective methodology. Beyond these external treatments, control may also be achieved through the careful use of additives such as antimicrobial agents, by the control of pH, and by the control of water activity.

The objective of many of these alternative techniques is to achieve control of microbial population and reduction of microbial loads while at the same time reduce the extent of chemical and physical change compared to that produced by the traditional thermal process. The characteristics of each approach will be discussed and compared with the conventional thermal process in terms of extent of change, and level of hazard. Before this, however, it is first necessary to identify those microorganisms which may lead to the safety hazard and also to identify the conditions under which these hazards may be produced.

3. FOOD POISONING MICROORGANISMS

A partial list of the over 40 microorganisms that have been identified as sources of food borne disease or illness includes verotoxigenic *Escherichia coli*, *Bacillus cereus*, *Clostridium perfringens*, *Vibrio parahemolyticus*, *Streptococcus*, *Staphylococcus aureus*, *Salmonella* spp., *Yersinia enterocolitica*, *Campylobacter jejuni*, *Clostridium botulinum*, and *Listeria monocytogenes*. Each of these organisms (Doyle, 1989) has its own particular conditions for growth, growth inhibition, and destruction. The control parameters for each are therefore different, and a process must be designed to control those organisms which are recognized to constitute a hazard in the particular product under consideration.

3.1. Conditions for Growth of Microorganisms

In order to grow and multiply, microorganisms require favorable conditions. There has to be sufficient water available to allow for growth. The temperature has to be within particular limits. At a sufficiently low temperature, growth does not take place. At some higher temperature, death of the organisms will occur. Somewhere between, there is a temperature range for optimal growth. Bacteria are classified according to their minimum, maximum and optimal temperatures for growth. The categories commonly identified are psychrotrophs, mesophiles, and thermophiles. In Table 1a-c some characteristic temperature ranges for growth are identified for selected organisms (Farber, 1989; ICMSF, 1996).

A source of nutrients is provided by the food. The exact composition of the growth medium can influence the capability for growth. In particular, there may be a need for specific nutrients. The presence of some compounds may inhibit growth. General conditions that can influence growth are the pH of the system, the presence of certain salts, and the control of water availability through increased solute concentration or decreased moisture content. This is discussed further when we consider control of microbiological growth

Table 1. Temperature ranges for growth of various hazardous microorganisms

Disease	Etiologic agent	Range of growth under ideal conditions (most strains)		Minimum water activity for growth	D values in various media (minutes @ temperature)
		Temperature	pH range		
A. Psychotropic organisms: organisms capable of growing at temperatures of less than 5 °C.					
Aeromonas hydrophila gastroenteritis (infection)	*Aeromonas hydrophila*	0–41°C	6.0–?	0.97	1.2–2.3 51°C
Botulism (intoxication)	*Clostridium botulinum* nonproteolytic types B, E, and F	3.3–45°C	5.0–9.0	0.97	4.4 95°C
Listeriosis (infection)	*Listeria monocytogenes*	-0.4–45°C	4.4–9.6	0.92	0.07–05 60°C
Yersiniosis (infection)	*Yersini enterocolitica*	1–44°C	4.6–9.0	0.96	0.07–0.5 60°C
B. Mesophillic organisms: organisms cpable of growing at 5 to 12 °C.					
Bacillus cereus diarrheal illness (infection)	*Bacillus cereus*	7–49 °C	4.3–9.3	0.93	1.5–36 95 °C
Bacillus cereus emetic illness	*Bacillus cereus*	7–49 °C	4.3–9.3	0.93	see above
Botulism (intoxication)	*Clostridium botulinum* proteolytic types A, B, and F	10–48 °C	4.6–9.0	0.93	0.3–13 100 °C
Clostridium perfringens gastroenteritis (infection)	*Clostridium perfringens*	10–52 °C	5.0–8.5	0.93	0.3–13 100 °C
Hemorrhagic colitis (infection)	*Escherichia coli* O157:H7	10–44.5 °C	3.8–9.0	0.95	0.8 60 °C
Salmonellosis (infection)	*Salmonella* spp.	5.2–45 °C	4.0–9.6	0.94	2.4–42 55 °C
Shigellosis (infection)	*Shigella* spp.	6–46 °C	4.9–9.3	0.97	similar to *E. coli*
Staphylococcal intoxication	*Staphylococcus aureus*	7–46 °C	4.0–10	0.83	4.9–12 54.5–55 °C
Vibrio parahaemolyticus gastroenteritis (infection)	*Vibrio parahaemolyticus*	5–44 °C	4.8–11	0.94	0.02–2.5 55 °C
Vibrio vulnificus septicemia (infection)	*Vibrio vulnificus*	5–42 °C	5–10	0.96	?
C. Mesophillic organisms: organisms incapable of growing below 12 °C.					
Campylobacteriosis (infection)	*Campylobacter jejuni*	31–45 °C	6.0–9.5	0.987	0.6–2.3 55 °C

through the use of additives or compositional adjustment. Certain organisms, under the appropriate conditions, may produce toxins within the food (Granum et al., 1995). Other organisms produce toxins as they grow within the host. Information about the characteristics of certain toxins is given in Table 2. Given the risk associated with toxins, the best strategy is to ensure that no toxin is produced during processing or storage.

Control of food borne diseases, through control of microbial contaminants, can be viewed at three levels. The first level of control is to take steps to prevent contamination of the food by microorganisms in the first place (this includes the prevention of recontamination of a previously processed material), or to have a food with a composition which does not allow for the growth of hazardous species.

The second level of control may be termed pasteurization, where treatment is applied which will inactivate vegetative pathogens. At the same time, spoilage organisms are reduced thereby extending the shelf life. Handling of a food subsequent to pasteurization requires control to prevent recontamination if the food is to remain adequately safe. Pasteurization is not a particularly severe treatment and it does not inactivate most spores. Under the appropriate conditions, in low acid foods, those spores may germinate, producing viable vegetative organisms which can then grow and spoil the food or produce harmful toxins. Storage conditions for pasteurized low acid materials must therefore both prevent recontamination and also prevent the germination of any pathogenic spores which are present, having survived the pasteurization treatment. Since in high acid foods, spore germination and outgrowth are not possible, the storage conditions may be less stringent.

Given the residual hazards associated with pasteurization of many foods, greater security may be required. This is provided by the third level of control, commercial sterilization. Commercially sterile foods have been rendered free of microorganisms capable of growing in the food under ambient storage conditions. A treatment is applied that is sufficient both to inactivate all the vegetative microorganisms which may be present, and also to render those spores present unable to germinate. This is, necessarily, a more severe treatment than pasteurization and consequently, it affects the other quality attributes to a greater extent. After sterilization it is necessary to protect the material from recontamination. Recontamination of a food, after the initial flora have been inactivated, can lead to a situation of higher hazard than the growth of the initial flora, since in the recontaminated system there are no competing organisms to the contaminant pathogen, and growth may be rapid. With the initial flora, a contaminating pathogen may not grow readily due to competition and competitive inhibition. The level of process necessary for appropriate preservation of a food is therefore determined by the particular microbiological hazard associated with the food. In some foods, compositional factors may remove the need for any

Table 2. Thermal stability of microbial toxins

Organism	Toxin	Site of production	Thermal stability
Salmonella	enterotoxin	host	to 60 °C
E. coli	enterotoxin LT	host	to 65 °C
Campylobacter	enterotoxin	host	?
E. coli	enterotoxin ST	host	> 100 °C
Yersinia enterocolitica	enterotoxin	host	> 100 °C
S. aureus	enterotoxin	food	> 100 °C
B. cereus	emetic toxin	food	>120 °C
C. botulinum	neurotoxin	food	to 65 °C
B. cereus	enterotoxin	small intestine	to 56 °C

other form of microbial hazard control. Bearing the preceding comments in mind, it is now appropriate to consider the various preservation methodologies available for the control of microbiological hazards in foods.

4. METHODS OF CONTROL OF MICROBIOLOGICAL HAZARD

4.1. Sterilization by Canning

The modern canning process, which is a sterilization process, has evolved since the initial development of the technique by Nicholas Appert in the early 1800s. The food is hermetically sealed into a robust container, and then a sufficient heat treatment applied to sterilize the contents. For most microorganisms, the extent of heat treatment that is necessary for effective inactivation of potentially hazardous spores has been quantified. The necessary treatment is usually expressed in D-values or F-values (Lewis 1987), and a wide range of tables exist which describe the conditions for inactivation of particular contaminants. Table 1 identifies some typical D-values for organisms of concern. The D-value, or decimal reduction time, is the time required to reduce a population of microorganisms by 90% or one log cycle. The composition of the food influences the necessary treatment for inactivation. Often a special configuration of apparatus is used to determine the required heat treatment for destruction. For example, thermal destruction may be tested in small samples sealed into easily heated tubes, or a specially designed flow-through system can be utilized to quantify the destruction rate at different temperatures (Cole and Jones, 1990). Since the real product will be in a container of some known geometry, the experimental results must be used to calculate the time-temperature experience of the thermal center, to ensure that this exceeds the requirements obtained from the characterization experiments. The thermal treatment necessary for sterilization to be guaranteed in a container produces a significant amount of chemical change in the product. In solid products, which heat by conduction, this is especially so for that portion close to the walls of the container, since the laws of heat transfer require that for an adequate process to occur at the thermal center there has to be significant over-processing at the outer regions of the container. More fluid products also experience heat transfer through convection, either natural or forced, so that the time required for the thermal center to attain the necessary process is reduced compared to that for a solid, conduction-heated product (Lewis, 1987). The thermal inertia of a can system and the non-uniformity of convection still result in some degree of over-processing with concomitant quality degradation. This has been one of the major incentives driving the development of newer preservation processes which can give some level of microbiological safety, while at the same time reduce the extent of change in the characteristics of the food from those of the fresh food.

4.2. Pasteurization

As indicated earlier, the term pasteurization is used rather loosely, and connotes a range of less severe processes which do not necessarily achieve commercial sterilization, but which do achieve the destruction or inactivation of targeted microorganisms. Where the extent of quality loss which accompanies commercial sterilization becomes an important issue, pasteurization may be an adequate treatment, providing that the hazards have been correctly identified, and that the pasteurization treatment does indeed properly destroy these organisms. Pasteurization results in a shorter shelf-life than canning, depending on the hazards which have been controlled. Also, maintenance of control requires conditions of preparation, formulation and storage which will not result in recontamination, growth of organisms other than those controlled, or in germination of spores within the product. The distribution system for such products therefore requires much more careful design than one which is adequate for the distribution of canned products. The demands on the distribution system are, as indicated earlier, much more severe for low acid products than for high acid products, and care must be taken to distinguish between the hazard levels associated with low acid and with high acid pasteurized products. Thermal pasteurization is a much less severe process than is thermal sterilization. Given the constraints of heat transfer, it is generally preferable that the thermal treatment be performed on an easily defined and controlled processing volume. These requirements are similar to the requirements for the processing unit in an aseptic process, and so the discussion of pasteurization will be incorporated into the discussion of aseptic processes, though aseptic processing has additional packaging and other constraints beyond those of pasteurization.

4.3. Aseptic Processing

Ideally, the thermal aseptic process is designed to provide the minimum necessary thermal treatment for sterilization (or pasteurization in appropriate foods) to all of the product without significantly exceeding this level of process for any part of the product. It requires that the heating process be carried out in appropriate equipment prior to the delivery of the product to the final, sealed container. A schematic diagram of such a process is given in Figure 1. The container itself is sterilized prior to being filled, which effectively prevents recontamination of the sterilized product as it is delivered into the container. The method of sealing the container must also be designed to obviate recontamination of the product, and the seal must have reliable integrity.

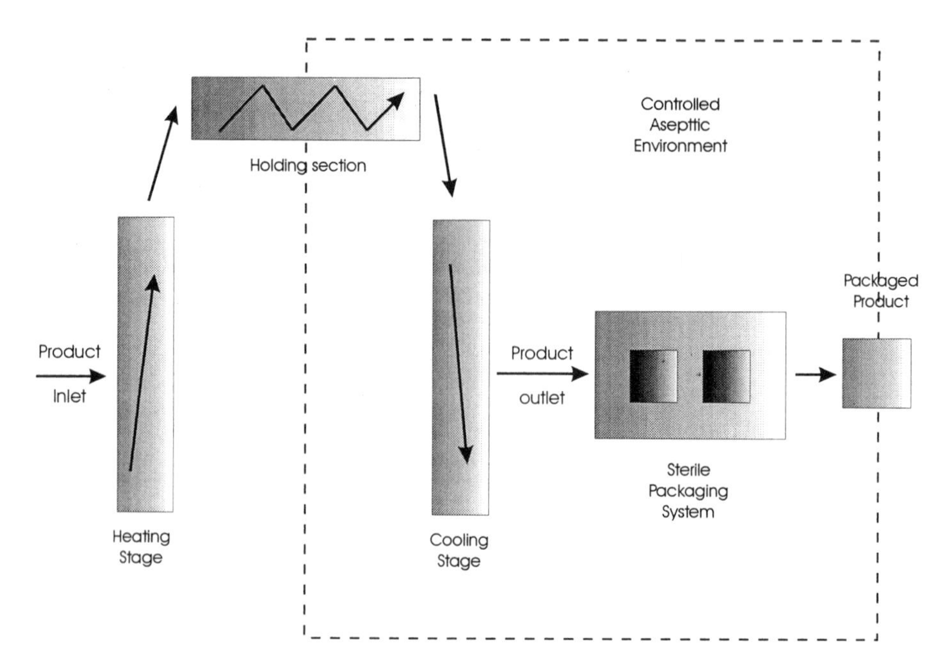

Figure 1. Schematic of thermal aseptic process.

Table 3. Apparent activation energies for various reactions relevant to thermal processing

Process	E_A (kcal mol^{-1})
Enzyme catalyzed reaction	0–8
Non-enzymic browning	9–40
General vitamin degradation	3–40
Lipid oxidation	10–25
Hydrolysis of disaccharide	10–15
Vegetative cell destruction	50–150
Spore destruction	60–80
Protein denaturation	80–120

Returning to consideration of the sterilization step, a variety of heating methods may used, and the zone where heating is produced can be of various geometries, and also of relatively small volume. Control of the temperature of all the product in this heating zone and the time of residence in the heating zone can be sufficiently precise to yield a uniform process to all parts of the volume of the product which occupies the final container. At one extreme, the container may be a single serving size, and at the other extreme may be a tank car, or a large holding tank. Note that sterilization of product in such a large container by the traditional methods of canning would be essentially impractical. The process time for sterilization at the thermal center increases with increasing container size. Hence aseptic processes are the only approach if large volumes are to be held in sterile storage.

The methods of heating the controlled volume of product vary. Fluid product can be passed through a heat exchanger of appropriate geometry which allows for precise and uniform control of the temperature—time history. This enables use of a variety of temperature—time profiles which can differentially influence the extent of chemical change, and the extent of microbial destruction (Lund, 1975). By the use of what are termed "high temperature—short time" (HTST) conditions, the appropriate level of microbial destruction can be attained while the extent of chemical change is decreased. This approach is not practical with traditional canning. The effect of temperature on the relative extent of these processes is indicated by comparing the apparent activation energies for the different reactions (Table 3). This approach, using a heat exchanger, and utilizing alternative temperature-time profiles to achieve the same level of microbial control with varied amounts of chemical change is also valid for pasteurization.

In addition to the use of conventional heat exchangers to rapidly raise product temperature to the required temperature, and then to rapidly cool it once the necessary holding time has been achieved, alternative methods have been developed to raise the temperature of the product. The influence of these methods on the detailed temperature-time history, as compared to conventional heat transfer, will influence the effectiveness of the sterilization or pasteurization procedure. Also, the method for generating heat within the product may of itself influence microbial survival, as it may for example, produce additional microbial destruction through alternative mechanisms. In some cases, microbial destruction may be achieved through entirely non-thermal means. It is now appropriate to consider some of these methodologies. Bear in mind that for a fluid product containing particulate material, the absolute requirement for safety is that the center of the largest particle has experienced a temperature-time history, or an equivalent experience, at least sufficient to produce the necessary lethality. Where heating is applied, this may require a careful analysis of the minimum residence time in the heating zone, and in the holding zone, which requires an analysis of flow patterns (Heldman, 1992).

4.3.1. Electrical Methods of Microbial Destruction. 4.3.1.1. Ohmic Heating. Ohmic heating involves the passage of electric current through a food. The food then heats through internal generation, acting as a resistor in which heat is generated through resistance heating. The important characteristics of the food are the electrical conductivities of the components. Particular attention has to be paid to the behavior of a system in which particles of lower electrical conductivity are suspended in a fluid phase of higher conductivity. This is a general description of many types of foods which are suitable for pumping through continuous process lines. Electrical models can be established to describe these ideal systems, and the thermal history of various particle configurations estimated (Sastry, 1992). The thermal profile can be quite complex. Successful ohmic heating systems have been designed and implemented for some products, but development is still necessary. Rapid heating of particulates can be achieved, more rapid than in the pure heat exchange through the convection process. The appropriate conditions for microbial safety of products have to be worked out and validated for specific systems, but for suitable products, the method promises precise control. The apparatus must be set up uniquely for each typical particle size system, and for each carrying fluid, since the balance of electrical properties between particle and carrier influences the thermal profile obtained within the particle during the heating stage.

4.3.1.2. Pulsed Electric Field. When microorganisms are exposed to a high intensity, pulsed electric field, they are inactivated. The mechanism of this inactivation is thought to involve the effects of electrical fields on cell membrane integrity. Castro et al (1993), and Qin et al. (1996) have identified the principal parameters to be considered as electrical field strength, pulse duration, number of pulses, shape of pulse, ionic strength and temperature of the food. Different types of pulsed field, involving exponentially decaying pulses, square waves, bipolar pulses, or oscillatory pulses, have different effects on the survival of microorganisms at the same field strength. Bipolar pulses have been found to be particularly effective in some situations. The reversal of field direction is thought to induce stresses in the membranes which cause their failure. The use of bipolar pulses also minimizes electrolytic effects and reduces the energy requirement for inactivation. The heating effect is not large and thus there is not a great influence upon the rates of most chemical reactions. Because this treatment can be carried out without the necessity of temperature rise, there is no need for a complex holding zone to provide an adequate time at some selected lethal temperature.

4.3.1.3. Dielectric/Microwave. In a high frequency electrical field, heating occurs through a variety of coupling mechanisms (Lewis, 1987). At the appropriate frequencies, energy can be very effectively transferred through resonance. As the radiation is absorbed, the energy is converted to heat. The efficiency of absorption influences the maximum depth of penetration of the electromagnetic radiation and therefore the depth of the heating zone. A simplistic view of the heating mechanism is that, at the appropriate frequency, polar molecules, particularly water, will vibrate in an attempt to align with the oscillating field. This results in frictional generation of heat. The rate of heating depends upon the amount of energy absorbed. This can be influenced by the design of the microwave chamber and the uniformity of the electrical field within the chamber. It is possible to design chambers for the heat treatment of product. Since heating takes place in a zone within the product, rapid heating is possible. Non-uniform heating can result both from inhomogeneous fields and from product inhomogeneities. This constitutes a challenge in the design of an effective process.

4.3.1.4. Pulsed Light Methods. Absorption of any radiation may lead to the release of the energy in the form of heat. High intensity light pulses can be an appropriate energy source. Depending upon the wavelength of the radiation and on the optical characteristics of the food under process, the energy can be absorbed in a variety of patterns. Should the absorption be by a reactive component, the extent of reaction can be influenced. Should the radiation preferentially be absorbed by molecules characteristic of microorganisms, selective destruction might be possible. This approach is in the early stages of development. Broad spectrum light pulses are suitable primarily for the sterilization or pasteurization of the surface material, since the light energy does not penetrate very far into the sample.

4.4. Alternative Processes for Microbial Destruction

4.4.1. Irradiation. When a biological material is exposed to high frequency radiation, such as X-rays, gamma-radiation, or an electron beam, this can produce microbial destruction due to damage to the constituent molecules and structures of the organism, in particular the DNA (Thorne, 1991) . In addition, free radicals may be produced throughout the product. Above some critical radiation dose this can cause many unwanted side effects, such as lipid oxidation, and the formation of potentially carcinogenic compounds. In foods where the side reactions lead to unacceptable characteristics, the extent of side reactions can be reduced by performing the procedure at sub-freezing temperatures. Unless an accelerator is used to provide the high energy radiation, a disadvantage of this method is that it utilizes radioactive emitters, which cannot be shut off. An irradiation facility must therefore be custom designed with appropriate shielding systems. This method does not lend itself to flexible process systems. In addition, irradiation does not effectively destroy many spores. High energy radiation easily penetrates the food, so that whole packages can be irradiated with uniform dose, and uniform lethality. In appropriate situations, irradiation can be an effective technique for enhancing safety and shelf-life of a product.

4.5. Processes Independent of Product Geometry

In the discussion up to this point, most alternatives to canning have performed the microbial inactivation process in a controlled volume, often prior to packaging. The techniques have been particularly appropriate to continuous processes, with product flowing through some form of "inactivation zone" in such a way as to experience a controlled extent of process appropriate to the safety requirements, and quality requirements, of the product. This is not always necessary. Procedures exist where the destructive agent is experienced uniformly throughout the volume. In such a case, there is no need to arrange for flow through a region of controlled geometry. Irradiation with high energy, ionizing radiation, which has already been discussed, is such a technique. Other such techniques exist.

4.5.1. High Pressure Processes. A major disadvantage of thermal processing for sterilizing a product which has been already sealed into its container is that the thermal process is not uniform throughout the container. In order to assure that all product has achieved the minimum safe process, much of the content is over-processed. Should a technique for microbial destruction exist which could provide a uniform result throughout the container, the need for the complex aseptic routines could be obviated. High hydrostatic pressures can result in microbial destruction (Knorr, 1993). Since hydrostatic pressure is uniform, the application of an appropriate pressure to a container could give a uniform destruction. The mechanism of microbial destruction by high pressure is thought to relate to the volumetric differences between membrane components in active and damaged forms, between native and denatured enzymes, and pressure effects on solvent characteristics (Hoover, 1993). Pressure influences mainly those properties mediated by the presence of non-covalent bonds, so that the effects on such attributes as flavor and color are slight. Studies have shown that high pressures can result in destruction of many vegetative microorganisms, but there is little in the way of systematic data on the effects of pressure and environmental conditions. Spores of *Clostridium botulinum* are resistant to high hydrostatic pressure, which means that high pressure processing is not a viable option where this is a hazard. It has been shown that the survival of spores can increase as the applied pressure increases. Additionally, there are indications that heat shock may increase the pressure resistance of some organisms to later exposure.

5. METHODS WHICH CONTROL THE MICROBIAL POPULATION

Discussions so far have concentrated on methods of microbial destruction. As mentioned in the introduction, alternative strategies entail the control or prevention of microbial growth. A variety of such methods exist and are important processes in widespread use (Gould, 1995).

5.1. Freezing

Freezing has been established for many years as a preservation process which gives long shelf-life, without necessarily changing the characteristics of the food, though there are characteristic alterations of many attributes which accompany the freezing process. It has long been recognized that the freezing process provides good control of biological hazard, providing that the preparation processes have followed good manufacturing practice (Mallett, 1995). Under frozen storage conditions, microbial growth is prevented, and there is often a reduction in viability. Some organisms are more capable of resisting freezing damage than are others, but in no case can freezing be considered to be a reliable means of reducing biological hazard. Freezing serves only to maintain the microbial contamination in stasis.

5.2. Refrigeration

Refrigeration, the maintenance of a product at controlled temperature ranges just above the freezing range, can be an entirely adequate method to provide an intermediate, safe shelf-life for many products. The growth characteristics of microbial contaminants are known, and so, given positive control of the initial microbial load, refrigerated storage conditions can be specified for an acceptable shelf life. Often, control of the composition of the internal atmosphere in a refrigerated package, or use of vacuum packaging, can lead to a further extension of the shelf-life. It must be realized that this route can lead to additional hazard in that without stringent control, in low acid foods, conditions may be encountered which allow the growth of anaerobic pathogens (exactly the hazard canning was developed to address). This puts major responsibility on producers and distributers of such foods to ensure close control of the conditions of the distribution chain. Producers do not always, however, wish to formulate to avoid this hazard, as this may make the achievement of a desired product attribute impossible. Products which require closely controlled conditions in distribution exist and can be of very high quality. Some question, however, whether consumer awareness of microbial hazard is adequate. In recent years, it has been realized that there are significant hazards which can increase at temperatures close to the freezing point invalidating the view which had been commonly held that materials which had been stored poorly would exhibit unacceptable spoilage flora long before any hazard could exist. The growth characteristics of *Listeria* render this complacent view entirely unacceptable.

5.3. Compositional Control

The use of composition to control microbiological hazard has been referred to several times. It is now appropriate to discuss such control in some more detail.

5.3.1. Chemical Additives. A variety of chemicals have been found to influence the ability of microorganisms to grow, multiply, and produce toxins in food systems without the chemical itself either being toxic, or imparting unacceptable properties to the food (Gould, 1989). Examples include many of the organic acids, such as lactic, acetic, citric, malic, or benzoic acid. These may function through general reduction of pH, reduction of the pH within the microbial cell, alteration of the cell membrane, or chelation of essential ions. For example, citric acid chelates metal ions, whereas benzoic acid diffuses in undissociated form through the cell membrane, and then dissociates within the cell. Bacteriocins, antimicrobial peptides or proteins produced by bacteria, which damage cell membranes of sensitive strains, may be incorporated into foods. This can be achieved by adding a preparation of the compound, a substrate in which the compound has already been expressed, or a bacteriocin-producing starter culture.

5.3.2. pH Control. Most microorganisms have a range of pH in which they will grow and an optimum pH for growth. The characterization of microorganisms always includes a determination of the pH range for growth in different media, the pH range for toxin production, if appropriate, and the pH ranges for inactivation or for suppression of growth. In addition, germination of spores is only possible in certain ranges of pH. It is not surprising therefore, that pH control is an important strategy for maintaining microbial safety. Some such products date back to prehistory. The appropriate pH may be natural to the food. For example, many fruits have low enough pH to limit the range of organisms which will grow. It may be produced by addition of acids (as described above), or various biological means may be utilized which cause alteration of the pH into a range which produces a stable, safe product. Many traditional fermented foods fall into this category.

5.3.3. Water Activity Control. In addition to pH influencing the capability for growth of many organisms, the availability of water, often quantified by the use of the term water activity, "a_w", is an important control parameter. A water activity of 0.85 or less is considered to be sufficient to control the growth of pathogenic microorganisms. Control of the state of water, e.g. in so-called intermediate moisture foods, can give important control of microbiological safety. A considerable body of work exists which identifies the ranges of a_w in which various organisms can grow under different conditions of pH and under other varied compositional factors. A useful compilation of data is contained in Troller and Christian (1978).

6. CONCLUSIONS

A variety of processing strategies exist which will influence the microbial safety of foods. Many of these have been discussed above. It is important to realize that to rely on one method for safety may be inappropriate, either in terms of risk, or in terms of inherent product quality. The use of multiple strategies to acquire microbial safety, often termed a hurdle strategy, may allow for the severity of the individual processes to be reduced compared to what would be necessary if that were the only control process. For example, in the presence of spores, alternative processes include sterilization, a severe heat treatment applicable in any food, or pasteurization, a lesser heat treatment, should the food pH preclude germination. The composition of a food is a major determinant of the necessary minimum process. Changing formulation may significantly influence the severity of the process necessary for stability. In this way it is possible to optimize the organoleptic impact of safety processing through careful process design and careful combination of safety-assurance strategies. The wide range of high quality, safe foods on the market serves as evidence of the successful application of alternative processing strategies by the food industry. The industry must never become complacent, however, as our recognition of new hazards, and new control requirements, is always evolving, and always requiring adjustment of process specifications to incorporate new knowledge.

REFERENCES

Barbosa-Canovas, G.V.; Pothakamury, U.R.; Swanson, B.G. State of the art technologies for the stabilization of foods by non-thermal processes: physical methods. In *Food preservation by moisture control*. Barbosa-Canovas, G.V.; Welti-Chanes, J., Eds,; Technomic Publishing: Lancaster, PA.,1995 pp 493–532.

Castro, A.J.; Barbosa-Canovas, G.V; Swanson, B.G. Microbial inactivation by pulsed magnetic fields. *J. Food Process Preserv.* **1993**, *17*, 47–73.

Cole, M.B; Jones, M.V. A submerged -coil heating apparatus for investigating thermal inactivation of micro-organisms. *Letters in Applied Microbiology* **1990,** *11*, 233–235.

Doyle, M.P. *Food borne Bacterial pathogens* Marcel Dekker, New York, NY 1989

Farber, J.M. Food borne pathogenic microorganisms: Characteristics of the organisms and their associated diseases I Bacteria. *Canad. Inst Food Sci Technol.* **1989,** *22 (4)* 311–21.

Gould, G.W. *Mechanisms of action of food preservation procedures.* Elsevier Applied Science; New York, NY. 1989

Gould, G.W. Homeostatic mechanisms during food preservation by combined methods. In *Food preservation by moisture control.* Barbosa-Canovas, G.V.,; Welti-Chanes, J. (Eds.); Technomic Publishing; Lancaster, PA., 1995, pp 397–410.

Granum, P.E.; Tomas, J.M.; Alouf, J.E. A survey of bacterial toxins involved in food poisoning: a suggestion for bacterial food poisoning toxin nomenclature. *International Journal of Food Microbiology*, **1995**, *28*, 129–44.

Heldman, D. Innovative concepts in equipment design for aseptic processing. In *Advances in Food Engineering*. Singh, R.P.; Wirakartakusumah, M.A., (Eds).; CRC Press, Boca Raton, FL, 1992 pp 309–320.

Hoover, D.G. Pressure effects on biological systems. *Food Technology* **1993,** *47(6)* 150–155.

ICMSF *Microorganisms in foods : Microbiological specifications of food pathogens*. Blackie Academic and Professional, New York and London, 1996.

Knorr, D. Effects of high hydrostatic pressure on food safety and quality. *Food Technology* **1993** *47(6)* 156–61.

Lewis, M.J. *Physical properties of foods and food processing systems*. VCH : Deerfield Beach, FL.1987 Chapter 9.

Lund, D.B. Heat transfer in foods. In *Principles of Food Science: Part II Physical Principles of Food Preservation.* Karel, M., Fennema, O.R., and Lund, D.B. Marcel Dekker, New York, NY, 1975.

Mallett, C.P. *Frozen Food Technology*. Blackie Academic and Professional, New York, NY and London , UK, 1993.

Qin, B.; Pothakamury, U.R,; Barbosa-Canovas, G.V.; Swanson, B.G. Nonthermal pasteurization of liquid foods using high-intensity pulsed electric fields. *Critical Reviews in Food Science and Nutrition,* **1996,** *36 (6)* 603–627.

Sastry, S.K. Advances in ohmic heating for sterilization of liquid—particle mixtures. In *Advances in Food Engineering.* Singh, R.P., and Wirakartakusumah, M.A., Eds.; CRC Press: Boca Raton, FL, 1992 pp 139–148.

Thorne, S. *Food irradiation* Elsevier Applied Science: London, UK, 1991.

Troller, J.A.; Christian, J.H.B. *Water activity and Food.* Academic Press: New York, NY, 1978.

3

FOOD PROCESSING AND LIPID OXIDATION

J. Bruce German

Department of Food Science and Technology
University of California
Davis, California 95616

1. ABSTRACT

Food lipids are principally triacylglycerides, phospholipids and sterols found naturally in most biological materials consumed as food and added as functional ingredients in many processed foods. As nutrients, lipids, especially triglycerides, are a concentrated caloric source, provide essential fatty acids and are a solvent and absorption vehicle for fat-soluble vitamins and other nutrients. The presence of fat significantly enhances the organoleptic perception of foods, which partly explains the strong preference and market advantage of fat-rich foods. As a class, lipids contribute many desirable qualities to foods, including attributes of texture, structure, mouthfeel, flavor and color. However, lipids are also one of the most chemically unstable food components and will readily undergo free-radical chain reactions that not only deteriorate the lipids but also: (a) produce oxidative fragments, some of which are volatile and are perceived as the off-flavors of rancidity, (b) degrade proteins, vitamins and pigments and (c) cross-link lipids and other macromolecules into non-nutritive polymers. Free-radical chain reactions are thermodynamically favorable, and as a result, evolutionary selection has strongly influenced the chemistry, metabolism and structure of biological cells to prevent these reactions kinetically. However, the loss of native structure and the death of cells can dramatically accelerate the deteriorative reactions of lipid oxidation. The effects of all processing steps, including raw product selection, harvesting, storage, refining, manufacturing and distribution, on the quality of lipids in the final commodity are considerable. Certain key variables now known to influence oxidative processes can be targeted to increase food lipid stability during and after processing. Retention of or addition of exogenous antioxidants is a well-known consideration, but the presence and activity of catalysts, the integrity of tissues and cells, the quantity of polyunsaturated lipids and the structural properties of the final food product, including total surface area of lipids, and the nature of surfactant materials all play important roles in final product stability.

Impact of Processing on Food Safety, edited by Jackson et al.,
Kluwer Academic / Plenum Publishers, New York, 1999.

2. INTRODUCTION

The term lipids is used to define a diverse group of organic compounds that are found in all living organisms. Lipids have the common functional property of being poorly soluble in water, and in water most will spontaneously form aggregates such as bilayers, liquid crystals and micelles. These multi-molecular aggregates are the building blocks of cell membranes and in essence define the physical, chemical and topological boundaries to aqueous compartments in all cells. This biological necessity for lipids around and in every cell means that ostensibly every food product will also contain some lipids. However, the bulk of lipids in foods are the storage lipids of biology. Lipids as triglycerides are an important energy storage form for many plants and most animals. The presence of large quantities of storage triglycerides confers many properties to these food commodities that are naturally rich in fat. Perhaps not surprisingly, with the recognition of the value of those commodities that are naturally rich in fat, a major processing success story of the food industries of this and past centuries has been to extract fats selectively from those commodities. The modern food industry has found triglycerides as fats and oils to be one of the most useful functional ingredients and processing media (especially as cooking oil) in the food supply. Arguably, the success of triglycerides as an industrial ingredient in foods and food processing has had a major impact on the food supply and the resulting overall diets consumed by the Western world. With the growing interest in the consequences of this food revolution, especially the lipid component of foods, and the proliferation of applications for lipids as isolated food ingredients, their stability and especially their susceptibility to oxidation reactions has become even more important. Understanding the key determinants of the susceptibility of lipids to oxidation is providing the means to process foods to minimize oxidation.

2.1. Classes of Lipids in Foods

Lipids that are the are most susceptible to oxidative free-radical reactions are those that contain polyunsaturated fatty acids (PUFA) and are primarily the class of molecules that includes the esters of glycerol with fatty acids, triacylglycerols and phospholipids. Another nutritionally important lipid is cholesterol, which is the main sterol synthesized by animals. Although sterols can oxidize, their oxidation is typically a later consequence of the oxidation of other lipids (Paniangvait et al., 1995). However, the altered biological activity of oxidized cholesterol implicates cholesterol oxidation as a potentially important consequence of lipid oxidation in cholesterol-containing foods.

Triacylglycerols, or triglycerides, play a major storage role in both plants and animals. Adipose tissue is the main storage form of fat in animals, in which specific cells, adipocytes, are the primary depository of triglycerides stored in phospholipid-delimited droplets within the cytoplasm. In those plants in which triglycerides are a storage form in seeds. the seed oils are similarly stored as phospholipid-delimited droplets in the cytoplasm of seed endosperm cells.

Phospholipids make up a smaller proportion of lipids than triacylglycerols in most food commodities, but they are structurally much more ubiquitous and biologically important compounds. The unique amphiphilic properties of phospholipids cause them to spontaneously form bilayer lamellae or align at the interface between lipid and aqueous environments, and as such are the major lipids in all biological membranes. Phospholipids, as powerful surfactants, can also facilitate the formation of food emulsions. For example, phospholipids are the major components of the surface of lipoproteins that transport lipids in the bloodstream of animals, and they are valuable to the preparation of food emulsions such as mayonnaise.

Both phospholipids and triglycerides are assembled from glycerol and activated fatty acids within the endoplasmic reticulum of cells. There is considerable variation in the fatty acid composition of both phospholipids and triglycerides depending on genetics, cell type and in the case of animals, diet. Certain structural principles appear to be retained within both plant and animal phospholipids. The three positions on the glycerol moiety are not esterified randomly, and since the sn-3 position is assigned to the phosphoryl moiety, the sn-1 and sn-2 positions tend to be acylated by saturated and unsaturated fatty acids, respectively. Thus, on average, biological membranes tend to be approximately one-half saturated and one-half unsaturated fatty acids. It is likely a requirement that PUFA occupy the sn-2 position to maintain the simple structural properties of the liquid crystal state of the phospholipids in a viable cellular membrane. This evolutionary decision to employ PUFA as an integral component surrounding every cell and cellular compartment renders the fluid matrix a highly unstable chemical entity relative to free-radical oxidation reactions. Evolution has developed a variety of preventive measures to maintain the oxidative stability of the membrane.

2.2. Composition of Lipids in Foods

The majority of lipids in foods is present as saturated, monounsaturated or polyunsaturated species of fatty acids esterified into triacylglycerides. Although triglycerides present in their natural biological condition are almost invariably liquid, extraction and concentration of lipids are frequently designed to attain a mixture that has a significant fraction of crystallized fat forming a semi-solid or plastic mass. These lipid materials are normally designed to contribute this solid or plastic functionality to foods at the temperature of consumption or processing and are referred to as fats. Triglyceride mixtures that remain liquid during processing and consumption are referred to as oils. Since all fats eventually melt depending on the temperature, the designation of fats and oils is admittedly contextual, nevertheless, there is a very important functionality implied by the terms, thus they will be used in this review to indicate the form and functions that they are likely to perform in foods. These arrangements are named according to the IUPAC stereochemical numbering system as the sn-1, sn-2 or sn-3 position of the triacylglycerol.

2.3. Functions of Lipids in Foods

Lipids in foods serve some very beneficial functions in the animal body. As nutrients, fats and oils provide a significant and perhaps even striking caloric density to the human diet. Lipids are the densest source of food calories, containing 9 kcal/g, which is about twice the caloric content of carbohydrates and proteins. This is especially important when comparing lipids to protein and carbohydrate when considering the relative volume or weight contribution of the three macromolecules to whole foods as consumed. Proteins and carbohydrates are accompanied by considerable water, obviously diluting the net calories per volume or weight. In contrast, fats and oils contain no water and as a result are by volume almost pure calorie vehicles. This is an important basis to their biological value as an energy storage form. However, in diets in which caloric density is high and nutrient densities per daily caloric requirement are low, diets with high levels of fats and oils are clearly problematic. Perhaps foremost in the minds of many is this contribution to total calorie intake. In addition, dietary fat in the form of triacylglycerides has been shown to exert effects on a variety of metabolic systems, most notably lipoprotein and cholesterol metabolism. The influence of fat on both lipoprotein and cholesterol metabolism is generally regarded as being extremely detrimental to risk factors for coronary disease, cancer and other chronic and degenerative diseases. However, these effects depend on the relative quantity of total fat in the diet, the presence of other dietary constituents, the fatty acid composition and the arrangement of fatty acids on the glycerol (for reviews see American Journal of Clinical Nutrition 1997 vol. 66 supplement). Lipids are not all bad. Lipids also provide essential nutrients. They are a source of essential fatty acids, not only linoleic and linolenic acids but also their metabolic products, such as arachidonic and docosahexaenoic acids. Lipids are a solvent of and delivery vehicle for fat-soluble vitamins and other non-essential but fat-soluble nutrients such as carotenoids. These various nutritional properties are not independent of either the commodity from which the fats were obtained, the processing that is applied or the form in which they are added to foods. Considerable care should be exercised in redesigning foods with altered fat contents for nutritional enhancement, lest the true value of the fat in the food be lost. Also, the beneficial properties of lipids in the diet are all susceptible to oxidative deterioration, and again, care must be taken in redesigning lipid systems for foods to ensure that oxidation does not become a significant problem to the very nutritional target of interest.

2.3.1. Organoleptic Properties of Food Lipids. The major organoleptic properties imparted to foods by lipids are flavor, as both taste and odor, and texture. As discussed by Love (1996), these properties are not always disassociated one from the other, and future advances relating chemical composition to flavor and texture will require an understanding of not only the structural basis of texture perception but the role of food matrices and their manipulation in the taste and olfactory perception of complex mixtures of molecules and compounds. The exact basis by which fats contribute positive sensation is still the subject of active research and speculation (Drewnowski, 1997).

While the role of lipids in positive flavor perception is debated, the contribution of oxidized lipids to food flavor deterioration is very well accepted. The contributions of volatiles from oxidized lipids to flavors of foods have long been recognized, and they often lead to consumer rejection of the food source. Early assessments of the organoleptic properties of soybean oils were made by flavor panels (Moser et al., 1950), and vegetables and fruit aromas (Buttery and Teranishi, 1961) and food product volatiles (Teranishi et al., 1962) were measured by gas chromatography. Recently, St. Angelo (1996) extensively reviewed the subject of lipid oxidation in foods, and Smouse (1996) reviewed the importance of lipid oxidation to food processors.

In relation to food quality, a number of the organoleptic qualities of fats contribute to the desirability of particular foods. Such foods are generally consumed by individuals because they judge the taste qualities as being pleasurable, and high-fat foods historically have been valued for their desirable flavor and texture. Thus, lipids contribute the desirable properties of flavor (Johnson et al., 1991), structure (German, 1989; Simoneau et al., 1992), texture (Drewnowski and Greenwood, 1983), satiety (Hetherington and Rolls, 1991) and high density calories (Warwick and Schiffman, 1992). Perhaps the primordial search by animals for the caloric value of fats led to the strongly positive flavor perception of fat-rich foods in modern humans. Recently the over-consumption of fats and fat-rich foods has been argued to be problematic to health (Anonymous, 1988). Nevertheless, it must be remembered that this consumption is a reflection of their apparent competitive advantage in a free-choice food marketplace. For centuries, given a choice, consumers have chosen fat-rich foods over their less expensive alternatives. The development of foods as organoleptically attractive as their full-fat competition has been a genuine challenge to the food industry. To date, these alternatives rarely emerge as less expensive.

An important consideration of the fat component of foods is their stability. Unsaturated lipids are highly susceptible to the deteriorative reactions of oxidative free-radical chemistry. These reactions, as summarized below (Section 3), give rise to the characteristic off-flavors of oxidative rancidity. Hydroperoxides produced in foods are themselves odorless. However, carbonyl compounds formed upon decomposition can impart to the food undesirable off-flavors. Oxidative deterioration and the production of off-flavors is one of the very distinctive quality attributes of virtually all foods. For example, the beaniness of poorly processed soybeans and soybean oil, the painty aroma of stored fried foods, the cardboard-like rancidity of wheat germ, the ëold sockí flavor of warmed-over red meat and the fishy off-flavor of stored fish products are all quite diagnostic and are the basis for rejection of these foods by even unsophisticated consumers. Interestingly, some of the same compounds that are recognized as off-flavors, when present in small amounts, are perceived as food-specific attributes and favorable. Nevertheless, in most cases lipid oxidation is a highly undesirable process and limits the shelf life and value of most foods. In fact, the relatively high flavor impact and low flavor threshold of these compounds generated by lipid oxidation are considered important safety aspects of foods in that they are rejected on an organoleptic basis before oxidative deterioration leads to significant health risk.

2.3.2. Safety and Health Implications of Oxidized Lipids. The products of oxidation are myriad and virtually all lipids are susceptible to some extent to oxidation and the formation of lipid-based free radicals, hydroperoxides and polymers between lipids and between lipids and other molecules. The hydroperoxides decompose into even more products, including short-chain aldehydes and ketones and alcohols (Frankel, 1991), as well as more radicals. The issues of oxidized lipids and health are therefore highly complex, and overall these molecules can compromise health a number of ways: (a) The direct oxidation of susceptible molecules can result in loss of normal biological function. For example, oxidation of membrane lipids alters membrane integrity, promotes red blood cell fragility and membrane leakage. The oxidation of proteins results in loss of enzyme catalytic activity and/or regulation. (b) Reaction of some of these products leads to adduct formation with loss of native functions of specific molecules. The oxidative modification of the apoB molecule on low-density lipoprotein (LDL) prevents uptake by the LDL receptor and stimulates uptake by the scavenger receptor. (c) Oxidation can cleave DNA, and cause point, frame shift, deletion and base damage. This oxidative cleavage impairs or destroys normal functionality. (d) Oxidative reactions can liberate signal molecules or analogs that elicit inappropriate responses, such as the activation of platelet aggregation and down-regulation of vascular relaxation by leukotoxin and eicosanoid analogs.

The susceptibility and overall rate of oxidation of a lipid molecule, whether in food or within the body, is related to the number of double bonds on the fatty acids. The rate of oxidation is determined by the ease of hydrogen abstraction. An increase in the number of double bonds increases the oxidation rate. These relative rates of oxidation as a function of number of double bonds may be important to rates of deterioration of various components in foods as well as biological molecules *in vivo*. Foods high in PUFA require more antioxidants to prevent oxidation and rancidity (Fritsche and Johnson, 1988). Consumption by animals, including humans, of foods with high amounts of PUFA appears to increase the antioxidant required to prevent tissue damage (Muggli, 1989). The molecular basis for this increased requirement is not known. Frequently, reports of increased *in vivo* oxidative damage are based on crude measures of lipid oxidation such as thiobarbituric acid-reactive substances. The thiobarbituric acid assay does not distinguish oxidation among different dietary fats as it responds differently to the same amount of oxidation in PUFA with different numbers of double bonds. A diet enriched in highly unsaturated fatty acids would appear to increase the tendency to oxidation and increase the incidence of oxidation-associated chronic degenerative diseases; however, this has not been observed. In fact, studies have shown that replacement of diets high in saturated fat with highly unsaturated fat diets frequently reduces atherosclerosis, thrombosis and other chronic diseases (Keen et al., 1991). Thus, when considering the myriad effects of food fats on subsequent oxidation within tissues, it is critical to understand all of the various biochemical and metabolic consequences as well. Since oxidative processes are initiated through a variety of chemical and enzymatic reactions (Kanner et al., 1987), the inhibition of oxidative biochemical and metabolic pathways by a variety of antioxidants may significantly alter their net effect on oxidative damage to tissues.

With the increasing interest in the public health implications of edible oils and the possibility that oxidation products of particular lipids may have uniquely detrimental properties, some emphasis has been placed on analyzing fats for the presence of oxidation products. Foremost among these are the oxides of cholesterol (Paniangvait et al., 1995). These molecules have been shown to be responsible for a variety of deleterious actions *in vivo* (Esterbauer, 1993; Morin and Peng, 1989; Sevanian et al., 1991). How much of the toxicity of cholesterol oxides *in vivo* is related to cholesterol oxides from ingested food is not known. Overall, the overt toxicity of all oxidized lipids ingested in foods appears to be remarkably low (Esterbauer, 1993). Nevertheless, the long-term influence of lipid peroxides and oxides of cholesterol, etc. may be deleterious, especially towards the development of chronic disease (Halliwell, 1993). In ongoing research attempting to elucidate the basis of LDL modification and the accumulation of atherosclerotic plaque, many studies have used cholesterol oxides as the index of LDL oxidation. This is a useful but not particularly sensitive barometer of the deterioration of LDL particles. The cholesterol molecule is not readily oxidized, the accumulation of the oxidation products of cholesterol likely reflects extensive decomposition of the particle. At the point at which LDL contain oxides of cholesterol, these particles can be readily shown to be taken up by the so-called scavenger receptor on macrophages. This is consistent with the conversion of native LDL to modified and atherogenic LDL (Steinberg et al., 1989). Cholesterol oxides then elicit serious changes in the functioning of the macrophages that accumulate them (Fielding et al., 1997). Although cholesterol oxides are toxic to a variety of biochemical processes and cells, especially macrophages, it is not yet clear that particular oxides of cholesterol found in foods are uniquely toxic or that their presence in foods contributes inordinately to chronic disease. Nevertheless, this research that is beginning to catalog the abundance of oxidized lipids in foods and edible oils has emphasized the need to stabilize oils against oxidation and has increased the rate of disappearance of animal-derived, cholesterol-containing cooking fats (Fontana et al., 1992; Morin and Peng, 1989; Zhang and Addis, 1990), all arguably with beneficial results. Coupled with an emphasis on dietary antioxidants and the broader protection of susceptible targets such as lipoproteins *in vivo*, the role of lipid protection is increasing in importance. On-going research is suggesting that such protection is involved in attenuating the risk of atherosclerosis, cancer and other degenerative diseases (Ames, 1989; Ames et al., 1993; Esterbauer, 1993; Halliwell, 1993). Thus, while the historic literature would conclude that oxidized lipids do not apparently pose grave acute risks, especially since most overtly-oxidized foods are unpalatable, both the chronic effects of consuming foods high in oxidized fats and low in antioxidants together with the possibility of processing foods to eliminate off-flavors but not to eliminate other products of oxidation argue that the health effects of lipid oxidation in foods are not sufficiently understood.

3. OXIDATION CHEMISTRY

The mechanism(s) of oxidative reactions leading to decreased quality of processed foods are the same mechanisms described for lipid oxidation in general chemistry. Lipid oxidation is a multi-step, multifactorial process, and in foods the variables encompassed include individual fatty acid susceptibility, molecular structure of lipids, physical state of lipids, initiation reactions, hydroperoxide decomposition catalysts (metals), presence of oxidized lipids and the amounts and selectivities of antioxidants present.

As described in general chemistry, thermodynamic equilibrium strongly favors the net oxidation of reduced, carbon-based biomolecules. The kinetic stability of all biological molecules in an oxygen-rich atmosphere results from the unique spin state of the unpaired electrons in ground state molecular (triplet) oxygen in the atmosphere. This property renders atmospheric oxygen relatively inert to reduced, carbon-based biomolecules. In effect, reactions between oxygen and protein, lipids, polynucleotides, carbohydrates, etc. proceed at vanishingly slow rates unless they are catalyzed. Catalysis generally takes the form of activating either the oxygen to an unpaired species, triplet oxygen or the organic molecule to a radical. Both reaction courses take place naturally, but the relative importance of these two modes of oxidation catalysis clearly differ depending on the food material and the conditions. The ease with which unsaturated fatty acids oxidize autocatalytically once initiated into a free-radical chain reaction means that this is the most important reaction to unsaturated fat-containing foods (Kanner et al., 1987). Singlet oxygen formation is an uphill reaction and thus highly dependent on the transfer of energy from an energetic donor. These are typically photosensitized reactions and thus important primarily in foods containing chlorophyll, a potent chemical photosensitizing pigment. Although these are very important reactions for chlorophyll-containing foods, they will not be discussed in detail. The basic reactions of autocatalytic free-radical lipid oxidations are summarized in Figure 1. The ability of the peroxy radical $ROO^{\bullet}$ to participate as an initiating single electron oxidant drives the very destructive self-perpetuating oxidation of unsaturated lipids. The free radicals generated rapidly propagate and interact directly with various targets and also yield hydroperoxides. These hydroperoxides are readily attacked by reduced metals, leading to a host of decomposition products. Some of these products cause further damage, some, formed through self-propagating reactions, are themselves free radicals; thus, oxidation is re-initiated. A large volume of literature points to several key participants in the reaction course (Frankel, 1991; Porter et al., 1995).

3.1. Initiation and Propagation of Lipid Oxidation

Initiators of oxidation eliminate the reactive impediments imposed by the spin restrictions of ground state oxygen by converting stable organic molecules, RH, to free radical-containing molecules, $R^{\bullet}$. Oxygen reacts readily with such species to form the peroxy radical, $ROO^{\bullet}$. Initiators of lipid oxidation are relatively ubiquitous, are primarily single electron oxidants and include trace metals, hydroperoxide cleavage products and high energy radiation. Unsaturated fatty acids, RH, are oxidized by the $ROO^{\bullet}$ species to yield another free radical, $R^{\bullet}$, and a lipid hydroperoxide, ROOH. This effectively sets up a self-propagating free-radical chain reaction, $R^{\bullet} + O_2 \rightarrow ROO^{\bullet} \rightarrow ROOH + R^{\bullet}$, that can lead eventually to the complete consumption of PUFA in a free-radical chain reaction (Kanner et al., 1987). The ability of the peroxy radical, $ROO^{\bullet}$, to act as an initiating, single-electron oxidant drives the destructive and self-perpetuating reactions of PUFA oxidation.

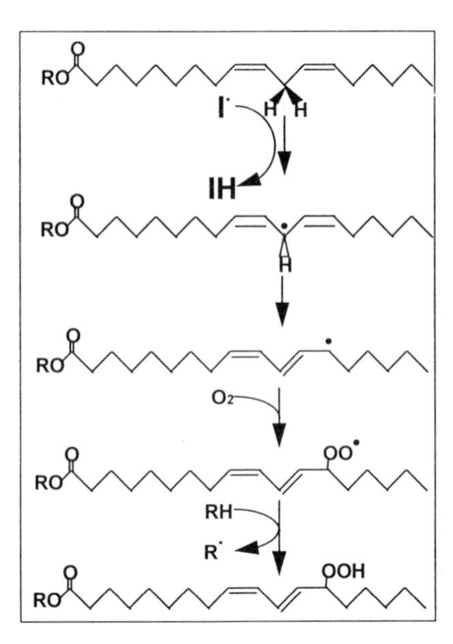

Figure 1. Initiation and propagation of single electron oxidation of a polyunsaturated lipid. The formation of a single hydroperoxide, 13-hydroperoxy linoleate is shown, however, the 9-hydroperoxy linoleate is produced in equal amounts by a free-radical reaction of linoleate-containing lipids. The internal hydroperoxides, 10-, 11- and 12-, are much less abundant products of free-radical oxidation reactions. In this scheme, a free-radical initiator designated I' is a single electron oxidant possessing a redox potential sufficient to couple with the methylene carbon in a methylene-interrupted double bond system and oxidize it, thus removing a hydrogen. This is illustrated to yield a reduced initiator, IH, and an alkyl radical, R$^{\cdot}$. The free-radical chain then propagates through the peroxy radical ROO$^{\cdot}$; ROO$^{\cdot}$ has sufficient redox potential to couple with and oxidize another methylene carbon within a double bond system. This autocatalytically propagates the free-radical chain reaction since there is no further need for exogenous initiators I'.

The overall rates of oxidation are affected by the ease of hydrogen abstraction afforded by the abundance of double bonds on fatty acids. Thus, oxidation of oils tends to increase dramatically with the content of PUFA. As the number of double bonds in a molecule increases, the number of methylenic hydrogens increases, which increases the rate of oxidation. The relative rate of oxidation as a function of number of double bonds has important practical consequences on the stability of edible oils. The relative oxidation rates for fatty acids with 1, 2, 3 and 4 double bonds are 1, 50, 100 and 200, respectively. This relative reaction rate is reconciled by the relative stability of the free radical formed by the abstraction reaction, which dictates the ease of abstraction. Two double bonds flanking a single methylene carbon confer the maximum stability to the free radical by delocalizing the radical over all 5 carbons of the 1,4-pentadiene system. This is illustrated by the 50-fold increase in rate of oxidation of linoleate over oleate. Further double bonds apparently neither affect the stability of the free radical formed nor its ease of abstraction. This is reflected in the increases in reaction rates for PUFA with more than two double bonds that reflect only the additional number of methylene-interrupted sites that do not affect the ease of hydrogen abstraction. The number of double bonds dramatically increases the number of possible hydroperoxide positions, however, and this further expands the possible outcomes during the breakdown pathways and the overall proliferation of products.

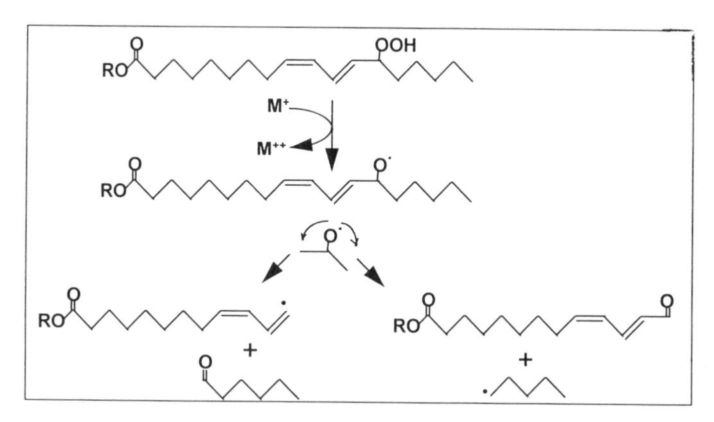

Figure 2. Decomposition of 13-hydroperoxy linoleate. Metal-catalyzed cleavage of the hydroperoxide yields a very reactive alkoxyl radical, RO$^{\bullet}$, and the reactivity of this radical is such that subsequent cleavage reactions are relatively non-specific, yielding two predominant aldehydes, in this case hexanal (left), which is liberated as a volatile product, and the core aldehyde, which remains attached as the fatty acid ester. The stoichiometric production of free-radical alkanes in these scission reactions can also promote further oxidations. These are just the predominant cleavage reactions. In actual oxidizing lipids, a substantial yield of a variety of less abundant products is also generated.

3.2. Decomposition Reactions of Lipid Oxidation

Hydroperoxides are the products of both free radical and photoxygenation reactions. Hydroperoxides are actually rather innocuous on their own, and they are neither volatile nor pigmented. However, their relative instability in the presence of reduced metals is the major basis of the deleterious properties of lipid oxidation to foods. The basic decomposition of a typical lipid hydroperoxide formed during oxidation of polyunsaturated lipids (in this case 13-hydroperoxy linoleate) is summarized in Figure 2.

As a result of the free-radical driven formation and breakdown of hydroperoxides (ROOH) of food lipids, short-chain aldehydes, ketones and alcohols are released (Frankel, 1991). These volatiles are sensed as off-flavors and lead to quality losses and ultimately to rejection due to the perceived rancidity of the fat or food. The voluminous literature that has gradually unraveled this chemistry in food lipids and more recently in biological lipids points to several key participants in the reactions. Interestingly, these same key participants are also important to the oxidation of lipid molecules in biological cells, and biology has evolved a considerable spectrum of preventive measures that focus largely on the same targets.

4. BIOLOGICAL PREVENTION OF OXIDATION

The overall response of living organisms to oxidation is highly sophisticated in keeping with the obvious catastrophic consequences of lipid oxidation to cell membranes. There are many complex biochemical pathways that have evolved to prevent, delimit or respond to and repair the consequences of oxidation.

4.1. Compartmentalization of Reactive Compounds

Within tissues, the reactions that produce free radicals are isolated and compartmentalized within subcellular organelles such as mitochondria and peroxisomes. This localization of stress allows a similar co-localization of both prevention and repair. In fact, this basic principle of topological protection applies similarly to intact tissues and whole bodies and is certainly not solely a function of oxidant protection. Nevertheless, the separation of oxidant production from sensitive tissues is an indication of rational tissue design for oxidant protection. Similarly, the distribution of molecules according to their varying physical properties is important to oxidation initiation and protection. Oxidants occur in all molecular compartments, so antioxidant protection must be equally ubiquitous. Membranes are examples of a discrete molecular assemblage that exists by virtue of the spontaneous assembly of primarily phospholipid molecules. The fatty acids of the membrane that are highly susceptible to oxidation are not accessible to the antioxidant protection of water-soluble antioxidants, yet there is a spectrum of membrane-soluble antioxidants of which the most important are the tocopherols. This principle of multiple protectants for multi-compartmental antioxidant protection to animals is exemplified by the severity of a deficiency of tocopherol as vitamin E in spite of an adequacy of water-soluble antioxidants.

4.2. Free-Radical Scavengers

Activated free-radical oxidants are scavenged by antioxidants. These are the classic actions of antioxidants and represent the key first line of defense against the potential ravaging effects of the chain reactions of free-radical oxidation. The molecules that are present in cellular and extracellular compartments in sufficient local concentration to participate significantly in free-radical scavenging include the tocopherols, and in animal tissues particularly the biologically retained isomer, α-tocopherol, ubiquinone, ascorbate, uric acid, certain amino acids and protein thiols. Present in plant tissues are phenolics, polyphenolics, various flavonoids and their polymers, carotenoids and diverse thiols. These compounds have been shown to exhibit a protective action *in vitro*, are proposed to be key to the stability of plant cells *in vivo* and also are capable of affecting oxidation in food material. In many cases, the free-radical scavenging actions of these molecules overlap, and levels of the integrated sum of these classes of compounds may be more important to oxidative protection than any single compound. Also, in living cells and tissues, the biosynthesis, location and redox state are all actively maintained. That is, oxidation of a protective molecule is rapidly followed by its re-reduction by the energy metabolism of the cell. As a result, estimates of the steady-state levels of particular free-radical scavenging antioxidants, especially when averaged over an entire tissue, may give an entirely underestimated view of the importance of an individual free-radical scavenging molecule to protection of a specific cellular site. The most obvious examples are the tocopherols, of which α-tocopherol is actively delivered to particular tissues and re-reduced from its oxidized state. These lipid-soluble molecules are particularly effective in protecting PUFA within membranes from free-radical chain reactions since they localize within the membrane itself. The inherent elegance and simplicity of design of these molecules is also evidenced by the specificity of their redox potential. These compounds effectively compete only for the peroxy-radical stage of oxidation, the one point at which the rate of reaction allows a kinetic mechanism of prevention. Because of this, one tocopherol per 1,000 lipid molecules is typically sufficient to provide adequate protection from uncontrolled chain reactions.

4.3. Detoxifying Enzymes

Enzyme systems reduce and inactivate reactive-oxygen species. Catalase, superoxide dismutases and peroxidases detoxify the active-oxygen species superoxide, hydrogen peroxide and acyl and other hydroperoxides. The production of activated oxygen species is an inevitable consequence of aerobic biology. It has been estimated that mitochondrial electron transport alone, a relatively efficient and error-free biochemical process, still produces in excess of 10^6 activated oxygen species per mitochondrion per day (Ames et al., 1993). This represents a substantial potential for damage within all cells. With this chronic oxidative load, the ubiquitous and clearly essential presence of enzymes to deactivate these active-oxygen species is perhaps the most important dimension of oxidant protection within an active, living cell. Cell death should then improve oxidative stability of foods by virtue of decreasing this contribution. Exactly how much of a decrease in the production of active-oxygen species accompanies cell death has not been well studied. However, at least in relatively fresh tissue, since substrates for oxidative metabolism remain, oxidant production by natural processes must be considered to be still proceeding with similar yields of active oxygen. Unfortunately, the stability of the protectant enzymes is not necessarily as high as the stability of the biosynthetic enzymes that produce oxidants.

4.4. Enzyme Repair Pathways for Oxidized Molecules

Enzymatic repair systems are both constitutive, that is present in cells all the time and able to immediately catalyze a necessary repair reaction, e.g., phospholipases and acyltransferases, and induced, that is, enzymes that are not present in cells until their genes are activated and the proteins actively translated in response to induction, typically by oxidation products. Damage to cellular molecules is inevitable. What makes life possible, and parenthetically what has made the search for the consequences of oxidation to living tissues so difficult to study scientifically, are the very active repair systems present in all cells. The sophistication of these repair systems is implicit in their function. That is, mechanisms must exist to distinguish a damaged macromolecule from a native molecule. Pathways must then selectively excise the defect, eliminate the unwanted products and replace them with either new, native components or the entire structure. Several examples of such pathways for repairing oxidized macromolecules have been described. For example, proteases, lipases, RNAases, etc. constantly turn over oxidized cellular constituents, and degradative enzymes often have substantially higher affinities for oxidatively-modified molecules. Alternatively, the substrate affinities of biosynthetic enzymes discriminate against oxidized forms of lipids, proteins and nucleotides. This net discriminatory process in a dynamic cellular environment constantly surveys and eliminates oxidatively-damaged molecules from the cell. The impairment of repair systems is devastating to cells, as is the potential for harm for those extracellular tissues that are not explicitly repaired. Low-density lipoproteins do not contain repair systems, and it is this lack of repair capability that appears to be an important factor underlying the development of atherosclerosis and coronary artery diseases in humans.

Perhaps one of the more interesting aspects of cellular response and repair mechanisms is the fact that biology has evolved enzymes that utilize the very same oxidative pathways to elicit a more aggressive and multi-cellular response to oxidation. The lipoxygenase class of enzymes is an example of enzymes that catalyze the direct oxidation of PUFA via a free-radical mechanism. These enzymes are virtually ubiquitous in higher eukaryotic organisms, both plants and animals. These enzymes are believed to constitute an

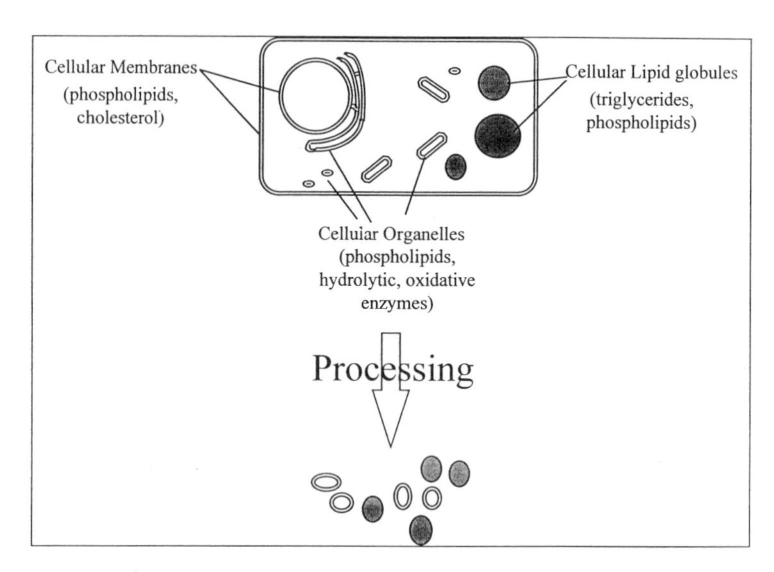

Figure 3. Overview of cellular complexity and structural distribution of lipids. The majority of this topological order of cells is lost on processing. Membrane phospholipids are sheared into random vesicles. Triglycerides and other neutral lipids are emulsified into smaller globules and acquire additional surface lipids and proteins. Organelles are sheared, liberating their contents of hydrolytic and oxidative enzymes. These enzymes catalyze down-hill reactions, which are prevented from proceeding spontaneously in cells by the separation of enzymes from substrates and cofactors. Processing releases these constraints and activates these enzymes. As a result, intact lipids are broken down into fatty acids and partial glycerides, further destabilizing the colloidal particles of intact lipids. Oxygenases are similarly exposed to their substrates, unesterified fatty acids, and oxidation proceeds rapidly on the newly freed fatty acids. Metals are contained in cells within specific proteins that form multi-coordinate ligands that chelate the metals and prevent them from participating in redox cycling and hydroperoxide decomposition reactions. The denaturation of proteins that invariably follows processing and the activation of hydrolases release the metals from these stabilizing ligand forms, and the released metals are then available for catalyzing oxidation.

ingredient in a communication pathway in which the oxygenated PUFA are signal molecules. While perhaps there is logic to adopting a biochemical pathway using free-radical oxidative chemistry as a means to cascade a response to oxidative damage, nevertheless, this seems to be one of biology's more boldly risk-taking strategies. The evolution of oxidative enzymes, however, and their constitutive presence in most tissues carries important implications to materials harvested for food.

4.5. Cellular Elimination

Perhaps the ultimate form of oxidative repair in intact organisms is whole cell elimination. Cells that are unrepairable are removed by the processes of 'programmed cell death' or apoptosis in animals and senescence in plants. These processes, many involving activation of oxygen species as triggers, are used by higher organisms to selectively remove cells undergoing subnecrotic stress. During apoptosis and senescence, cells are disassembled in a highly-regulated and coordinated fashion. This regular disassembly of cells has the huge advantage of limiting the damage that would inevitably coincide with the release of reactive and toxic compounds from lysosomes, peroxisomes, etc. The discovery of programmed cell death and the ways that biological organisms have evolved such passive and benign ends for themselves has highlighted just how devastating uncontrolled death or necrosis can be. Cells contain a variety of hydrolytic and oxidative catalysts and reactive intermediates whose presence is only tolerable by virtue of strict compartmentalization and separation of substrates from enzymes and reactants. Catastrophic cell death or necrosis, such as occurs when tissues are converted to food, destroys cellular integrity, activates hydrolytic and oxidative catalysts, releases potent reactants, overwhelms protectants and uncouples reduction and repair systems. In essence, all of the exquisite protection incorporated into biological cells by billions of years of aerobic evolution are bypassed by the conversion of tissue to food (Figure 3).

In summary, the macromolecules of life are discouragingly unstable relative to oxidation. Lipids in particular carry an Achilles heel in the ease of hydrogen abstraction of the hydrogens on carbons methylene to two double bonds and in the potential for free-radical chain reactions. In the face of this thermodynamic and kinetic reality, biology has assembled an elaborate battery of defenses from oxidative damage. Yet the complexity and interdependence of these multiple protectant systems is highly reliant on a cell's structural integrity and the biochemical energy needed to maintain protection and repair. The disruption of cells and tissues associated with food processing abrogates the majority of oxidant defenses in natural tissues. Therefore, the challenge for food processing is to determine (a) how to optimize the condition of the tissues at harvest in preparation for post-harvest conditions, (b) how to minimize the effects of processing on the natural instability of cellular lipids and, finally, (c) how to augment the remaining natural protection so as to maximize the acceptable shelf life of the products obtained.

5. EFFECT OF PROCESSING ON OXIDATION STABILITY

5.1. Raw Food Commodities

Living organisms are the basis of the food supply. Harvesting starts an inevitable cascade of cellular responses within the cells of the harvested material. While scientists are still studying the various processes that take place as a consequence of cellular and tissue death, it is certainly clear that these are neither passive nor unchangeable. Cell death is a continuous, ongoing process for all organisms, and the tolerance for dying cells by a tissue depends strongly on the means by which cell death is accomplished. Similarly, when an organism is harvested for food, the tendency of the tissues to maintain normal biochemical processes will have substantial effects on the subsequent oxidative events as a food commodity. Since oxidation of lipids is successfully prevented or repaired in living cells, the oxidative deterioration of lipids in harvested biomaterials occurs as a result of one of three basic catastrophic changes brought about by harvesting: (a) oxidative enzymes are released that catalyze lipid oxidation, (b) non-enzymatic but catalytically-active reduced transition metals are released that promote lipid oxidation and (c) depletion of antioxidant enzymes, protectants and scavengers in the immediate molecular vicinity of the lipids abrogates their natural protection. While all three of these basic means of instability are important in most harvested foods, there are various examples in which one in particular is overwhelming. The solution to this problem substantially improves the subsequent stability of the food material. The off-flavor of soybean oil due to the lipoxygenase enzyme of soybeans is an example of the liberation of an endogenous enzyme that accelerates lipid oxidation in soybeans, and the warmed-over flavor associated with the liberation of hematin iron in muscle tissue is an example of the release of activated transition metals that accelerate oxidation in red meat.

While all raw commodities experience an alteration in the stability of their lipids as a result of processing, the most vivid example of this and the commodity for which lipid oxidation is most problematic is isolated edible oils. Their processing and the points at which oxidative stability are most sensitive will be summarized.

5.2. Processed Foods

5.2.1. Modification of Edible Fats during Processing. The modification of edible oils has been pursued for centuries to convert the relatively unstable raw materials into more functional commodities and food ingredients. Thus, chemical modification of edible oils should be considered as a continuum from the centuries-old separation and clarification of butterfat to modern techniques of hydrogenation, interesterification and enzymatic modification. Similarly, while public perception frequently tends to view edible fat modification as invariably negative from a nutritional standpoint, many benefits have resulted from modifications of the raw materials of edible oils.

Recently, Smouse (1996) discussed numerous cause-and-effect relationships of processing steps on the quality and stability of oil products. Details of the following factors were reviewed: oil seed quality; seed storage; antioxidants; free fatty acids; metals, especially those that derive from tanks, fittings and other containers used for oil processing; phospholipids; pigments; fatty acid composition of the triglycerides in oils; type of clay used for removal of pigments such as chlorophyll; deodorizer time and temperature; metal sequestrants; and light and use of inert gases to reduce oxygen in the oil storage atmosphere. The following summarizes the general points in oil processing that influence oxidation and stability of lipid-containing food products.

5.2.2. Refining and Degumming. Various processes have been developed to clarify the triacylglycerol fraction from edible oils and to remove the various polar components extracted from plant and animal tissues during edible oil pressing, rendering or solvent extraction (Norris, 1982). Most of these polar components are fatty acids, glycerides and phospholipids from membrane material and the various amphipathic lipids dissolved in the membranes, including tocopherols, pigments, chlorophylls, etc. As a result of the degumming of edible oils, the stability, color, flavor and clarity of the resulting, largely triacylglycerol product is improved for most applications. Thus, considerable refining of domestic oils is pursued to produce a highly bleached, colorless and essentially flavorless oil from whichever oil source is used. In contrast, certain plant oils are produced with a minimum of refining. Prototypical of these is olive oil, for which any processing beyond cold pressing is considered to detract from the quality and market value. The reception of such ‘virgin’ edible oils by the American consumer, however, still requires a significant period of education since their relatively strong flavor and lower stability tends to be unacceptable to Americans more familiar with highly refined vegetable oils.

5.2.3. Hydrogenation. Among the major chemical advances in the edible oils industry in the past century were the developments in catalytic hydrogenation of the double bonds of unsaturated fatty acids (Allen, 1982). These developments permitted technologists to control the stability, plasticity and melting properties of liquid plant oils. These processes allowed plant oils to compete effectively with rendered animal fats for various food applications requiring plastic fats. Originally, catalytic hydrogenation, which is the spontaneous addition of hydrogen across the double bonds of fats, was applied non-specifically, leading to complete hydrogenation and fully-saturated fatty acids. More detailed understanding of selective catalysis in the 1940s led to processes that controlled the conversion of PUFA to mixtures of saturated and monounsaturated fatty acids. One of the consequences of this selectivity, however, was the isomerization of double bonds due to non-productive interactions between double bonds on the fatty acids and the surface of the catalysts. Thus, catalytic hydrogenation of PUFA such as linolenic acid gave rise not only to oleic acid but also to various positional and *trans* isomers. The negative nutritional properties of *trans* isomers have been the basis of concern by edible oil processors for decades, and hydrogenation methods have been continuously optimized to minimize formation of *trans* isomers. As a result, the total content of *trans* isomers continues to decline with time. Nevertheless, depending on the product applications, the content of *trans* isomers can be a significant, though not principal component, of partially-hydrogenated vegetable oils.

One of the important consequences of hydrogenation of plant oils is the production of triacylglycerols with saturated or *trans* fatty acids on the sn-2 position. As described above, the acyltransferases of plants are highly specific and do not form this particular arrangement of fatty acids on triacylglycerols. Thus, the hydrogenation process has important effects both on the composition of fatty acids and their positioning on the glycerol backbone. This is done industrially to prepare oil materials with functionalities designed for particular applications. The formation of triglyceride species with saturated or *trans* fatty acids on all three glycerol positions is necessary to the functionality of plasticity and the industrial production of edible fats as shortenings, margarines and spreads. To date, there has not been a definitive study to determine if there are important differences in positioning due to hydrogenation methods or what the precise post-hydrogenation consequences are to oxidation of the arrangement of fatty acids.

5.2.4. Interesterification. Interesterification is the process of rearranging the fatty acids on the glycerol backbone either chemically or enzymatically. Normally, chemical methods randomize the arrangement since they are not capable of strongly favoring one of the positions over another. These methods are used to control the melting properties of particular fat and oil mixtures but they are not currently widely used for edible oils. A variety of specialized oils is emerging, however, in which interesterification is pursued for nutritionally targeted oils. Enzymatic methods typically rearrange fatty acids on the sn-1 and sn-3 position and retain the distribution on the sn-2 position. The biological specificity associated with positioning of fatty acids on the glycerol backbone has been altered for specific effects in relatively few edible oils. The most notable example is the lipolysis of fish oils to enrich products with n-3 PUFA. Fish oils typically contain 30% or less n-3 PUFA. This maximum is largely due to the fact that fatty acids are not randomly distributed on the glycerol in fish oils, and essentially all of the n-3 PUFA are on the sn-2 position. Controlled lipolysis of triacylglycerol molecules at positions sn-1 and sn-3, however, yields a monoglyceride that is highly enriched in the n-3 PUFA. Subsequent purification and re-esterification yields a fish oil supplement with greater than 80% n-3 PUFA. Similarly, palmitic acid is primarily on the sn-2 position of human milk but on the sn-1 and sn-3 positions of vegetable oils. Controlled interesterification of oils for infant formulae has been studied. Again, the oxidative stability of these triglycerides in which positional specificity is changed is not well understood.

5.2.5. Lipolysis. One of the main quality defects in edible oils is the process of hydrolysis of triacylglycerols and the liberation of free fatty acids. This is most problematic in certain oil-bearing plants that contain active and/or stable lipases. Rice bran is the classic example. In fact, although rice bran constitutes the largest reservoir of plant oil in the world, most is not utilized as edible oil due to the instability afforded by lipase-catalyzed lipolysis. This defect is typically monitored by the acid degree value as a standard quality attribute. Most commercial oils are rejected at 1–2% free fatty acids in raw oils.

6. LIPID OXIDATION DURING STORAGE OR HEATING

In most practical applications of polyunsaturated oils, oxidative stability is an important limitation to its consumption. Nevertheless, a variety of chemical changes occur in edible oils as a result of processing, storage and final application, especially if the oil is used as a frying or cooking medium. These changes can lead to the development of a host of breakdown products, volatiles and polymers. Considerable interest has focused on these products and their toxicity. Deleterious effects have been studied with respect to overt toxicity, mutagenicity, loss of essential fatty acids and formation of oxides of important molecules, especially cholesterol. The overt toxicity of products of oxidative deterioration of edible oils has been shown only with high doses of these products relative to those found in normal food oils (Dhopeshwarkar, 1980; Alexander, 1981). Nevertheless, these results argue that post-use processing that seeks to reuse oil needs to avoid concentrating products of deterioration.

The oxidation products formed during high temperature cooking have frequently been shown to be mutagenic (Billek, 1985). Although the mutagenicity is frequently associated with protein constituents added during the frying process (Osman et al., 1983), there does appear to be a host of potentially mutagenic compounds formed, though their abundance and activity would not appear to be high. Interestingly, due to their mutagenicity in the lung (Qu et al., 1992), the volatiles released during the cooking process have been suggested to be a more important hazard than their consumption. The prolonged oxidation of cooking oils can lead to the eventual loss of most of the PUFA, and if this is the sole fatty acid fed to animals, essential fatty acid deficiency can develop (Gere, 1982). However, it is unlikely that this would occur in normal conditions of human consumption.

Due to the rapid development of objectionable palatability in slightly oxidized oils, the risks of accumulating potentially toxic peroxides, oxidation products and indigestible polymers due to oxidative deterioration in edible oils appear to be minor in normal conditions. However, it has been demonstrated that frying oils gradually polymerizing over time can accumulate significant quantities (up to 20%) of polymeric material in normal usage . Although the precise molecular species that are developed are not known, inferential evidence suggests that these are nutritionally non-absorbable.

7. ANTIOXIDANT INHIBITION OF OXIDATION

Oxidation of oils can be slowed or limited by a variety of mechanisms, including preventing initiation; inactivating catalysts, such as by metal chelators; removing substrates, e.g., removing oxygen; altering substrates such as hydrogenation of PUFA; eliminating reactive intermediates, especially peroxides; or scavenging propagating radicals. All of these and many more have net antioxidant mechanisms, but it is clear that applying the term antioxidant to such a variety of different molecules and reactive strategies has little scientific or chemical meaning, and it unfortunately has become more and more a marketing slogan. This is analogous to using the term catalyst when referring to protein enzymes. It is no longer of sufficient value to the understanding of oxidation inhibition to refer to all processes that slow oxidation by the sole term antioxidant. Thus, in this review, the term antioxidant will refer to the overall effect of slowing oxidation, but attempts will be made to specify each mode by which different molecules act as antioxidants. The original use of the term antioxidant referred to oxidizable substrates that scavenge free radicals; i.e., they donate an electron to lipid free-radical species, but their reactivity is such that their presence slows subsequent free-radical propagation and initiation reactions. There is a host of free-radical scavenging molecules, from ascorbate to tocopherols, phenolics and polyphenols, to tannins and carotenoids. This discrete mode of oxidation inhibition has several common features. Free-radical scavenging antioxidants slow oxidation by interfering with the slowest step in the chain reaction. By contributing a single electron and reducing the hydroperoxy radical, these antioxidants substitute a less reactive radical, the antioxidant radical, $A^{\bullet}$, for the more reactive hydroperoxy radical, $ROO^{\bullet}$. The overall chain reaction will then proceed at the rate at which the antioxidant radical, $A^{\bullet}$, abstracts an electron from an unsaturated lipid, $RH \rightarrow R^{\bullet}$, thus propagating the chain reaction. For most phenolic antioxidants and conditions, this is quite slow relative to the reaction that occurs in the absence of the scavenging antioxidant. The limitation to this class of antioxidants is that since their mechanism of action results in a net oxidation of the antioxidant molecule, eventually all of the antioxidant is oxidized and its ability to interfere with the chain reaction is lost. At this point, the lipid oxidation chain reactions continue at the same rate as in the absence of antioxidant.

The second most important group of antioxidants is probably the metal chelators that bind to sufficient available ligands to inactivate transition metals from participating in either single-electron oxidations or reductive-cleavage reactions of peroxides. These molecules thus act both to prevent initiation reactions and to prevent hydroperoxide decomposition reactions. In many highly labile lipid systems, chelating antioxidants are absolutely essential to stability. These chelating antioxidants occur either naturally within raw commodities or are added explicitly during processing (Frankel, 1989). Citrate is the most common metal-chelating antioxidant added to foods.

Antioxidants thus may act prior to or during a free-radical chain reaction, at initiation, propagation and termination, as well as at the decomposition stages or at points where the subsequent reactions of oxidation products attack sensitive targets. Antioxygenic compounds participate in several of the protective strategies described above for higher animals. Differences in point of activity are not trivial. They not only influence the efficacy of a given compound to act as a net antioxidant or protectant, but also affect the specific oxidation products formed. The steps at which different molecules act on oxidation inhibition can also affect food functionality of lipids and have obvious consequences on flavor, color, texture, nutrient content and stability. Although the processes of oxidation are clearly more complex than a simple two-stage approach, let alone a single perspective, inhibition of oxidation will be viewed for the purposes of this review from the two quite discrete stages of hydroperoxide formation and hydroperoxide decomposition.

7.1. Inhibition of Hydroperoxide Formation

As described above, the hydroperoxide formation process via free-radical chain reactions is classically viewed as a three-stage process, initiation, propagation and termination. Initiation invariably involves the formation of a single-electron oxidant capable of abstracting an allylic hydrogen from an unsaturated fatty acid. Since the vast majority of these single-electron oxidants in foods are likely to be products of oxidative decomposition reactions (see below), considerable controversy still surrounds the identity of the truly initiating species in non-oxidized oils (Kanner et al., 1987). Therefore, it is difficult to evaluate the nature of the most effective initiation antioxidants since it is not clear what is being inhibited. This is likely a moot point in most food applications since the presence of trace quantities of hyderoperoxides and metals is inevitable. The true success of an antioxidant must be achieved during the propagation phases. The alkyl radical, $R^{\bullet}$, is too reactive in an oxygen-rich environment for any competing species to successfully re-reduce $R^{\bullet}$ to RH before oxygen adds to form the peroxy radical, $ROO^{\bullet}$. At this point, however, $ROO^{\bullet}$ is a relatively stable free radical that reacts with comparative slowness with targets such as PUFA. This $ROO^{\bullet}$ is the most widely accepted point of action for free-radical scavenging antioxidants such as the phenolic tocopherols. This basically points to a kinetic form of inhibition, i.e., the oxidation is slowed by virtue of competing for a rate-determining step in the reaction. Thus, it is appropriate to review the basic kinetics of oxidation:

$$-d\left[O_2\right]/dt = [RH](k_i)^{1/2} k_p / (2k_t)^{1/2}$$

where the rate law for oxygen consumption is shown to be a linear function of the substrate concentration, RH, the square root of the initiation rate constant, ki, and the propagation rate constant, k_p, and an inverse function of the root of the termination rate constant, k_t. Under normal conditions of oxidation, the termination rate is quite low. However, it is the preferential interaction of antioxidants with existing free radicals that provides their kinetic advantage. Thus, the basic rate law equation, assuming that k_{inh}, the rate of reaction $ROO^{\bullet} + AH \rightarrow ROOH + A^{\bullet}$, is much greater than the spontaneous termination reaction, $ROO^{\bullet} + ROO^{\bullet} \rightarrow$ non-radical products and O_2 becomes:

$$-d[O_2]/dt = [RH]k_i k_p / n2k_{inh}[AH]$$

The inhibition rate constant, k_{inh}, is favorable for certain antioxidants such as the tocopherols that can reduce $ROO^{\bullet}$ to ROOH with such ease that tocopherols are competitive with other more-sensitive targets such as unsaturated lipids, RH, even at 10,000-fold lower concentration. The tocopheroxyl radical, $A^{\bullet}$, is in general a poor oxidant and reacts significantly more slowly than $ROO^{\bullet}$. Conversion of $ROO^{\bullet}$ to ROOH and formation of $A^{\bullet}$ effectively impart a kinetic hindrance on the propagating chain reaction. The tocopheroxyl radical can be either re-reduced by reductants such as ascorbate, dimerize with another radical or be further oxidized to a quinone. These free-radical scavenging functions of tocopherols and other synthetic and natural antioxidants are documented (Larson, 1995; Buettner, 1993; Burton and Ingold, 1981).

The simple rate law approach described above, however, assumes one important property of oxidizing lipids and antioxidants. The rate law assumes that all of the substrates are mutually and equally soluble, thus [RH] and [AH] are simply the concentration of the substrates and antioxidants present. However, lipids, being insoluble molecules, tend to exist in most food systems in colloidal form as droplets bounded by a surfactant emulsifier. Similarly, most antioxidants are only partially soluble and tend to partition selectively into the different phases of colloidal particles. Under these conditions, the concentration of substrates, initiators and antioxidants can no longer be assumed to be homogeneous, and the actual concentration of antioxidants at the site of oxidation depends significantly on the physical properties of the particular antioxidant and the colloidal properties of the food system (Schwarz et al., 1996; Frankel et al., 1994). In practice, foods consist of various multiple phases, and the partitioning of lipids and antioxidants into these phases is quite complex. For example, cells consist of membranes composed of surfactant phospholipids in the form of a bilayer and proteins, bounding various aqueous compartments in the interior of which can also exist insoluble lipids consisting primarily of triglycerides. These triglycerides are themselves contained as discrete globules bounded by a single monolayer of phospholipids. Even more complexity is produced by the harvesting of these cells, which invariably disrupts the cell architecture, remixing and separating the various lipid compartments further. Since the distribution of antioxidant materials is not homogeneous in the various cellular phases prior to harvesting, it is unlikely that the distribution of these molecules achieves equilibrium in the multiple phases at any subsequent processing step. Thus, predicting the precise consequences of processing on the colloidal behavior of antioxidants in foods remains at best a somewhat empirical exercise.

Many phenolic plant constituents other than tocopherols, broadly referred to as phytochemicals, that are present in the food supply have been shown to be capable of interfering with and inhibiting free-radical chain reactions of lipids. Plant phenolics inhibit lipid hydroperoxide formation catalyzed by metals, radiation and heme compounds (Buettner, 1993; Hanasaki et al., 1994). The mechanisms appear to be similar in that the ability of most of these compounds to compete kinetically for the peroxy radical is key to their antioxidant actions. However, tocopherols have a long history of research that has described their stability in foods, their partitioning into biological membranes where they are most effective, their re-reduction by ascorbate and their final disposition as quinones. Considerably less information is available with respect to other plant phenolics, especially on their varying stability, their ability to be reduced by other cellular reductants, their partitioning properties into cellular and membrane compartments and the anti- or pro-oxidant properties of their oxidized products.

The information gathered to date indicates that there are fundamental differences in the ability of different phenolic compounds to act as antioxidants. This was first recognized as a difference in the stability of different raw commodities with respect to oxidation. The ability of different sources of polyphenolics to act as transferable antioxidants has been recognized empirically for centuries, as some Greek fisherman apparently wrapped their daily catch in rosemary leaves. Only recently have the compounds carnosol, carnosic acid and rosemarinic acid been identified as potent antioxidants within rosemary leaves (Das et al., 1992; Hopia et al., 1996). Rosemary extracts have been both actively studied and applied to food protection as an example of natural polyphenolics as antioxidants. However, many naturally-occurring polyphenolics possess free-radical scavenging activities that may be transferable as antioxidant actions to other commodities. And, while considerable interest is focusing in the industrial application of such natural antioxidants, in most cases, these materials are contained within crude extracts that also carry both colors and flavors into the products in which they are added as potential protectants.

7.2. Inhibition of Hydroperoxide Decomposition

Hydroperoxide formation is typically modeled and studied as the net result of lipid oxidation reactions. It is generally assumed that subsequent decomposition reactions are an inevitable and invariant part of the overall chain reaction of autoxidation. The rapid decomposition of hydroperoxides, however, is true only when reduced metals are abundant or at elevated temperatures. Unfortunately, while these conditions (abundant contaminating metals and/or high temperatures) are usually employed in assay systems, such is not the case in most autoxidizing foods! Differences between hydroperoxide formation and decomposition have become apparent as the relative actions of different antioxidants have been more fully explored. For example, it has been shown that some antioxidants are more effective inhibitors of hydroperoxide formation while others are more effective inhibitors of hydroperoxide decomposition (Huang et al., 1994). Even tocopherol isomers differ with respect to their ability to prevent decomposition of hydroperoxides (Huang et al., 1994; Huang et al., 1995). The classic example of such behavior is ascorbic acid. This compound is an electron-donating, scavenging antioxidant towards free-radical chain reactions and hydroperoxide formation, and it is also a metal-reducing, redox-cycling promoter of decomposition reactions. The overall effect is that ascorbic acid in foods can range from a potent antioxidant to a potent pro-oxidant depending on its final concentration, the concentration of hydroperoxides and the concentration of contaminating metals.

Hydroperoxide decomposition reactions depend very strongly on several different factors, and these are quite often ignored, especially when establishing methods for evaluating antioxidants. Not only are rates of decomposition affected by such variables as temperature, but the entire mechanisms of decomposition change. Thus, at low temperature, reduced metals are the most important factor promoting the homolytic decomposition of hydroperoxides. In such circumstances, the availability of reactive, transition metals is extremely important. Alternatively, at high temperatures approaching 100°C, hydroperoxides decompose spontaneously and metal contamination is not as important. Under these conditions, those antioxidants that effectively compete for and scavenge alkoxy radicals and prevent both cleavage reactions and re-initiation of free-radical chain reactions are more important. Similarly, whereas strategies to limit oxygen contents are viable for inhibiting hydroperoxide formation, in foods in which hydroperoxides have accumulated, oxygen barriers will have little effect on preventing the subsequent deterioration of quality.

The activity of different antioxidants on the decomposition reactions tend to vary depending on several additional factors. The importance of reduced metals to the decomposition of lipid hydroperoxides at low temperature emphasizes the compartmentalization of hydroperoxides, catalysts and antioxidants. Because metal-binding sites tend to concentrate at surfaces, the ability of different antioxidants to partition into the different chemical or colloidal phases of foods becomes quite important to their actions as inhibitors of decomposition reactions (Huang et al., 1995). This has been proposed to be an explanation for the paradoxical behavior of antioxidants in foods and oils. The paradox, in essence, is that water-soluble molecules are better antioxidants in oil and oil-soluble antioxidants are better in water!. More precisely, it has been observed that among antioxidants whose redox activity is similar, the hydrophilic, water-soluble molecules are more successful antioxidants in bulk oils whereas oil-soluble molecules tend to be better antioxidants in oils emulsified in water (Frankel et al., 1994).

Polyphenolics from plants also scavenge peroxy, alkoxy and hydroxy radicals and singlet oxygen (Hanasaki et al., 1994; Laughton et al., 1991; Tournaire et al., 1993). These compounds that are relatively ubiquitous in plant-based food commodities, however, differ substantially in their structures in the native commodities and perhaps even more importantly differ in their response to processing. In many cases, the tendency of polyphenolics to oxidize and/or polymerize during processing and storage has been an underlying rationale to eliminate them from processed foods. More recently, however, their value as protectants has led to a renewed interest in the ability of polyphenolics to inhibit oxidation in foods, especially in the context of natural or otherwise less apparently processed foods.

Plant phenolics vary in their ability to interrupt a free-radical chain reaction with differences detectable among different lipid systems, oxidation initiators and other antioxygenic components (Hopia et al., 1996) Polyphenolics have other benefits as well. Tocopherols in oxidizing lipid systems are spared by flavonoids (Terao et al., 1994; Jessup et al., 1990). If α-tocopherol is an essential antioxidant that acts where no other compound can, the sparing effect of non-essential antioxidants may be one of their more important actions.

7.3. Antioxidants Added to Foods

Soluble chain-breaking antioxidants used in foods include ascorbate as either the naturally-occurring free acid or as synthetic ascorbate, and various soluble and insoluble ester forms. The acid form is an excellent electron donor in foods. This property leads to its excellent antioxidant activity at low levels, but at high levels, its ability to reduce metal initiators can actually lead to a pro-oxidant effect (Frankel, 1989).

In response to a perceived desire by consumers for less chemically-processed food ingredients, several naturally-occurring chain-breaking antioxidants are being introduced to accomplish essentially the same effects as substituted phenols such as butylated hydroxyanisole and butylated hydroxytoluene (Aruoma et al., 1992). The natural antioxidants are primarily extracts of herbs or plant materials with inordinately high levels of particular polyphenolics that have good electron-donation and chain-breaking properties. Rosemary extract is perhaps the most widely known of these natural antioxidants, although a variety of novel materials is being pursued.

Since once initiated, lipid oxidation of PUFA tends to proceed autocatalytically, breaking this chain reaction is a critical step in affording stability. This stability is afforded both *in vivo* and in food lipids by the presence of scavengers of the peroxy radical oxidant. The abundance of scavengers of oxidants and peroxyl radicals is therefore a critical variable limiting the progress of lipid oxidation.

8. PROCESSING STRATEGIES TO ENHANCE PROTECTION FROM LIPID OXIDATION

A variety of strategies have developed over the history of food harvesting and manufacturing to improve the oxidative stability of acquired commodities. These strategies have taken many forms, from the obvious (enclosing pigmented foods in light restricted containers) to the technologic (one of the first applications of the chemistry of isolating individual gases was the incubation of unsaturated vegetable oils in a hydrogen atmosphere to make stable margarines), to the more sublime (Greek fisherman had wrapped their catches in rosemary leaves for centuries before modern science recognized the antioxidant properties of carnosol and carnosic and rosemarinic acids in rosemary). Many of these approaches have now been more fully explored and refined as science has described the precise mechanisms of action, nevertheless, the basic approaches are those that were recognized historically.

8.1. Minimize Cellular Destruction

The considerations summarized above all make it clear that not only are the natural protections from oxidation dependent on cellular structure, but various pro-oxidant systems exist in cells that are liberated by cell destruction. In general, harvesting and processing methods should be designed to maintain as much as possible the native integrity of the tis-

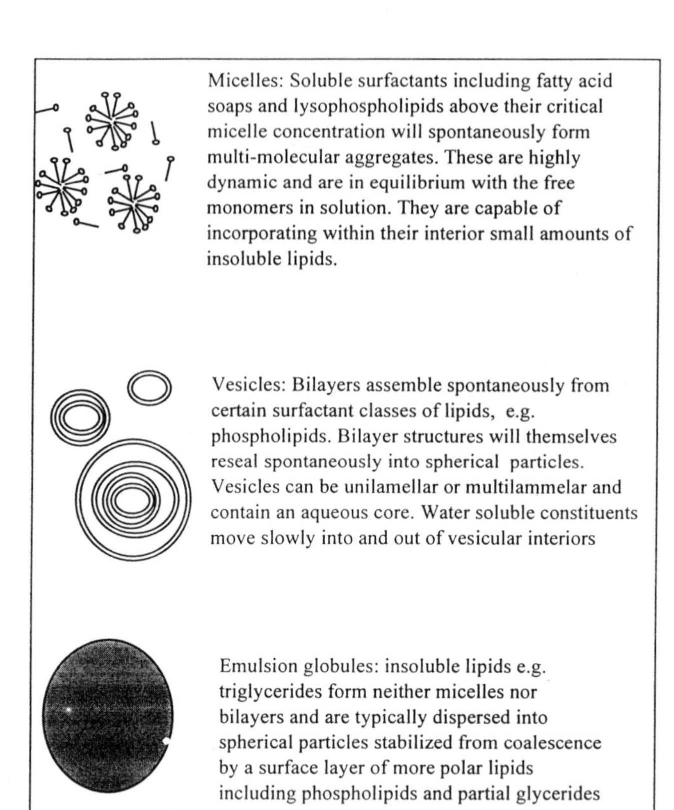

Figure 4. Colloidal phases that are formed during the processing of lipid-containing foods (not drawn to scale). The relative proportion of each of these phases will depend on the types of lipids present, the extent of cellular damage, hydrolysis of lipids, the temperature, pH, etc. Similarly, as the figures suggest, the overall surface composition and surface areas will differ substantially depending on the relative proportion of each of these phases.

sues being harvested. The natural surfactant lipids in cells, including phospholipids, partial glycerides and sterols, are readily disassembled from their native structures in cells since these are held together by non-covalent forces. This not only destroys the native structure of the membranes but provides new surfaces and access of metals, oxidants, etc., to these surfaces. The membrane lipids will reform into a variety of colloidal structures as a function of their concentration and the concentration of other components in the matrix (Figure 4).

8.2. Inactivate Cellular Enzyme Catalysts

For many raw food commodities, the liberation of endogenous enzymes that is inevitable during harvest is catastrophic to the final product quality. Examples include the soybean lipoxygenases and the lipase in rice bran. These enzymes are sufficiently active that their presence in the tissue can overwhelm other considerations for future stability. Inactivating these enzymes becomes a priority in the initial processing. Usually the incorporation of a high-heat step early in processing and ideally at the same time as tissue destruction is optimum for inactivating these enzymes.

8.3. Remove Endogenous Catalysts

Again, depending on the raw commodity, certain components in the material prior to harvest will have a significant effect in subsequent processing stages and must be dealt with as soon as possible. Examples of catalysts that are present in the commodity at harvest include chlorophylls in green plant tissue that are photosensitizers to photooxidation, metals liberated by hemolysis of blood in red meats and, ironically, in soybeans the extremely high levels of tocopherol in the raw material are net pro-oxidant. In such commodities, it is vital to know exactly the basis of the instability and process accordingly. Chlorophyll contamination must be dealt with by selective extraction, bleaching or packaging in light barriers. Metal contamination must be complexed with effective chelating agents. The excessive tocopherol content of soybean oils is largely solved by the degumming process. Interestingly, the excessive tocopherols of soybean and the need to remove them has led to the largest industrial source of tocopherols as antioxidants and supplements.

8.4. Exclude Exogenous Substrates and Catalysts

Oxidation requires unsaturated lipids, oxygen and initiation and decomposition catalysts. While the first is usually a valuable component of the food material, the latter three are not. Oxygen is a necessary substrate to the oxidation reactions of lipids. Oxygen barriers, such as air-tight containers, have been employed with considerable success for centuries to improve the stability of many lipid-containing foods. This basic principle is being pursued somewhat more broadly in modern processing as new technologies emerge. Unusual packaging materials, oxygen-scavenging systems and the availability of inert gases as blanketing atmospheres have all been applied to food materials, especially those containing unstable lipids. The negative nutritional perception of hydrogenated oils has led to a significant challenge for the fried snack food industry. Unsaturated vegetable oils are highly unstable under frying conditions and their stability during storage is even worse. The frying process produces a host of problems for the long-term stability of these products. One of the organoleptic targets of fried snack foods is a crisp, aerated food structure. This translates into very high surface areas in the final product, all coated with a very thin film of the frying oil. This is clearly a potentially disastrous situation for the stability of the oil and the subsequent quality of the product. The availability of air-tight polymeric films and nitrogen gas as an inert atmosphere has made it possible to utilize unhydrogenated oils in an increasingly large spectrum of snack products.

Metals are the key initiation and decomposition catalysts present in raw food materials, but they are also potential additives from various exogenous sources including processing equipment, flavorants, colorants and packaging materials. Two obvious strategies have been applied successfully to this problem. Great strides have been made in recognizing sources of metals and carefully excluding them during processing. As an example, copper contamination of processing lines was the bane of the dairy industry in the early half of the century, but now is unheard of. Alternatively, metals that cannot be excluded are inactivated by the inclusion of successful inactivating chelates. An antioxidant-acting chelate is a chemical that occupies more than one ligand field of a transition metal, in this case rendering it incapable of participating in redox reactions with lipids or oxygen. Citric acid is the most widely-used inactivating chelator, although there are many alternatives that have been used in specific products. Finally, protecting light-sensitive food materials from light has a dramatic effect in reducing the rate of singlet oxygen production in the presence of photosensitizers.

8.5. Modify Substrate Oxidizability

The inherent oxidizability of commodities varies depending on the composition of their oxidizable molecules. For example, fish are extremely susceptible to oxidation due to the high content of long-chain n-3 PUFA. These fatty acids are not only highly susceptible chemically due to the large number of double bonds on a single fatty acid, but the spectacular number of possible products of oxidation of these fatty acids leads to a very distinctive spectrum of volatile off-flavors. Many of these volatiles are detectable at parts per billion or less, and as a result, the thresholds for off-flavor rejection are also quite low. Similarly, any commodity containing long-chain PUFA will exhibit increased oxidation and increased rates of deterioration due to this fact alone. Finally, the distribution of fatty acids among different lipid classes varies among tissues, and this can alter the subsequent stability. Green leafy tissues of plants that perform photosynthesis contain photosynthetic membranes that are highly enriched in α-linolenic acid (18:3n-3). Contamination of the processed commodity by leaf tissue, therefore, can increase the susceptibility to oxidation by this means as well.

Solutions to the inherent oxidizability of substrate molecules have been pursued for decades, if not centuries because this principle remains important and evident in even the most processed final product. Thus, the final stability of any soybean product is influenced by the content of 18:3n-3. The types of solutions that have been pursued span the range from crop and variety selection (all of the major crops have been selected in part for their stability, leading to the substantial overall reduction in n-3 PUFA in the food supply), to extensive processing (including degumming to remove phospholipids and partial glycerides from edible oils), to hydrogenation, which chemically eliminates double bonds (the majority of soybean, cottonseed and canola oils used in industrial applications have been partially hydrogenated explicitly to reduce the levels of 18:3n-3 to produce oils that can tolerate the temperatures needed for cooking).

These are the basic strategies that in principle have been pursued for decades if not centuries. However, as our understanding of the various strategies used by living organisms to protect themselves against oxidation expands, similar strategies can be applied to the processing of foods for enhanced stability.

8.6. Modify Food Microstructure for Enhanced Stability

Cells maintain stability by considerable control of the topological location of potential initiators, oxidants, substrates and antioxidants in cells. In essence, an antioxidant that is located far from the site of oxidation is of no value, and an antioxidant that is concentrated at the sites of oxidation is far more potent than its simple overall concentration would imply. Moving this concept to food product design, however, requires an appreciation of the sites of oxidation initiation in foods, the physical properties of the substrates of oxidation and the physical properties of antioxidant molecules. While this information base is still developing, certain aspects are known. Metals are not soluble and in most foods are associated with binding and activating ligands. The distribution of metals in foods is thus more dependent on the metal-binding molecules present than on the actual metals. In most cases in which it has been determined, metals tend to associate not with lipids but with the interfaces between lipids and water. Thus, the most important target locations for oxidation inhibition are the same interfaces. The properties of lipid-water interfaces in foods are most influenced by the interfaces present in the raw commodity. They can be modified during processing (a) by the composition of the surfactants in the raw material and those added, (b) by the type and amount of energy put in to disrupt the phases originally present and (c) by the stabilizing ingredients added to maintain the structures that develop. These are the basic dimensions that can be accessed to design foods for optimal structural stability.

The tools to develop food structure are increasing rapidly. Novel surfactants and stabilizing systems for producing and maintaining discrete phases in foods is one of the most active areas in food process design. Even more variation is appearing for the future. The production of edible films is an old practice, but a new generation of edible film materials and applications are making the stability of novel food structures more and more possible. The concept of explicitly designing the composition and properties of the barriers to different phases in final food products is in principle what biology does for its own cells. Including oxidative stability to the range of advantages of edible films is obvious. Thus, edible films that prevent the migration and diffusion of oxygen into a lipid-rich compartment of foods and that also include antioxidant molecules in the film material are being developed (Miller and Krochta, 1997).

8.7. Modify Antioxidant Properties to Target Lipid Compartments

Since cells elaborate multiple and overlapping antioxidant strategies to ensure adequate protection, it is not unreasonable to apply this multiple compartment approach to complex multi-phase food systems and their processing. Figure 4 illustrates the very simplest overview of the colloidal complexity of lipid-containing foods, nevertheless, it is clear from this picture that there are multiple phases of lipids that contain unsaturated fatty acids and thus multiple compartments into which antioxidant protection must be dissolved. Not only lipids but antioxidants as well partition differently into these phases or compartments (Frankel et al., 1994; Huang et al., 1997; Schwarz et al., 1996). The notion of developing a premier antioxidant that would adequately cover all such compartments is fundamentally flawed. The inability of surfactant antioxidants such as tocopherol to stabilize bulk oils is such an example. Instead, multiple antioxidants are much more effective at an overall lower total concentration. These principles have already been developed from the perspective of chemical synthesis. For example, ascorbyl palmitate is an example of a redox-active center (ascorbate) tethered to a physical location-directing component (palmitate) to generate a final antioxidant that locates where the parent compound would not. As in all applications of ascorbate, however, the need for metal-inactivating chelators in the presence of the redox-recycling catalyst ascorbate remains important. As the enthusiasm for chemically-synthesized antioxidants has diminished, the search for naturally-occurring antioxidants that provide a similar functionality has accelerated. Again, while this is a relatively new field, experience has proven that mixtures of antioxidants are more successful than single purified compounds.

An intriguing direction for an albeit small potential to alter oxidative stability during processing is to generate antioxidant activities by the processing steps themselves. The most notable example of such a strategy is the formation of antioxidant activities from Maillard browning products (Eriksson and Na, 1995). Interestingly, this material shows antioxidant properties towards a variety of oxidizing lipid systems. The reaction mechanism appears to be similar to that of ascorbate in that antioxidant effects are reversed to pro-oxidant effects in the presence of active redox-cycling metals such as iron and copper.

8.8. Recognize and Repair

The true secret to the success of biology in an oxidizing environment is the investment in cellular repair. From simple bacteria to humans, the ability to recognize and repair oxidative damage is key to successful life. Thus, it seems appropriate to apply the concept of repair to food stability. The principle of recognition and repair is crudely applied to many commodities in such practices as product shelf-life estimation. Times to oxidative deterioration are estimated, and when that time is expired, remaining products are discarded. This principle could be used much more efficiently, however, by the development of more accurate and predictive sensors. For example, to continue the existing strategy, substantial advantage could be taken of discarding products as spoiled only when they are indeed spoiled. Instead, the practice of shelf-life dating discards all products at the point at which the least stable product is likely to be spoiled. Simply by discarding according to a true test rather than an inferred test of deterioration would be valuable. Very few products are actually repaired in any meaningful sense. The degumming and deodorization of edible oils during refining is perhaps the only example of true product repair after oxidative damage. Free fatty acids, volatiles and oxidation products are removed by the aggressive chemical processing of raw oils after extraction from the commodity of origin. While this has several drawbacks, including the elimination of much of the protecting components from edible oils, the improvement in product quality is undeniable.

There is considerable potential to expand on the principle of product repair in the future. The elimination of hydroperoxides by selective catalysis is one example, however, regeneration of natural antioxidants is a possibility, as is the selective partitioning of oxidized products out of the parent product. Although unsuccessful to date, one of the more actively pursued targets over the years has been the purification of spent frying oils. While the bulk of oxidized lipids, polymers and polar material can be removed by various adsorbents, the oil that is recovered is invariably much less stable than the original product, and the gain in value by clarifying is negligible.

ACKNOWLEDGMENTS

The author acknowledges support from BARD United States Israel Binational Agricultural Research and Development fund and the California Dairy Research Center.

REFERENCES

Alexander, J. C.; Chemical and biological properties related to toxicity of heated fats, *J. Toxicol. Environ. Health* **1981**, *7*, 125–138.

Allen, R. R. Hydrogenation. In *Bailey's Industrial Oil and Fat Products*; Vol. 2; Swern, D., Ed.; J. Wiley: New York, 1982; pp 1–90.

Ames, B. N. Endogenous oxidative DNA damage, aging, and cancer. *Free Radical Res. Commun.* **1989**,*7*, 121–128.

Ames, B. N.; Shigenaga, M. K.; Hagen, T. M. Oxidants, antioxidants, and the degenerative diseases of aging. *Proc. Nat. Acad. Sci. (USA)* **1992**,*90*, 7915–7922.

Anonymous. *The Surgeon General's Report on Nutrition and Health. U.S. Department of Health and Human Services, Publication No. 88–50210.* U.S. Government Printing Office: Washington, DC, 1988.

Aruoma, O. I.; Halliwell, B.; Aeschbach, R.; Loligers, J. Antioxidant and pro-oxidant properties of active rosemary constituents: carnosol and carnosic acid. *Xenobiotica* **1992**,*22*, 257–268.

Billek. G., Heated fats in the diet, in *The Role of Fats in Human Nutrition*, Padley, F. B.; Podmore, J., Eds.; Horwood: Chichester, UK, 1985; pp 163–172.

Buettner, G. R. The pecking order of free radicals and antioxidants: lipid peroxidation, alpha-tocopherol, and ascorbate. *Arch. Biochem. Biophys.* **1993**, *300*, 535–543.

Burton, G.; Ingold, K. I. Autoxidation of biological molecules I. The antioxidant activity of vitamin E and related chain breaking phenolic antioxidants in vitro, *J. Am. Chem. Soc.* **1981**, *103*, 6472–6477.

Buttery, R. G.; Teranishi, R. Gas-liquid chromatography of aroma of vegetables and fruits. Direct injection of aqueous vapors. *Anal. Chem.* **1961**,*33*, 1439–1441.

Das, N. P.; Ramanathan, L. Studies on flavonoids and related compounds as antioxidant in food. In *Lipid-Soluble Antioxidants: Biochemistry and Clinical Applications*; Ong, A. S. H.; Packer, L., Eds.; Birkhauser: Basel, 1992; 295–306.

Dhopeshwarkar, G.A., Naturally occurring food toxicants: toxic lipids. *Prog. Lipid Res.* **1980**,*19*, 107–118.

Drewnowski, A.; Greenwood, M. R. C. Cream and sugar: human preferences for high fat foods. *Physiol. Behav.* **1983**,*30*, 629–633.

Drewnowski, A. Taste preferences and food intake. *Ann. Rev. Nutr.* **1997**,*17*, 237–253.

Eriksson, C. E; Na, A. Antioxidant agents in raw materials and processed foods. *Biochem. Soc. Symp.* **1995**, *61*, 221–234.

Esterbauer, H., Cytotoxicity and genotoxicity of lipid-oxidation products. *Am. J. Clin. Nutr.* **1993**,*57 (Suppl. 5)*, 779S-786S.

Fielding, C. J.; Bist, A.; Fielding, P. E. Caveolin mRNA levels are up-regulated by free cholesterol and down-regulated by oxysterols in fibroblast monolayers. *Proc. Natl. Acad. Sci. USA* **1997**, *94*, 3753–3758.

Fontana, A.; Antoniazzi, F; Cimino, G.; Mazza, G.; Trivellone, E.; Zanone, B. High-resolution NMR detection of cholesterol oxides in spray dried egg yolk. *J. Food Sci.* **1992**,*57*, 869–872.

Frankel, E. N. The antioxidant and nutritional effects of tocopherols, ascorbic acid and beta-carotene in relation to processing of edible oils. *Bibl. Nutr. Dieta* **1989**,*43*, 297–312.

Frankel, E. N. Recent advances in lipid oxidation. *J. Sci. Food Agric.* **1991**, *54*, 495–511.

Frankel, E. N.; Huang, S. W.; Kanner, J.; German, J. B. Interfacial phenomena in the evaluation of antioxidants: bulk oils versus emulsions. *J. Agric. Food Chem.* **1994**, *42*, 1054–1059.

Fritsche, K. L.; Johnston, P. V. Rapid autoxidation of fish oil in diets without added antioxidants. *J. Nutr.* **1988**,*118*, 425–426.

Gere, A. Decrease in essential fatty acid content of edible fats during the frying process. *Z. Ernaehrungswiss* **1982**, *21*, 191–201.

German, J. B. Muscle lipids. *J. Muscle Foods* **1989**, *1*, 339–361.

Halliwell, B. The role of oxygen radicals in human disease, with particular reference to the vascular system. *Haemostasis* **1993**, *23 (Suppl. 1)*, 118–126.

Hanasaki, Y.; Ogawa, S.; Fukui, S. The correlation between active oxygen scavenging and antioxidative effects of flavonoids. *Free Radical Biol. Med.* **1994**,*16*, 845–850.

Hetherington, M. M.; Rolls, B. J. Eating behavior in eating disorders: response to preloads. *Physiol. Behav.* **1991**, *50*, 101–108.

Hopia, A. I.; Huang, S.-W.; Schwarz, K.; German, J. B.; Frankel; E. N. Effect of different lipid systems on antioxidant activity of rosemary constituents carnosol and carnosic acid with and without α-tocopherol. *J. Agric. Food Chem.* **1996**, *44*, 2030–2036.

Huang, S.-W.; Frankel, E. N.; German, J. B. Antioxidant activity of alpha- and gamma-tocopherols in bulk oils and in oil-in-water emulsions. *J. Agric. Food Chem.* **1994**, *42*, 2108–2114.

Huang, S.-W.; Frankel, E. N.; German, J. B. Effects of individual tocopherols and tocopherol mixtures on the oxidative stability of corn oil triglycerides. *J. Agric. Food Chem.* **1995**,*43*, 2345–2350.

Huang, S. W.; Frankel, E. N.; Aeschbach, R.; German J. B. (1997) Partition of selected antioxidants in corn oil-water model systems. *J. Agric. Food Chem.* **1997**, *45*, 1991–1994.

Jessup, W.; Rankin, S. M.; De Whalley, C. V.; Hoult, J. R.; Scott, J.; Leake, D. S. Alpha-tocopherol consumption during low-density-lipoprotein oxidation. *Biochem. J.* **1990**, *265*, 399–405.

Johnson, S. L.; McPhee, L.; Birch, L. L. Conditioned preferences: young children prefer flavors associated with high dietary fat. *Physiol. Behav.* **1991**,*50*, 1245–1251.

Kanner, J.; German, J. B; Kinsella, J. E. Initiation of lipid oxidation in biological systems. *Crit. Rev. Food Sci. Nutr.* **1987**, *25*, 317–364.

Keen, C. L.; German, J. B.; Mareschi, J. P.; Gershwin, M. E. Nutritional modulation of murine models of autoimmunity. *Rheum. Dis. Clin. North Am.* **1991**, *17*, 223–234.

Larson, R. A. Antoxidant mechanisms of secondary natural products. In *Oxidative Stress and Antioxidant Defenses in Biology*; Ahmad, S., Ed.; Chapman and Hall: New York, 1995, pp 210–233.

Laughton, M. J.; Evans, P. J.; Moroney, M. A.; Hoult, J. R.; Halliwell, B. Inhibition of mammalian 5-lipoxygenase and cyclo-oxygenase by flavonoids and phenolic dietary additives. Relationship to antioxidant activity and to iron ion-reducing ability. *Biochem. Pharmacol.* **1991**, *42*, 1673–1681.

Love, J. Mechanism of iron catalysis of lipid oxidation in warmed-over flavor of meat. In *Food Lipids and Health*; McDonald, R. E.; Min, D. B., Eds.; Marcel Dekker: New York, 1996, pp 269–286.

Miller, K. S; Krochta, J. M. Oxygen and aroma barrier properties of edible films: A review. *Trends Food Sci. Tech.* **1997**, *8*, 228–237.

Morin, R. J.; Peng, S. K. The role of cholesterol oxidation products in the pathogenesis of atherosclerosis. *Ann. Clin. Lab. Sci.* **1989**, *19*, 225–237.

Moser, H. A.; Dutton, H. J.; Evans, C. D.; Cowan, J. C. Conducting a taste panel for the evaluation of edible oils. *Food Technol.* **1950**, *4*, 105–109.

Muggli, R. Dietary fish oils increase the requirement for vitamin E in humans. In *Health Effects of Fish and Fish Oils*; Chandra, R. K., Ed.; ARTS Biomedical Publishers and Distributors: St. John's, Newfoundland, 1989; pp 201–210.

Norris, F. A. Extraction of fats and oils. In *Bailey's Industrial Oil and Fat Products*; Vol. 2; Swern, D., Ed.; J. Wiley: New York, 1982; pp 178–245.

Osman, A., M. Wootton, R.S. Baker, A. Arlauskas, and T.M. Bonin, Mutagenic Activity of Heated Potato/Oil Systems, *Nutr. Cancer* **1983**, *5*, 146–151.

Paniangvait, P.; King, A. J.; Jones, A. D.; German, J. B. Cholesterol oxides in foods of animal origin. *J. Food Sci.* **1995**, *60*, 1159–1174.

Porter, N. A.; Caldwell, S. E.; Mills, S. A. Mechanisms of free radical oxidation of unsaturated lipids. *Lipids* **1995**, *30*, 277–290.

Qu, Y. H.; Xu, G. X.; Zhou, J. Z.; Chen, T. D.; Zhu, L. F.; Shields, P. G.; Wang, H. W.; Gao, Y. T. Genotoxicity of heated cooking oil vapors. *Mutat. Res.* **1992**, *298*, 105–111.

Schwarz, K.; Frankel, E. N.; German, J. B. Partition behavior of antioxidative phenolic compounds in heterophasic systems. *Fett/Lipid* **1996**, *98*, 115–121.

Sevanian, A.; Berliner, J.; Peterson, H. Uptake, metabolism, and cytotoxicity of isomeric cholesterol-5,6-epoxides in rabbit aortic endothelial cells. *J. Lipid Res.* **1991**, *32*, 147–155.

Simoneau, C.; McCarthy, M. J.; Reid, D. S.; German, J. B. Measurement of fat crystallization using NMR imaging and spectroscopy. *Trends Food Sci. Technol.* **1992**, *3*, 208–211.

Smouse, T. H. Significance of lipid oxidation to food processors. In *Food Lipids and Health*; McDonald, R. E.; Min, D. B., Eds.; Marcel Dekker: New York, 1996; pp 269–286.

St. Angelo, A. J. Lipid oxidation in foods. *Crit. Rev. Food Sci. Nutr.* **1996**,*36*, 175–224.

Steinberg, D.; Parthasarathy, S.; Carew, T. E.; Khoo, J. C.; Witztum, J. L. Beyond cholesterol. modifications of low-density lipoprotein that increase its atherogenicity. *New Eng. J. Med.* **1989**, *320*, 915–924.

Teranishi, R.; Buttery, R. G.; Lundin, R. Gas chromatography-direct vapor analyses of food products with programmed temperature control of dual column with dual flame ionization detectors. *Anal. Chem.* **1962**, *34*, 1033–1035.

Terao, J., Piskula, M.; Yao, Q. Protective effect of epicatechin, epicatechin gallate, and quercetin on lipid peroxidation in phospholipid bilayers. *Arch. Biochem. Biophys.* **1994**, *308*, 278–284.

Tournaire, C.; Croux, S.; Maurette, M. T.; Beck, I.; Hocquaux, M.; Braun, A. M.; Oliveros, E. J. Antioxidant activity of flavonoids: efficiency of singlet oxygen (1 delta g) quenching. *J. Photochem. Photobiol. B, Biol.* **1993**, *19*, 205–215.

Warwick, Z. S.; Schiffman, S. S. Role of dietary fat in calorie intake and weight gain. *Neurosci. Biobehav. Rev.* **1992**, *16*, 585–596.

Zhang, W. B.; Addis, P. B. Prediction of levels of cholesterol oxides in heated tallow by dielectric measurement. *J. Food Sci.* **1990**, *55*, 1673–1675.

4

IMPACT OF PROCESSING ON FORMATION OF *TRANS* FATTY ACIDS

J. M. King[1] and P. J. White[2]

[1]Department of Food Science
Louisiana State University
Baton Rouge, Louisiana 70803
[2]Department of Food Science and Human Nutrition
Iowa State University
Ames, Iowa 50011

1. ABSTRACT

Trans fatty acids are formed during hydrogenation which is done to improve the functionality and oxidative stability of oils. Several process conditions affect the content of *trans* fatty acids in hydrogenated oil. There is conflicting evidence as to whether intake of *trans* fatty acids, in foods such as margarine, affects the types and levels of cholesterol produced in the blood. Epidemiological studies have shown associated increases in total cholesterol and low density lipoproteins, as well as decreased levels of high density lipoproteins in the blood. It is unknown whether these effects are related directly to *trans* fatty acids or to the decrease of unsaturated fatty acids in the diet. This chapter will cover the recent nutritional status of *trans* fatty acids and the effect of processing on the levels of *trans* fatty acids in foods.

2. INTRODUCTION

The issue of *trans* fatty acids (f.a.) in the human diet has been an area of debate for food scientists and nutritionists worldwide. There is conflicting evidence as to whether intake of *trans* f.a., in foods such as margarine, affects the types and levels of cholesterol produced in the blood. Epidemiological studies have shown associated increases in total cholesterol and low density lipoproteins, as well as decreased levels of high density lipoproteins in the blood. It is unknown whether these effects are related directly to *trans* f.a. or to the decrease of unsaturated f.a. in the diet. There are two main ways in which *trans* f.a. can

Impact of Processing on Food Safety, edited by Jackson et al.,
Kluwer Academic / Plenum Publishers, New York, 1999.

enter into the food system: through biohydrogenation of dietary lipids in ruminant animals and through chemical hydrogenation of oils by using catalysts. Biohydrogenation produces more monoenoic isomers with the *trans* bond at the 11 position (vaccenic acid or 11-*trans*-octadecenoic acid), whereas chemical hydrogenation produces more isomers with the *trans* bond at position 9 (elaidic acid or 9-*trans*-octadecenoic acid) (O'Donnell, 1993).

3. BIOHYDROGENATION

Biohydrogenation occurs through the action of bacteria in the rumen of animals, following the general pathways shown in Figure 1 (Kellens et al., 1986). Several factors affect biohydrogenation and the formation of *trans* isomers. Biohydrogenation was facilitated by the presence of small food particles because microorganisms were attached to the surface of these particles (Harfoot, 1978). In *in vitro* studies, the presence of cell-free rumen fluid resulted in increased biohydrogenation in an incubation mixture containing yeast-based media, a cell suspension and 1 mg/ml of linoleic acid (9-*cis*-12-*cis*-octadecadienoic acid) as a serum albumin complex (Kellens, 1986). The amount of vaccenic acid formed from linoleic acid after 7 hours in a standard yeast-based media was 38.6% of the f.a. composition, whereas that formed in a standard media with 10% rumen fluid added was 67.3%. The addition of more linoleic acid to the media resulted in less biohydrogenation to vaccenic acid and an increase in the formation of 9-*cis*-11-*trans*- octadecadienoic acid isomers. If 0.01 mg/ml of linoleic acid was added instead of rumen fluid, then the vaccenic acid content was 25.3% and the 9-*cis*-11-*trans*-octadecadienoic acid isomer content was 35.2% (Kellens et al., 1986). When the standard media contained additional linoleic acid and rumen fluid, the vaccenic acid content increased to 59.7% and the 9-*cis*-11-*trans*-octadecadienoic acid content decreased to 20.7%. Without additional linoleic acid, the 9-*cis*-11-*trans*- octadecadienoic acid isomer content was 12.9% and 18.5%, respectively, in the rumen fluid-media mix and media alone. The presence of rumen fluid caused more of the 9-*cis*-11-*trans*- octadecadienoic acid to transform into vaccenic acid. Age of the culture also affected biohydrogenation. The older the

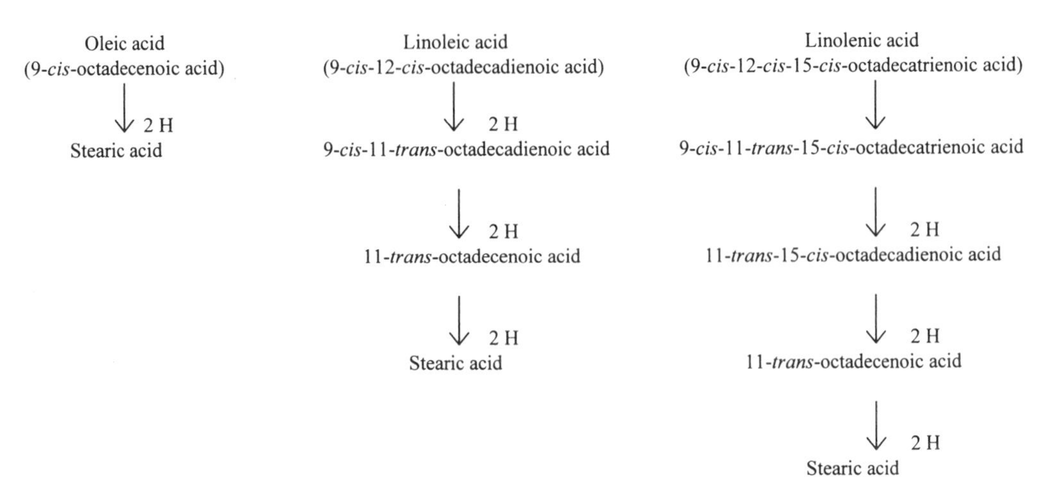

Figure 1. General pathways of biohydrogenation of unsaturated fatty acids by a mixed culture of microorganisms. Reprinted with permission from Kellens et al. (1986).

mixed rumen culture, the more vaccenic acid formed. During 18 hours of aging, 29.6% vaccenic acid was formed in a standard media with rumen fluid, whereas the same culture aged 24 hours resulted in 67.3% vaccenic acid (Kellens et al., 1986).

When linoleic acid was used in *in vitro* experiments at levels greater than 1.0 mg/ml of rumen contents, the major end product formed was vaccenic acid (Harfoot et al., 1973), as a result of the irreversible inhibition by linoleic acid of biohydrogenation of vaccenic acid to stearic acid. If a continuous supply of easily fermented substrate such as sucrose was provided, then the inhibitory effects of linoleic acid were reduced (Harfoot et al., 1973). Also, if less than 1 mg/ml of linoleic acid was used, then the main biohydrogenation product was stearic acid. Both of these steps resulted in less *trans* isomer formation. A diet containing 1.7% nitrogen and 44% total starch and soluble sugars, compared to lesser levels of carbohydrate (down to 30.5%) and greater levels of nitrogen (up to 3.72%), when fed to sheep, resulted in the lowest amount of esterified *trans* f.a. formation in the rumen, a value of 1.9% (Gerson et al., 1983). Unesterified *trans* f.a. content in the rumen was lowest for a diet containing 3.72% nitrogen, 30.5% starch and 3.8% soluble sugars.

In vitro experiments showed that incubation of diets with a blend of animal and vegetable fat resulted in greater formation of *trans* f.a. than diets containing calcium soaps of palm f.a. (Wu and Palmquist, 1991). This result was because of a greater content of linoleic acid in the animal and vegetable blend than in the calcium soap diet. Another factor was the availability of the f.a. for biohydrogenation (Wu and Palmquist, 1991). The animal and vegetable blend diet, however, still showed a higher level of *trans* f.a. formation even if the linoleic acid contents were equalized to those of the calcium soap diet. When linoleic acid was continuously added to an *in vitro* fermentation of cow ruminal contents to maintain a steady state level, there also was an increase in oleic acid (9-*cis*-octadecenoic acid) and linoleic acid, in addition to the increase in vaccenic acid (Fellner, 1995).

When cows were fed diets containing oil supplements, the amount of fat produced in their milk decreased and the amount of *trans* isomers formed during biohydrogenation increased. There was an inverse relationship between the amount of *trans* f.a. formed and the level of fat produced *in vivo*. *Trans* f.a. tended to inhibit the synthesis of short and medium chain f.a. which in turn caused milk-fat depression (Selener and Schultz, 1980).

In other studies, the objective was to protect polyunsaturated f.a. from biohydrogenation in order to decrease the saturated and *trans* f.a. content of animal fat. Fotouhi and Jenkins (1992) found that when linoleoyl methionine was included in the diet of sheep, the loss of unsaturated f.a. was 69.8% compared to 92.9% and 94.6% for free linoleic acid and calcium linoleate, respectively. There were fewer *trans* f.a. in the duodenum of the sheep fed linoleoyl methionine. The resistance of linoleoyl methionine to biohydrogenation may be because of the size of the amide bond substituents (Fotouhi and Jenkins, 1992).

Cows, goats and sheep were fed linseed oil particles encapsulated with formaldehyde-treated casein. The unsaturated f.a. composition of milk fat or depot fat from these animals was greater than for those fed normal diets (Scott, 1971). The level of linolenic acid in the abomasum (the true stomach) was 31.9% for goats fed the diet with formaldehyde-treated casein particles of linseed oil and 1.05% for goats fed the diet with untreated casein particles of linseed oil. The level of linolenic acid in milk lipids of goats fed the diet with formaldehyde-treated casein particles of linseed oil was 23.1%, whereas that of the normal diet was 1.45%. Similar results were found for linoleic acid contents of sheep depot fats. The formaldehyde treatment prevented the biohydrogenation of oil in the rumen, but the resulting complex was broken down by acid in the abomasum so the lipid could be absorbed. Therefore, the encapsulation of oil supplements with formaldehyde-treated casein should result in less *trans* f.a. formation, and the levels of unsaturated f.a. in milk fat, depot fat and plasma should be increased (Scott, 1971).

In summary, the overall factors affecting biohydrogenation and the formation of *trans* isomers include 1) the level and form of linoleic acid in the animals' diets, 2) the availability of hydrogen donors such as sucrose, 3) the presence of food particles, 4) the presence of rumen fluid, and 5) the age of the rumen culture.

4. CHEMICAL HYDROGENATION

4.1. General Information

Hydrogenation is used to improve the oxidative stability and functionality of fats and oils found in foods. Hydrogenation can be done in a batch process, which is used commercially, or in a continuous operation. There is more control over pressure and temperature in batch processes, but a continuous method saves time and money. Batch hydrogenation can be done in two different ways. The oil can be sprayed into an atmosphere of hydrogen: this type of hydrogenation is known as the Wibuschewitsch process. The reverse also may be done where the hydrogen is sparged into the oil. This method is known as the Normann process and it is preferred in the United States (Edvardsson and Ivandoust, 1994). Batch reactors can be recirculating, where the hydrogen is continuously removed from the headspace and then sparged back in after purification, or dead-end, where there is a static headspace hydrogen content (Edvardsson and Ivandoust, 1994). The dead-end reactor provides better process control of temperature and pressure which, in turn, helps the selectivity of the process. The equipment also is simpler, cheaper and easier to maintain than continuous reactors.

Continuous reactors can be one of two types: tubular or flow (Edvardsson and Ivandoust, 1994). Flow reactors have several disadvantages. It is hard to maintain uniform contact between gas and liquid phases and to maintain their residence times. There also is the possibility of back-mixing of the liquid phase. There are several experimental pilot-plant scale reactors, each with their own advantages and disadvantages (Edvardsson and Ivandoust, 1994).

The experimental variables that can be manipulated in chemical hydrogenation include the type and concentration of catalyst, the type of oil used, the pressure, the temperature, the time and the agitation level. In general, if the hydrogenation process proceeds for a long enough period of time, fewer *trans* isomers will be found in the final product because all of the unsaturated f.a. become fully saturated. Also, decreased agitation will result in less hydrogen circulation and a slower rate of hydrogenation and, therefore, more isomer formation. Several studies have been done to determine the specific parameters for obtaining the lowest final content of *trans* isomers as well as maintaining a high catalytic activity. One way the formation of *trans* f.a. during hydrogenation can be controlled is by varying the type of catalyst used. It is important that the catalyst be easily removed from the oil and that the greatest selectivity for hydrogenation of specific f.a. can be obtained. Selectivity is most important during processing of partially hydrogenated oil, where monounsaturated f.a. production is one of the desired goals. Selective hydrogenation tends to result in increased *trans* f.a. formation, and *trans* f.a. provide a quicker mouth melt for margarine and confectionery fats (Patterson, 1983).

The main catalyst utilized in commercial hydrogenation is nickel. It is low cost and has high activity, but it causes the formation of *trans* f.a. more than other types of catalysts. Other catalysts include those with palladium such as palladium on carbon, palladium on polystyrene and palladium on aluminum sulfate or barium sulfate. Also available are the arene chromium carbonyl complexes such as methyl benzoate-$Cr(CO)_3$, benzene-$Cr(CO)_3$, and toluene-$Cr(CO)_3$, and dichlorodicarbonylbis (triphenylphosphine) ruthenium (II), gold and copper chromite or mixtures of catalysts. Catalytic transfer hydrogenation also has been done using formate as a hydrogen donor with palladium on carbon as the catalyst. This prccedure is simple and requires neither hydrogen gas nor high pressures and temperatures.

4.2. Palladium Catalysts

Catalysts have been studied in comparison to each other and in several types of reactors. Heldal et al. (1989) found that, in a fixed-bed continuous reactor during hydrogenation of soybean oil, palladium on polystyrene catalyst caused the formation of fewer *trans* isomers than palladium on carbon. Increased temperature had no effect on isomerization, and the continuous process resulted in less isomerization than would a batch system (Heldal et al., 1989). The activity of these catalysts increased with increased temperature to a certain extent, but a main drawback was that the selectivity for linoleate and linolenate was lower than that for batch hydrogenation. In comparison, adding nickel as the catalyst with an increase in temperature resulted in increased *trans* contents and hydrogenation activity (Heldal et al., 1989).

Hsu et al. (1989) found that at higher temperatures, during batch hydrogenation, palladium on carbon catalyst caused increased *trans* formation, but the effect of temperature was less at higher pressures. *Trans* isomer formation was favored at lower pressures and increased catalyst concentration (Hsu et al., 1989). The selectivity for linoleic acid and the amount of *trans* isomer formation with palladium-alumina pellets was similar to that found with palladium on carbon, but both were higher than those observed for 5% palladium on alumina (Hsu et al., 1988). Hsu et al. (1988) also found that canola oil had a lower *trans* content than soybean oil at the same pressure of hydrogenation. The *trans* isomer content of canola oil hydrogenated at 90°C and 750 pounds per square inch was 13.5 %, whereas that for soybean oil under the same conditions was 16.7%. The *trans* isomer formation doubled from 19.0% to 37.8%, for canola oil hydrogenation at a pressure of 100 pounds per square inch, with a change in temperature from 50°C to 90°C. Increases in the amount of catalyst did not affect the content of *trans* isomers in soybean oil (Hsu et al., 1988). Five percent palladium on carbon produced less than half of the *trans* isomer content formed at higher pressures of hydrogenation using nickel (Hsu et al., 1988). It was possible to use 50 to 150 times less palladium than nickel as a catalyst, but palladium was 150 to 250 times more expensive than nickel in 1986, so the economics were not favorable (Hsu et al., 1986).

Smidovnik et al. (1992) used 10% palladium on carbon in batch and continuous forms of catalytic transfer hydrogenation of soybean oil. In the batch system, sodium formate was dissolved in water and triethylammonium formate or formic acid was dissolved in organic solvent. There was less isomerization in the aqueous system: 33.0% *trans* isomer formation after 24 hours, as compared to 42.5% from a system containing acetone and triethylammonium formate (Smidovnik et al., 1992).

4.3. Nickel Catalysts

Variations of nickel catalysts in hydrogenation also have been studied. Grompone and Moyna (1986) found when a commercial catalyst containing 20.5% nickel was used in the presence of carbon dioxide gas instead of hydrogen gas, isomerization of pure oleic acid to the *trans* isomer occurred. After 19 hours, 45.6% of the oleic acid was converted to elaidic acid when the weight of catalyst used was 10% of the oil weight. Generally for nickel during batch hydrogenation, greater pressures and higher temperatures resulted in increased hydrogenation, with selectivity being affected more by pressure than temperature (Koseoglu and Lusas, 1990). Other studies showed that increased temperature caused increased formation of *trans* isomers, and pressure and catalyst concentration had a minimal effect on *trans* formation (Koseoglu and Lusas, 1990). Sulfur has a poisoning effect on nickel and causes the formation of nickel-sulfur compounds that can cause increased formation of *trans* isomers (Koseoglu and Lusas, 1990).

Nickel has been tested in various hydrogenation systems. Electrocatalytic hydrogenation of soybean oil with Raney nickel as the cathode resulted in less *trans* isomer formation than traditional hydrogenation (Yusem and Pintauro, 1992). Hydrogen gas was formed *in situ* by the reduction of electrolytic solvent containing tetraethylammonium p-toluenesulfonate salt. Changes in the electrolyte butanol composition from 0 to 50% did not affect *trans* formation. Ultrasonic energy increased the rate of hydrogenation without increasing the amount of *trans* isomerization, in contrast to batch hydrogenation (Moulton, 1987). Although pressure changes did not affect the formation of *trans* isomers during ultrasonic hydrogenation, greater catalyst concentration and lower temperatures resulted in more *trans* isomers.

4.4. Other Catalysts

Krishnaiah and Sarkar (1990) and Rubin et al. (1986) tested a mixed catalyst system with nickel and chromium. Chromium was used in two forms: chromia (Cr_2O_3) and methyl benzoate-chromium tricarbonyl for the hydrogenation of cottonseed and canola oils, respectively. A molar ratio of chromia chromium to nickel of 0.17 gave the highest concentration of oleic acid, 52.2%, whereas a molar ratio of nickel to chromium, from the methyl benzoate tricarbonyl form, of 0.89 gave the lowest *trans* isomer formation (Krishnaiah and Sarkar, 1990; Rubin et al., 1986). Higher concentrations of nickel or methyl benzoate-chromium tricarbonyl alone, without added nickel, resulted in more *trans* isomers (Rubin et al., 1986).

Other chromite catalysts have been tested. Szukalska and Drozdowski (1982) used copper-chromite as a catalyst in the hydrogenation of rapeseed oils with various erucic acid (13-*cis*-docosenoic acid) concentrations. Not only did copper-chromite produce 2 to 2.5 times fewer *trans* isomers than nickel in a dead-end reactor method, but the greater the erucic acid level in the oil, the slower the selective hydrogenation. Erucic acid itself formed very limited amounts of *trans* isomers, less than 0.5% after 4 hours of hydrogenation. High erucic acid oil (51.2% erucic acid) has most of its linolenic acid in position 2 on the triglyceride so linoleic acid is sterically hindered from hydrogenation by the erucic acid in positions 1 and 3 (Szukalska and Drozdowski, 1982).

Arene complexes of chromium tricarbonyl $(CrCO)_3$ had decreased formation of *trans* isomers in the order of methyl benzoate>benzene>toluene. This decrease was because of increased stability of the arene-Cr bond by electron-donating groups (Bernstein, 1989). Chromium phosphine as homogeneous, supported and heterogeneous catalysts prepared from chromium also have been tested. Homogeneous triphenylphosphine chromium pentacarbonyl ($Cr(CO)_5PPh_3$) produced *trans* isomer content similar to that produced from chromium hexacarbonyl (Bernstein, 1989). Silica-supported chromium catalysts produced low amounts of *trans* isomer. Precipitated heterogeneous chromium on silica catalysts with chromium in a zero oxidation state gave the greatest *trans* isomer concentration, 9.3%, whereas chromium in the +2 or +3 states gave very low levels of *trans* isomer, 0.8% and 1.5%, respectively (Bernstein, 1989). The problem with these chromium catalysts is that their activity is low.

Two other catalysts tested were gold and dichlorodicarbonyl bis(triphenylphosphine) ruthenium (II) ($RuCl_2(CO)_2(PPh_3)_2$ (Koseoglu and Lusas, 1990). Gold supported on silica or alumina was more stable than unsupported gold, was easy to separate from oil and was a good candidate for continuous hydrogenation, but the lower the iodine value needed, the greater the resulting *trans* isomer concentration. The ruthenium catalyst concentration did not affect the level of *trans* isomers formed during hydrogenation of canola oil. A greater temperature and lesser pressure resulted in increased *trans* isomer formation with ruthenium complex catalysts. At a pressure of 50 pounds per square inch and a temperature of 140°C, the *trans* isomer content was about 60%, whereas the *trans* isomer content at a pressure of 750 pounds per square inch and a temperature of 110°C was 10% (Koseoglu and Lusas, 1990). The negative side of ruthenium catalysts is that they are hard to separate from the oil.

In summary, the overall factors that can be adjusted to regulate the formation of *trans* f.a. during chemical hydrogenation are: 1) the type of hydrogenation process, 2) the type and concentration of catalyst, 3) the type of oil used, 4) the pressure, 5) the temperature, 6) the time, 7) the agitation level and 8) varying combinations of these factors.

5. EFFECT OF HYDROGENATION AND *TRANS* F.A. ON FUNCTION OF FATS IN FOODS

Hydrogenation makes fats more stable to rancidity because of the resulting decrease in the number of double bonds available for oxidation. *Trans* double bonds also are more stable to oxidation than *cis* double bonds. Selective hydrogenation conditions can be varied to produce fats with different amounts of saturation, resulting in fats with different melting points and functionality as well as lower *trans* f.a. contents. Table 1 lists the effects of hydrogenation temperature on the functionality of the oils (Patterson, 1983). Hydrogenation at 150°C provides fat with a prolonged melting range, whereas hydrogenation at 180°C provides a fat with a quick melting range. Hydrogenation at 160°C results in equilibrium formation of *trans* f.a., whereas lower temperatures form fewer *trans* f.a.

Table 1. Effect of hydrogenation temperature on the functionality of oils

Temperature (°C)	Effect
100 to 115	Partial hydrogenation of a vegetable oil with minimum formation of *trans* isomers.
c. 120	The first two stages in hydrogenation, resulting in minimum solids content and flavor stability.
150	Level at which completely hydrogenated vegetable shortening is formed with prolonged melting.
160	Above this temperature there is an increased effect of poisoning of nickel and formation of *trans* isomers is encouraged to reach an equilibrium level.
180	The usual level for edible oil hydrogenation. If a relatively quick melting range is needed, this temperature should be used as much as possible after any other control requirements have been met.
200	Should not be exceeded for edible product hardening. Above this temperature color defects as well as increased free fatty acid formation occur.

Adapted and reprinted with permission from Patterson (1983).

Table 2. Concentration of *trans* fatty acids in US oil products

Type of fat	*Trans* fatty acids (range % of fatty acids)	Reference
Shortening	13.0 to 42.4	Smith et al., 1986, Enig et al., 1983
Stick margarine	16.1 to 36.0	Slover et al., 1985, Carpenter and Slover, 1973
Tub margarine	10.6 to 29.8	Enig et al., 1983, Slover et al., 1985
Partially hydrogenated	4.9 to 13.4	Enig et al., 1983, Scholfield et al., 1967
Butter	3.4	Enig et al., 1983
Animal fat	0.2 to 7.8	Slover et al., 1987, Parodi, 1976

Table 2 shows the range of *trans* f.a. as a percentage of total f.a. content found in U.S. oil products (Smith et al., 1986; Enig et al., 1983; Slover et al., 1985; Carpenter and Slover,1973; Scholfield et al., 1967; Slover et al., 1987; Parodi, 1976). Hydrogenation is used to make salad and cooking oils, shortenings and margarine. Partial hydrogenation of soybean oil to <3 % linoleic acid content provides some stability against oxidation for oils in salad dressings or mayonnaise (Dupont, 1991). For cooking oils, partial hydrogenation provides some stability to both oxidation and hydrolytic breakdown, hence reducing the likelihood of polymerization. Polymerization causes the oil to become more viscous and results in fried foods becoming more greasy. Partially hydrogenated oils have *trans* f.a. contents ranging from 4.9% to 13.4% (Table 2). Shortenings are used in baked foods such as breads, cakes and doughnuts to add richness, enhance aeration and flavor, and in icings and fillings to give a light and fluffy structure (Dupont, 1991). Shortenings made by blending partially hydrogenated oil and fully hydrogenated oil are used for making baked goods. These blends have a wide melting range to enhance mixability. The *trans* f.a. content of shortenings ranges from 13.0% to 42.4% (Table 2).

Selective hydrogenation is used to make margarine. It is necessary to have the correct ratio of polyunsaturated, monounsaturated and saturated f.a. as well as to control the amount of *trans* f.a. in the product so that margarine has a quick mouth melt without a waxy mouth feel. Elaidic acid has a higher melting point, 45°C, than oleic acid, 16°C, and stick margarine has a greater *trans* content than tub margarine with ranges of 16.1% to 36.0% for the former and 10.6% to 29.8% for the latter (Table 2).

In a comparison of several available commercial nickel catalysts for the hydrogenation of soybean oil, the solid fat fraction had a greater *trans* content and lower flavor scores than did the liquid oil fraction of hydrogenated, winterized soybean oil. The *trans* content of the solid fat fraction ranged from 29.0% to 33.9%, whereas that for the liquid fat fraction ranged from 25.3% to 29.3% (Chu and Lin, 1991). The oil flavor score, on a scale of 0 for strong to 10 for bland, for the solid fat fraction was 4.25 and for the liquid oil fraction was 5.85. Therefore, not only can *trans* isomers affect the nutritional attributes and texture of fats, but they also may influence the flavor of fats (Chu and Lin, 1991).

6. *TRANS* F.A. CONTENTS IN THE U.S. DIET

There are several ways to estimate the amounts of *trans* f.a. available in the human diet including: 1) availability based on the total U.S. population using fat disappearance data, 2) availability based on the total U.S. population using adipose tissue data, 3) intake based on the adult U.S. population using adipose tissue and actual fat intake data, and 4) intake based on the adult U.S. population using published fats and oils data and actual fat

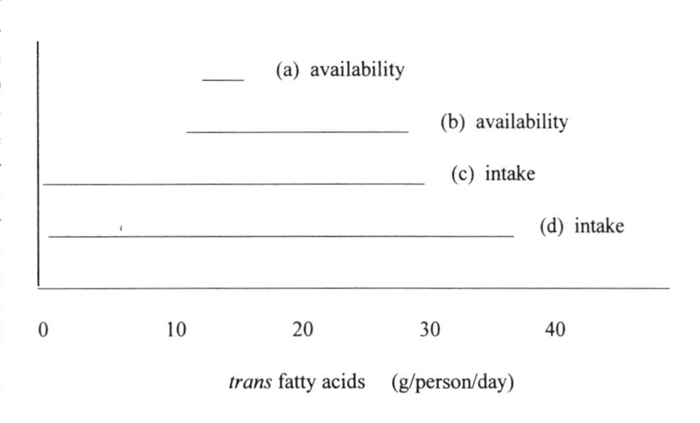

Figure 2. Estimated range of per capita *trans* fatty acids availability/intake (consumption) based on different methods of calculation: (a) estimated availability for total population based on fat disappearance data, (b) estimated availability for total population based on adipose tissue data, (c) estimated intake for the adult population based on adipose tissue data and actual fat intake data, (d) estimated intake for the adult population based on published fats and oils data and actual fat intake data. Reprinted with permission from Enig et al. (1983).

intake data (Figure 2, Enig et al., 1990). To make these estimates the following must be known: the amounts of fats and oils in the food supply that are sources of *trans* f.a., the amounts of fats and oils used in edible products, production levels of the main types of fats and oils, the amount of *trans* f.a. in each type of fat/oil and edible product, the amount of wastage of fats and oils, dietary history of fat consumption of various age groups and adipose tissue levels of *trans* fatty acids in humans.

There are two main sources of fats; vegetable and animal. Vegetable fats and oils were used in edible products at a level of 12,505 million pounds in 1984–1985 with a total source of fat of 62.9 g/person/day based on the total U.S. population (Enig et al., 1990). Based on estimates of a weighted average of 23% *trans* f.a. in margarine (20% tub margarine and 80% stick margarine), 10.2% *trans* f.a. in oils and 25.3% *trans* f.a. in shortenings, the result is an availability of 11.72 g *trans* f.a./person/day (Enig et al., 1990). A total of 12.83 g *trans* f.a./person/day is obtained when the availability of animal and dairy *trans* f.a. is included, with a calculated wastage of 15% for shortenings and salad and cooking oils as well as 72.5% wastage for beef fat (Figure 2). Hunter and Applewhite (1991) estimated *trans* f.a. availability to be 8.1 g/person/day in 1989 based on market size data, measured amounts of *trans* f.a. found in products, 50% wastage for deep-frying fats and the total U.S. population in 1989.

Enig et al. (1990) found a significant correlation between dietary linoleic acid and adipose tissue elaidic acid contents in rats and mice in the literature. A graph of these data gave an equation with which estimates of human dietary intake could be made from existing data on human adipose tissue *trans* f.a. levels. These calculations suggested a range of 2.4% to 11.1% *trans* f.a. in the human diet. This concentration represents 0.7 to 28.7 g *trans* f.a./person/day (Figure 2). When utilizing fat intake data from the Lipid Research Clinic ranges of 40 to 258 g/person/day for men at 8% *trans* f.a. concentration, Enig et al. (1990) estimated the range of *trans* f.a. intake as 2.4 to 20.6 g/person/day. For women, the fat intake ranged from 31 to 179 g with an estimated *trans* f.a. intake of 1.9 to 14.3 g/person/day. Enig et al. (1990) found ranges of 6% to 12% *trans* f.a. of the total f.a. in diets analyzed by their laboratory, so the complete range of possible intake of *trans* f.a. could be 1.6 to 38.7 g/person/day, calculated by using intake data (Figure 2). Figure 2 summarizes these findings (Enig et al., 1990). The results vary overall, depending on whether all or part of the population is used in the calculations and whether the calculation is based on market size data, fat disappearance data, fat intake data or adipose tissue data.

7. EFFECT OF DIETARY *TRANS* F.A. ON HEALTH

7.1. Studies on Blood Plasma and Serum Cholesterol Levels

There also are discrepancies in studies on the effects of *trans* f.a. on health depending upon the method used, as well as the types of f.a. consumed in the diets and the specific isomer involved. Three different studies on the effect of dietary *trans* f.a. on lipoprotein (a) levels in humans were published in the same volume of the Journal of Lipid Research in 1992 (Mensink et al., 1992; Zock and Katan, 1992; Nestel et al., 1992). Blood plasma cholesterol measurements were done on subjects after they consumed randomized, balanced diets with different contents of saturated, *cis*-unsaturated and *trans*-unsaturated f.a. Mensink et al. (1992) performed three separate experiments on healthy normacholesterolemic men and women. In the first experiment, diets consisting of 17 days of highly saturated f.a. were consumed followed by 36 days of 6.5% of the total energy from saturates replaced by either a combination of monounsaturates and polyunsaturates or polyunsaturates alone. Neither of these diets significantly affected serum lipoprotein (a) levels.

In the second experiment, 10% of the energy intake from saturated f.a. was replaced by oleic acid or *trans* monounsaturated f.a. mainly elaidic, for a period of 3 weeks (Mensink et al.,1992). The diet high in elaidic acid resulted in a significantly ($P<0.020$) greater serum lipoprotein (a) level than the diets high in saturated f.a. or oleic acid. Median levels of serum lipoprotein (a) ranged from 26 mg/liter for the diet high in saturated f.a. to 32 mg/liter for the diet high in oleic acid to 45 mg/liter for the diet high in elaidic acid. Median low density lipoprotein (LDL)-cholesterol levels ranged from 2.67 mmol/liter for the diet high in oleic acid to 3.04 mmol/liter for the diet high in elaidic acid to 3.14 mmol/liter for the diet high in saturated f.a. (Mensink et al., 1992).

Eight percent of the energy intake of the 3-week diet in a third experiment was obtained from stearic acid, linoleic acid or elaidic acid. Both the stearate and linoleate diets resulted in median lipoprotein (a) levels of 69 mg/liter, but the elaidic acid diet resulted in a significantly greater ($p<0.020$) median lipoprotein (a) level of 85 mg/liter (Mensink et al., 1992). The elaidic acid diet also resulted in a significantly greater ($p<0.020$) median serum LDL-cholesterol level of 3.07 mmol/liter, compared to 3.00 mmol/liter for the stearic acid diet and 2.83 mmol/liter for the linoleate diet (Mensink et al., 1992; Zock and Katan, 1992). The overall conclusion of the three experiments of Mensink et al. (1992) was that diets high in *trans* monounsaturated f.a. may increase serum levels of lipoprotein (a). No overall conclusion was given concerning LDL-cholesterol. Zock and Katan (1992) found that average serum high-density lipoprotein (HDL)-cholesterol was significantly lower ($p<0.0001$) for a diet high in elaidic acid, 1.37 mmol/liter, compared to a diet with high linoleic acid levels, 1.47 mmol/liter. The average HDL/LDL ratios also were significantly different ($p<0.02$), with a ratio of 0.55 for the diet high in linoleic acid and a ratio of 0.47 for the diet high in elaidic acid (Zock and Katan, 1992).

Nestel et al. (1992) examined the effects of four different diets on plasma lipids: 1) butter fat with lauric, myristic and palmitic acids (1% of the energy intake from *trans* f.a.); 2) oleic acid-rich (2 % of the energy from *trans* f.a.); 3) elaidic acid-rich (7% of the energy intake or 20 g *trans* f.a./day); and 4) palmitic acid-rich (0 % of the energy intake from *trans* f.a.). Twenty-seven mildly hypercholesterolemic men participated in the study. All participants began with a diet consistent with their own eating habits, followed by the diet rich in oleic acid and then, in random order, the diets rich in elaidic and palmitic acid. The entire feeding regimen took 11 weeks. Average plasma total cholesterol ranged from 215 mg/dl for the diet rich in oleic acid to 226 mg/dl, 228 mg/dl and 229 mg/dl for the diets rich in palmitic acid, butter fat and elaidic acid, respectively (Nestel et al., 1992). Average total cholesterol levels and LDL-cholesterol levels resulting from the latter three diets were significantly greater ($p<0.001$) than levels resulting from the diet rich in oleic acid. The average HDL-cholesterol level was 38 mg/liter for the diets rich in butter fat, oleic acid and elaidic acid, but the diet rich in palmitic acid resulted in a significantly greater ($p<0.001$) HDL-cholesterol level of 42 mg/dl. The average lipoprotein (a) level of 296 U/liter (1 U/liter=0.7 mg/liter) resulting from the diet rich in elaidic acid was significantly greater ($p<0.001$) than levels from the other three diets (Nestel et al., 1992). The overall conclusion in the study was that a diet rich in elaidic acid resulted in LDL-cholesterol levels similar to those resulting from palmitic acid-rich or butter fat-rich diets. HDL-cholesterol was not lowered by a diet rich in elaidic acid, but lipoprotein (a) significantly increased with a diet rich in elaidic acid

All of these studies showed that diets with about 7% of the energy from *trans* f.a., mainly elaidic acid, resulted in a greater average serum LDL-cholesterol level relative to oleic or linoleic acid and a greater average lipoprotein (a) level relative to oleic acid, linoleic acid or saturated fatty acids (Mensink et al, 1992; Nestel et al., 1992). Whereas, Zock and Katan (1992) found lower average serum HDL-cholesterol levels after consumption of elaidic-rich diets relative to linoleic acid, Nestel et al. (1992) found that HDL-cholesterol did not decrease in an elaidic acid-rich diet relative to an oleic acid-rich diet. Another balanced, randomized study found no significant differences in plasma lipoprotein (a) levels between diets rich in *trans*-monoenes and saturated or oleic acid-rich diets (Clevidence et al., 1995). Kris-Etherton and Nicolosi (1995) noted that there is a large variation in the HDL cholesterol levels and lipoprotein (a) levels among individuals, so these studies may not have been large enough to "clearly define effects." Also noted was the fact that individuals with high levels of lipoprotein (a) may show more of an effect of *trans* f.a. (Kris-Etherton and Nicolosi, 1995).

In an older study, the diets were not completely randomized in regard to a palm oil diet, which was fed either first or last after an equilibrium period (Laine et al., 1982). Corn oil and unhydrogenated soybean oil diets resulted in similar significant ($p<0.001$) decreases in LDL-cholesterol and total cholesterol from those levels found from the palm oil diet. Decreases of 27.7 mg/dl and 30.3 mg/dl were found for the diets rich in corn oil and the diet rich in unhydrogenated soybean oil, respectively. The diet high in lightly hydrogenated soybean oil resulted in a significantly ($p<0.01$) lesser decrease, 10.8 mg/dl, in LDL-cholesterol than the palm oil diet. The *trans* isomer content of the lightly hydrogenated oil was 15.5% of the total f.a. content. *Trans* isomer contents in the other oils were non-determinable by the method used. There were no significant differences in HDL-cholesterol between the palm oil diet and any of the other diets (Laine et al., 1982). In calculated overall averages of the LDL-cholesterol data from each diet, corn oil had the lowest level at 90.6 mg/dl, with values of 93.8 mg/dl, 97.7 mg/dl and 116.3 mg/dl, for unhydrogenated soybean oil, lightly hydrogenated soybean oil and palm oil, respectively. What the reader does not know about these studies is whether there were significant changes in cholesterol levels from the original levels in the blood plasma.

7.2. Risk Assessment Studies

7.2.1. Adipose Tissue Data. Another method for determining health effects of *trans* f.a. is through risk assessment studies. Three studies, utilizing adipose tissue levels of *trans* f.a., found no overall associated risk of cardiovascular disease, sudden cardiac death and myocardial infarction with *trans* f.a. Hudgins et al. (Hudgins et al.,1991) found a range of 0.99% to 6.15% *trans* f.a. in adipose tissue triglyceride of 76 U.S. adult males, which represents consumption of 1.3 to 7.6 g/day. Correlation analysis was done to determine which specific *trans* f.a. may be associated with risk factors for coronary heart disease. Vaccenic acid was negatively correlated with total cholesterol and LDL-cholesterol levels, whereas the total level of f.a. isomers in adipose tissue was not significantly correlated with cardiovascular risk factors (Hudgins et al., 1991).

Two studies determined adipose tissue levels of *trans* f.a. in people who had died from coronary heart disease or who had acute myocardial infarction compared to healthy controls. Roberts et al. (1995) found significantly ($p<0.05$) lower levels of total *trans* f.a. (C18:1 and C18:2) of 2.68% from all adipose tissue f.a., in subjects who had died from coronary heart disease, than in controls with *trans* f.a. levels of 2.86% in adipose tissue. *Trans* forms of oleic acid were negatively associated with risk of sudden cardiac death, but all of the *trans* forms of linoleic acid were not associated in any way with sudden cardiac death. In the EURAMIC study by Aro et al. (1995), no overall differences in adipose *trans* f.a. levels were found between men with acute myocardial infarction and healthy controls from several European countries. There was a non-significant increased risk of acute myocardial infarction for subjects with median levels of *trans* monoenes at 1.98 % or higher.

7.2.2. Intake Data. Two major studies were done to determine the risk of coronary heart disease associated with *trans* f.a. intake. Willett et al. (1993) analyzed data collected from the Nurse's Health Study begun in 1976 to develop a baseline group of women who answered a questionnaire in 1980 on food intake and medical history. The subjects were divided into five groups depending on their *trans* f.a. intake level, which ranged from 2.4 g/day to 5.7 g/day. Sixty percent of the *trans* f.a. intake was from vegetable sources and 40% was from beef and dairy fat. Every 2 years, for a total of 8 years, subjects filled in questionnaires on changes in their health and in dietary intake. Proportional hazards models were used to determine the risks for coronary heart disease after adjustment for other risk factors such as smoking or age. The relative risk after adjustment for age was 1.5 for the highest *trans* f.a. intake, compared to the lowest *trans* f.a. intake, which was assigned a risk of 1 (Willett et al., 1993). Adjustments for other risk factors such as weight, alcohol intake and menopausal status resulted in a slightly lower risk factor of 1.35 for the *trans* f.a. intake, whereas adjustments for intake of saturated and monounsaturated fat and linoleic acid did not significantly change the risk factor. Specific foods also were analyzed for their associated risk factors. Margarine intake at levels greater than 4 teaspoons (tsp)/day resulted in a risk of 1.66 relative to that of less than 1 tsp/month, which was assigned a risk factor of 1. Two or more cookies or bread slices per day resulted in risk factors of 1.55 and 1.43, respectively, whereas intake of beef, pork or lamb as the main dish at a frequency of 1 serving per day or higher resulted in a risk factor of 1.22, not different ($p<0.86$) from other intake levels (Willett et al., 1993).

Willett et al. (1993) suggested that the risk for coronary heart disease associated with intake of *trans* f.a. was because of isomers from vegetable fats, with significant differences ($p<0.009$) in risk between the levels of intake. There were no differences among the risk factors for the levels of intake from animal sources of *trans* f.a. such as beef, pork or lamb, but there was a significantly greater risk of coronary heart disease with consumption of cookies and white bread (Willett et al., 1993). Willett et al. (1993) stated that butter intake also was not associated with risk of coronary heart disease, but did not give a risk factor or level on intake. Willett et al. (1993) stated that the difference in structure of the animal source of *trans* f.a., double bond in position 11 (*trans*-vaccenic acid), compared to the vegetable source of *trans* f.a., double bond in position 9 (elaidic acid) may be the reason for the difference in risk associated with coronary heart disease. Elaidic acid affects f.a. synthesis more than vaccenic acid.

Kris-Etherton and Nicolosi (1995) noted that the lowest risk factor in the study by Willett et al. (1993) was found for the subjects consuming intermediate levels of *trans* f.a.

This fact indicated that there was no dose-response relationship between intake of *trans* f.a. and risk of coronary heart disease. Also, subjects in these kinds of studies may have increased intake of *trans* f.a. because they believe they are at greater risk for coronary heart disease. The belief that margarine products are more healthful than butter because they have lower amounts of saturated f.a. has led to increased margarine consumption in such populations. Thus, perhaps individuals predisposed to coronary heart disease have self-selected a diet high in *trans* f.a. intake. It also was pointed out that studies using data from adipose tissue assays showed no significant relationship to coronary heart disease risk, which was in contrast to conclusions drawn from intake studies.

Gillman et al. (1997) studied male subjects from the Framingham Study, which began in 1948. Baseline data on dietary intake was collected from 1966 to 1969, and subjects were examined biennially by physicians. Proportional hazards analysis was used to determine relative risk for coronary heart disease. Subjects were divided into three groups based upon butter and margarine intake levels of 0 tsp/day, 1–4 tsp/day and 5 tsp/day or above. Margarine intake levels significantly ($p<0.04$) affected the incidence of coronary heart disease, with increased incidences for increased level of intake, but increased intake of butter did not ($p<0.58$) (Gillman et al., 1997). There was no significant change in risk after adjustment for factors such as fat and alcohol intake, cigarette smoking and physical activity. This increased incidence of coronary heart disease was not significant for the first 10 years of the study, but was significant ($p<0.006$) for the second 10 years. The overall adjusted risk ratio for the first 10 years of the study was 0.99, whereas that for the second 10 years was 1.12 (Gillman et al., 1997). The authors concluded that intake of margarine, which contains *trans* f.a., may increase the risk for developing coronary heart disease. The authors also stated that margarine produced in the 1960s is not the same as margarine used now. Margarine manufactured today should have lower levels of *trans* f.a.

8. FOOD LABELING

The final question in the *trans* f.a. debate is whether to change food labeling requirements to account for *trans* f.a. and if so, how to change them. Should *trans* f.a. be included in the total for saturated f.a. percentage or should they be listed separately, or should they not be included at all? The argument for inclusion in the saturated f.a. total was supported by Longnecker (1997) on the basis that *trans* f.a. have physiological effects similar to saturated f.a. The effects are still being debated. The Institute of Food Technologists, the American Society for Clinical Nutrition, the American Institute of Nutrition and the British Nutrition Foundation all agree that, until more succinct evidence is available on the harmful effects of *trans* f.a., label regulations should *not* be changed to include *trans* f.a. (Blackburn et al., 1995; Schaley, 1995).

ACKNOWLEDGMENTS

Journal Paper No. J-17354 of the Iowa Agricultural and Home Economics Experiment Station, Iowa, project No. 3396, and supported by Hatch Act and State of Iowa funds.

REFERENCES

Aro, A.; Kardinaal, A.F.M.; Salminen, I.; Kark, J.D.; Riemersma, R.A. Delgado-Rodriguez, M.; Gomez-Aracena, J.; Huttunen, J.K.; Kohlmeier, L.; Martin, B.C.; Martin-Moreno, J.M.; Mazaev, V.P.; Ringstad, J.; Thamm,

M.; van't Veer, P.; Kok, F.J. Adipose tissue isomeric *trans* fatty acids and risk of myocardial infarction in nine countries: the EURAMIC study. *Lancet* **1995**, 345, 273.

Blackburn, G.L.; Nettleton, J.A.; Milner, J.A. Nutrition societies urge FDA not to change labeling regulations on *trans* fatty acids. "News Release". *IFT Science Communications.* Institute of Food Technologists. Chicago, IL, July, 1995.

Bernstein, P.A.; Graydon, W.F.; Diosady. L.L. Hydrogenation of canola oil using chromium catalysts. *J. Am. Oil Chem. Soc.* ***1989***, 66, 680.

Carpenter, D.L.; Slover, H.T. Lipid composition of selected margarines. *J. Am. Oil Chem. Soc.* **1973**, 50, 372.

Chu, Y.H.; Lin, L.H. An evaluation of commercial nickel catalysts during hydrogenation of soybean oil. *J. Am. Oil Chem. Soc.* **1991**, 68, 680.

Clevidence, B.A.; Judd, J.T.; Schaefer, E.J.; McNamara, J.R.; Muesing, R.A.; Whittes, J.: Sunkin, M.E. Plasma lipoprotein (a) levels in subjects consuming *trans* fatty acids. *FASEB J.* **1995**, 9; A579.

Craig-Schmidt, M.C. Fatty acid isomers in foods. In *Fatty Acids in Foods and Their Health Implications*, Chow, C.K., Ed.; Marcel Dekker, Inc.: New York, 1992; pp 365–398.

Dupont, J.; White, P.J.; Feldman, E.B. Saturated and hydrogenated fats in food in relation to health. *J. Amer. Coll. Nutr.* **1991**, 10, 577.

Edvardsson, J.; Ivandoust, S. Reactors for hydrogenation of edible oils. *J. Am. Oil Chem. Soc.* **1994**, 71, 235.

Enig, M.G.; Atal, S.; Keeney, M.; Sampugna, J. Isomeric *trans* fatty acids in the U.S. diet. *J. Am. Coll. Nutr.* **1990**, 9, 471.

Enig, M.G.; Pallansch, L.A.; Sampugna, J.; Keeney, M. Fatty acid composition of the fat in selected food items with emphasis on *trans* components. *J. Am. Oil Chem. Soc.* **1983**, 60, 1788.

Fellner, V.; Sauer, F.D.; Kramer, J.K.G. Steady-state rates of linoleic acid biohydrogenation by ruminal bacteria in continuous culture. *J. Dairy Sci.* **1995**, 78, 1815.

Fotouhi, N.; Jenkins, T.C. Resistance of fatty acyl amides to degradation and hydrogenation by ruminal microorganisms. *J. Dairy Sci.* **1992**, 75, 1527.

Fotouhi, N.; Jenkins, T.C. Ruminal biohydrogenation of linoleoyl methionine and calcium linoleate in sheep. *J. Anim. Sci.* **1992**, 70, 3607.

Gerson, T.; John, A.; Sinclair, B.R. The effect of dietary n on *in vitro* lipolysis and fatty acid hydrogenation in rumen digesta from sheep fed diets high in starch. *Agri. Sci. Camb.* **1983**, 101, 97.

Gillman, M.W.; Cupples, L.A.; Gagnon, D.; Millen, B.E.; Ellison, R.C.; Castelli, W.P. Margarine intake and subsequent coronary heart disease in men. *Epidemiology.* **1997**, 8, 145.

Grompone, M.A.; Moyna, P. Geometric isomerization of fatty acids with nickel catalysts. J. *Am. Oil Chem. Soc.* **1986**, 63, 550.

Harfoot, C.G. Lipid metabolism in the rumen. *Prog. Lipid Res.* **1978**, 17, 21.

Harfoot, C.G.; Noble, R.C.; Moore, J.H. Factors influencing the extent of biohydrogenation of linoleic acid by rumen micro-organisms *in vitro*. *J. Sci. Food Agric.* **1973**, 24, 961.

Heldal, J.A.; Moulton, K.J., Sr.; Frankel, E. N. Fixed-bed continuous hydrogenation of soybean oil with palladium-polymer supported catalysts. *J. Am. Oil Chem. Soc.* **1989**, 66, 979.

Hsu, N.; Diosady, L.L.; Rubin, L.J. Catalytic behavior of palladium in the hydrogenation of edible oils. II. Geometrical and positional isomerization characteristics. *J. Am. Oil Chem. Soc.* **1989**, 66, 232.

Hsu, N.; Diosady, L.L.;Rubin, L.J. Catalytic behavior of palladium in the hydrogenation of edible oils. *J. Am. Oil Chem. Soc.* **1988**, 65, 349.

Hsu, N.; Diosady, L.L.; Graydon, W.F.; Rubin, L.J. Heterogeneous catalytic hydrogenation of canola oil using palladium. *J. Am. Oil Chem. Soc.* **1986**, 63, 1036.

Hudgins, L.C.; Hirsch, J.; Emken, E.A. Correlation of isomeric fatty acids in human adipose tissue with clinical risk factors for cardiovascular disease. *Am. J. Clin. Nutr.* **1991**, 53, 474.

Hunter, J.E.; Applewhite, T.H. Reassessment of *trans* fatty acid availability in the U.S. diet. *Am. J. Clin. Nutr.* **1991**, 54, 363.

Kellens, M.J.; Goderis, H.L.; Tobback, P.P. Biohydrogenation of unsaturated fatty acids by a mixed culture of rumen microorganisms. *Biotechnology and Bioengineering.* **1986**, 28, 1268.

Koseoglu, S.S.; Lusas, E.W. Recent advances in canola oil hydrogenation. *J. Am. Oil Chem. Soc.* **1990**, 67, 39.

Kris-Etherton, P.M ; Nicolosi, N.J. *Trans* fatty acids and coronary heart disease risk. *Am. J. Clin. Nutr.* **1995**, 62, 651S.

Krishnaiah, D.; Sarkar, S. Kinetics of liquid phase hydrogenation of cottonseed oil with nickel catalysts. *J. Am. Oil Chem. Soc.* **1990**, 67, 233.

Laine, D.C.; Snodgrass, C.M.; Dawson, E.A.; Ener, M.A.; Kuba, K.; Frantz, I.D. Lightly hydrogenated soy oil versus other vegetable oils as a lipid-lowering dietary constituent. *Am. J. Clin. Nutr.* **1982**, 35, 683.

Longnecker, M.P. Food labels, *trans* fatty acids and coronary heart disease. *Epidemiology.* **1997**, 8, 122.

Mensink, R.P.; Zock, P.L.; Katan, M.B.; Hornstra, G. Effect of dietary *cis* and *trans* fatty acids on serum lipoprotein (a) levels in humans. J. Lipid Res. **1992**, 33, 1493.

Moulton, K.J.; Koritala, S.; Warner, K.; Frankel, E.N. Continuous ultrasonic hydrogenation of soybean oil. ii. operating conditions and oil quality. *J. Am. Oil Chem. Soc.* **1987**, 64, 542.

Nestel, P.; Noakes, M.; Belling, B.; McArthur, R.; Clifton, P.; Janus, E.; Abbey, M. Plasma lipoprotein lipid and Lp (a) changes with substitution of elaidic acid for oleic acid in the diet. *J. Lipid Res.* **1992**, 33, 1029.

O'Donnell, J.A. Future of milk fat modification by production or processing: integration of nutrition, food science and animal science. *J. Dairy Sci.* **1993**, 76, 1797.

Parodi, P.W. Composition and structure of some consumer-available edible fats. *J. Am. Oil Chem. Soc.* **1976**, 53, 530.

Patterson, H.B.W. *Hydrogenation of Fats and Oils.* Applied Science Publishers: New, York; 1983; P. 52.

Roberts, T.L.; Wood, D.A.; Riemersma, R.A.; Gallagher, P.J.; Lampe, F.C. *Trans* isomers of oleic and linoleic acids in adipose tissue and sudden cardiac death. *Lancet.* **1995**, 345, 278.

Rubin, L.J.; Koseoglu, S.S.; Diosady, L.L.; Graydon, W.F. Hydrogenation of canola oil in the presence of nickel and the methyl benzoate-chrome carbonyl complex. *J. Am. Oil Chem. Soc.* **1986**, 63, 1551.

Schaley, T.L. Corrected alert: BNF and CSPI action on *trans* fatty acids. *IFT Science Communications.* Institute of Food Technologists. Chicago, IL, July, 1995.

Scholfield, C.R.; Davidson, V.L.; Dutton, H.J. Analysis for geometrical and positional isomers of fatty acids in partially hydrogenated fats. *J. Am. Oil Chem. Soc.* **1967**, 44, 648.

Scott, T.W.; Cook, L.J.; Mills, S.C. Protection of dietary polyunsaturated fatty acids against microbial hydrogenation in ruminants. *J. Am. Oil Chem. Soc.* **1971**, 48, 358.

Selener, D.R.; Schultz, L.H. Effects of feeding oleic acid or hydrogenated vegetable oils to lactating cows. *J. Dairy Sci.* **1980**, 63, 1235.

Slover, H.T.; Thompson, R.H., Jr.; Davis, C.S.; Merola, G.V. Lipids in margarines and margarine-like foods. *J. Am. Oil Chem. Soc.* **1985**, 62, 775.

Slover, H.T., Thompson, R.H., Jr.; Davis, C.S.; Merola, G.V. The lipid composition of raw and cooked fresh pork. *J. Food Comp. Anal.* **1987**, 1, 38.

Smidovnik, A.; Stimac, A.; Kobe, J. Catalytic transfer hydrogenation of soybean oil. *J. Am. Oil Chem. Soc.* **1992**, 69, 405.

Smith, L.M.; Clifford, A.J.; Hamblin, C.L.;Creveling, R.K. Changes in physical and chemical properties of shortenings used for commercial deep-fat frying. *J. Am. Oil Chem. Soc.* **1986**, 63, 1017.

Szukalska, E.; Drozdowski, B. Selective hydrogenation of rapeseed oils with copper-chromite catalyst: influence of erucic acid. *J. Am. Oil Chem. Soc.* **1982**, 59, 134.

Willett, W.C.; Stampfer, M.J.; Manson, J.E.; Colditz, G.A.; Speizer, F.E.; Rosner, B.A.; Sampson, L.A.; Hennekens, C.H. Intake of *trans* fatty acids and risk of coronary heart disease among women. *Lancet.* **1993**, 341, 581.

Wu, Z.; Palmquist, D. L. Synthesis and biohydrogenation of fatty acids by ruminal microorganisms *in vitro*. *J. Dairy Sci.* **1991**, 74, 3035.

Yusem, G.J.; Pintauro, P.N. The electrocatalytic hydrogenation of soybean oil. *J. Am. Oil Chem. Soc.* **1992**, 69, 399.

Zock, P.L.; Katan, M.B. Hydrogenation Alternatives: Effects of *trans* fatty acids and stearic acid versus linoleic acid on serum lipid and lipoproteins in humans. *J. Lipid Res.* **1992**, 33, 399.

5

IMPACT OF HIGH-TEMPERATURE FOOD PROCESSING ON FATS AND OILS

Kathleen Warner

Food Quality and Safety Research
National Center for Agricultural Utilization Research
Agricultural Research Service, U.S. Dept. of Agriculture
Peoria, Illinois 61604

1. ABSTRACT

Fats and oils are heated at high temperatures during baking, grilling and pan frying; however, deep fat frying is the most common method of high temperature treatment. Deep fat frying is a popular food preparation method because it produces desirable fried food flavor, golden brown color and crisp texture. For example, in the U.S. in 1994, approximately 12 billion pounds of fats and oils were used with 5.5 billion pounds used for frying and baking (USDA, 1995). Fried snack foods accounted for 2.9 bilion pounds of oil, whereas 2 billion pounds were used for frying in restaurants (USDA, 1995). Because of such large consumption of frying oils and fats, the effects of high temperatures on these oils and fats is of major concern both for product quality and nutrition. This chapter will discuss the process of frying and the chemical and physical reactions that occur. The products formed from these reactions will be reviewed as well as information on the effects of the products and the control of these deteriorative reactions.

2. INTRODUCTION

Toxicants that are detected in food can be present naturally or can occur from changes during harvesting, processing, or preservation. They can be further catagorized as 1) naturally occurring compounds such as nutmeg; 2) compounds that can be removed by processing such as trypsin inhibitors or aflatoxin; 3) compounds that cannot be removed such as in some seafood and 4) compounds produced by preservation and processing such as in cured meats and in fried food (Morton, 1977). Thermal processing of foods can have positive and negative effects. For example, trypsin inhibitors in soybeans are inactivated

Impact of Processing on Food Safety, edited by Jackson et al.,
Kluwer Academic / Plenum Publishers, New York, 1999.

during a steaming process to produce products that are safe to consume. In addition, high temperature processing can contribute desirable flavors to foods such as roasted coffee, caramel, or fried food. On the other hand, high temperatures may also cause excessive formation of compounds that negatively affect color and flavor in foods such as canned vegetable and fried foods.

3. CHANGES IN OILS AND FOOD DURING DEEP-FAT FRYING

During frying, at approximately 190°C, as oils thermally and oxidatively decompose, volatile and nonvolatile products are formed which alter functional, sensory, and nutritional qualities of oils. Scientists have extensively reported on the physical and chemical changes that occur during frying and on the wide variety of decomposition products formed in frying oils. Physical and chemical changes in oils that occur during heating and frying are presented in Table 1. Specific methods exist to quantitatively measure degradation processes and products, for example, free fatty acids, carbonyl compounds, and high molecular weight products. In addition, decreases in unsaturation, flavor quality, and essential fatty acids can be monitored. However, some physical, qualitative changes in the oil can also be determined subjectively by visual inspection such as increased viscosity, color, and foaming as well as decreased smoke point. Some frying operations, such as in restaurants, discard frying oils when frying causes excessive foaming of oil, when the oil tends to smoke excessively, or when the oil color darkens. In addition, abused oil increases in off-odors such as acrid and burnt and fried food develops off-flavors. There are five stages in the life cycle of a frying oil that generally correspond to the five phases of frying oil deterioration—induction, peroxide formation, peroxide decomposition, polymerization, and degradation—that are based on the chemical reactions that occur during frying. The first stage of the cycle begins when the oil is fresh and is chemically known as the induction phase. Oils in this phase provide little browning and in fact, the food may look undercooked. Fried food flavor intensity is also low. The oil is actually at peak performance during the second phase of the cycle which is the peroxide formation stage. Food has a desirable golden brown color; is fully cooked; and has moderate (optimum) fried flavor. During the third part of the cycle, peroxides decompose and the oil is lower in quality than at the second stage. Food has a darker brown color and a lower fried food flavor intensity than at the previous stage. Off-flavors may be detectable at this phase. By the fourth stage, the oil has begun to polymerize and the oil quality is marginal. Food has a dark brown color and off-flavors; and the oil has begun to foam. By the time an oil reaches phase five, severe oil degradation is occurring and the oil should be discarded. Food has an unacceptable flavor and may not be fully cooked in center because foaming of the oil has limited the direct contact of oil and food. Nonvolatile decomposition prod-

Table 1. Effects of physical and chemical changes during deep fat frying

Physical changes	
Increased:	viscosity, color, foaming
Decreased:	smoke point
Chemical changes	
Increased:	free fatty acids, carbonyl compounds, high molecular weight products
Decreased:	unsaturation, flavor quality, essential fatty acids

ucts eventually produce these physical changes in frying oil—increases in viscosity, color, and foaming (Perkins, 1967). Chemical changes during frying increase free fatty acids, carbonyls, and polymeric compounds and decrease fatty acid unsaturation.

4. PHYSICAL AND CHEMICAL REACTIONS OCCURRING DURING HEATING AND FRYING

Deep fat frying is a complex process with many physical and chemical reactions occurring simultaneously. Frying oils not only transfer heat to cook foods but also help produce distinctive fried food flavor and unfortunately, undesirable off-flavors if the oil is deteriorated. During deep-fat frying, various deteriorative chemical processes such as hydrolysis, oxidation, and polymerization take place and oils decompose to form volatile products and nonvolatile compounds (Figure 1). As heat is transferred from the oil to the food, water is evaporated from the food and oil is absorbed by the food. In addition, the oil is aerated with oxygen as food is added. This process helps enhance one of the major chemical reactions occurring during frying—oxidation. Primary oxidation products—hydroperoxides—are rapidly formed and cleave to alkoxy and hydroxy free radicals that are very unstable at 190°C (Figure 2). Free radicals will react with other compounds to form secondary oxidation products such as aldehydes, alcohols, ketones and hydrocarbons. As water is added to the oil, usually through the addition of food, hydrolysis occurs. Free fatty acids are formed in addition to diglycerides and monoglycerides as the triglyceride decomposes (Figure 3). Polymerization of the oil takes place with the formation of many compounds including dimers, trimers and polymers (Figure 4). The complex process of formation and degradation of volatile and nonvolatile compounds is shown in Figure 5 along with some of the physical changes in the frying oil. With continued heating and frying, these compounds further decompose until breakdown products accumulate to the level that the oil is no longer suitable for use because high levels of these compounds produce off-flavors and potentially toxic effects.

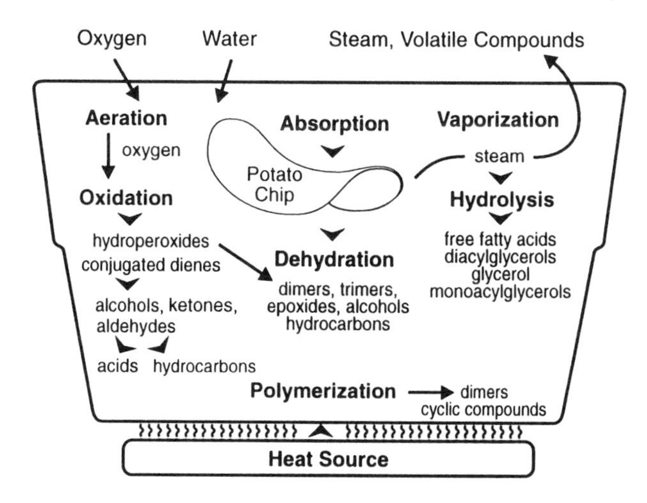

Figure 1. Physical and chemical reactions and products during deep fat frying.

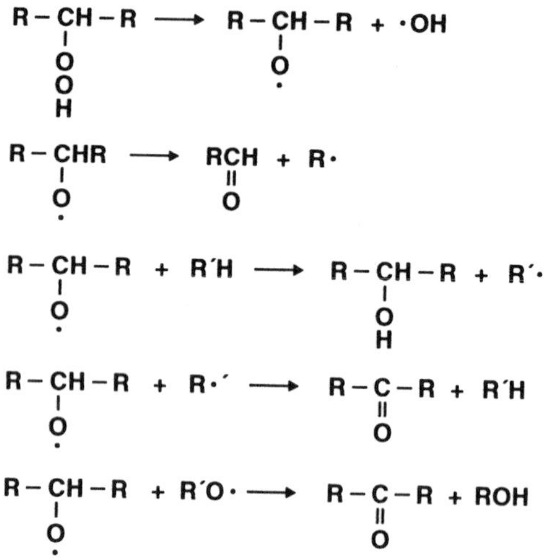

Figure 2. Oxidation reactions and products during deep fat frying.

4.1 Hydrolysis

As food is fried in oil, air and water initiate a series of interrelated reactions. Water and steam hydrolyze triglycerides which produces monoglycerides and diglycerides, and eventually free fatty acids and glycerol (Figure 3). The extent of hydrolysis is a function of oil temperature, interface between oil and aqueous phases, and amount of water and steam since water will hydrolyze oil more quickly than steam (Pokorny, 1989). Free fatty acids and low-molecular weight acidic products from oxidation enhance hydrolysis in the presence of steam during frying (Pokorny, 1989). Hydrolysis products decrease the stability of frying oils and can be used as one measure of oil fry life.

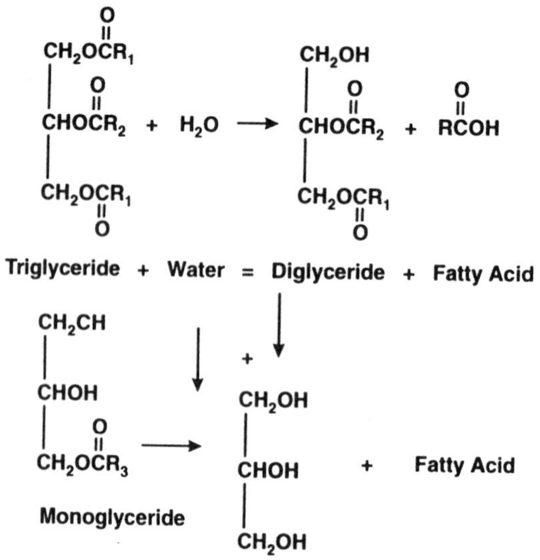

Figure 3. Hydrolytic reactions and products during deep fat frying.

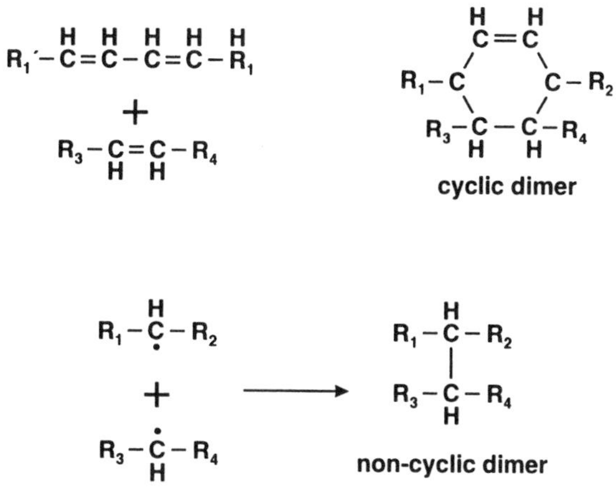

```
   H   H   H   H   H                        H   H
R1'-C = C - C = C - R1                       C = C
                                            /     \
        +                               R1-C       C-R2
                                            \     /
R3-C = C-R4                             R3-C - C-R4
   H   H                                   H   H
                                        cyclic dimer


     H                                     H
R1 - C - R2                           R1 - C - R2
     •                                     |
     +          ----------->          R3 - C - R4
     •                                     H
R3 - C - R4
     H                                non-cyclic dimer
```

Figure 4. Polymerization reactions and products during deep fat frying.

4.2 Oxidation

Oxygen that is in the oil or that is incorporated with food causes reactions that form volatile and nonvolatile decomposition products. The oxidation mechanism in frying oils is similar to autoxidation at ambient temperature; however, unstable primary oxidation products—hydroperoxides—decompose rapidly at 190°C into secondary oxidation products such as aldehydes (Figure 2). These volatile secondary oxidation products can significantly contribute to the odor of the oil and flavor of the fried food. Analysis of highly volatile products such as hydroperoxides at any one point in the frying process provides

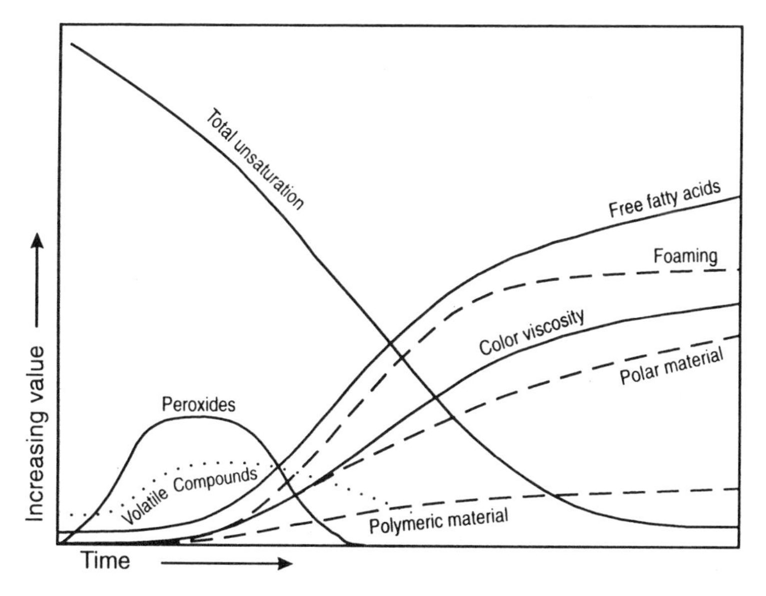

Figure 5. Formation and degradation of compounds in frying oils.

little information since their formation and decomposition fluctuate quickly. During frying, oils with polyunsaturated fatty acids such as linoleic acid have a distinct induction period of primary breakdown products—hydroperoxides—followed by a rapid increase in peroxide values, then a rapid destruction of peroxides (Perkins, 1967; Wessels, 1983). Therefore, monitoring peroxides is not a good indication of the state of the oil. Oxidative degradation produces oxidized triglycerides containing hydroperoxide-, epoxy-, hydroxy-, and keto- groups and dimeric fatty acids or dimeric triglycerides (Wessels, 1983). Volatile degradation products are usually saturated and monounstaurated hydroxy-, aldehydic-, keto-, and dicarboxylic- acids; hydrocarbons; alcohols; aldehydes; ketones; and aromatic compounds (Perkins, 1996).

4.3. Polymerization

Frying produces compounds with high molecular weight such as polymers that can form from free radicals or triglycerides by the Diels-Alder reaction (Figure 4). Cyclic fatty acids can form within one fatty acid; dimeric fatty acids form between two fatty acids, either within or between triglycerides; and polymers are obtained as these molecules cross-link. Oil viscosity increases as the amount of polymerized material increases. Polymerization products decrease the stability of frying oils and can be used to measure oil fry life.

5. FORMATION OF NONVOLATILE AND VOLATILE DEGRADATION PRODUCTS

The extent of thermal degradation of frying oil is affected by unsaturation of fatty acids, frying temperature, oxygen absorption, metals, and food type (Arroyo et al., 1992). Other factors affecting hydrolysis, oxidation, polymerization and frying oil deterioration are presented in Table 2. The type of food being fried can affect the resulting composition of the frying oil as fatty acids are released from fat-containing foods such as chicken. Breaded/battered food can degrade frying oil more quickly and decrease stability compared to uncoated food. Accumulation of degradation products in the frying medium and their incorporation in fried foods is of concern when frying is conducted under abusive conditions (Clark and Serbia, 1991). Combinations of these degradation factors (Table 2) determine the rate of reactions, for example, in one operation, the rate of hydrolysis may be twice that of the rate of oxidation, whereas in another operation with different conditions, the reverse may occur (Fritsch, 1981).

Table 2. Factors affecting frying oil degradation

Oil/food	Process
Unsaturation of fatty acids	Oil temperature
Type of oil	Frying time
Type of food	Aeration / oxygen absorption
Metals in oil / food	Frying equipment
Initial oil quality	Continuous or intermittent heating or frying
Degradation products in oil	Frying rate
Antioxidants	Heat transfer
Anti-foam additives	Turnover rate; addition of makeup oil, Filtering of oil / fryer cleaning

Table 3. Volatile compounds in french fried potatoes and frying oils

Frying oil		French fried potatoes	
Butanal	t2 t4-Heptadienal	Hexanal	Decanal
Hexane	2t 4-Heptadienal	Methyl pyrazine	2-Decenal
1-Butanol	2-Octenal	2-Hexenal	2,c4-Decadienal
Pentanol	Nonanal	2-Heptanone	Undecanal
Heptane	2-Nonenal	Nonane	2, t4-Decadienal
Hexane	Decanal	Heptanal	Nonanal
2-Hexenal	1-Decene	2,5 Dimethylpyrazine	2-Octenal
2-Heptanone	3-Octanone	2-Heptenal	t2,t4-Heptadienal
Nonane	2-Decenal	2-Pentylfuran	Octanal
Heptanal	2,c 4-Decadienal		
2-Heptenal	Undecanal		
2-Pentylfuran	2,t4-Decandienal		
Octanal	2-Octen-1-ol		
2-Undecenal	Dodecanal		

5.1. Volatile and Nonvolatile Degradation Products

Frying oils degrade to form volatile and nonvolatile decomposition products (Figure 5). Although volatile compounds are primarily responsible for flavor—both positive and negative, thermal polymers do not affect flavor directly. Foods fried in these deteriorated oils may contain a significant amount of decomposition products to cause potential adverse effects to safety, flavor, oxidative stability, color and texture of the fried food. Conditions that produce polymers are not usually encountered in well-managed commercial operations because of practices such as make-up oil addition and monitoring of frying conditions.

Perkins (1996) found several hundred volatile compounds in frying oil and french fried potatoes. The major compounds, listed in Table 3 in the order of elution on a nonpolar capillary column, include aldehydes, ketones, alcohols and hydrocarbons. At lower levels, many of these compounds can contribute to a positive flavor in fried foods; however, at higher levels they may contribute to undesirable off-flavors. Selke et al. (1977) identified volatile compounds and their precursors from heated soybean oil, using triglycerides (triolein, 25% triolein/75%tristearin, and a randomly esterified triglyceride of stearic and 25% oleic acids) heated at 192°C in air for 10 minutes. Each lipid system produced the same major compounds (heptane, octane, heptanal, octanal, nonanal, 2-decenal, and 2-undecenal) that were unique to the oxidation of the oleate fatty acid in each triglyceride sample. Selke et al. (1980) also analyzed pure trilinolein and mixtures of trilinolein-tristearin, trilinolein-triolein, and trilinolein-triolein-tristearin heated at 192°C in air and found pentane, acrolein, pentanal, 1-pentanal, hexanal, 2- and/or 3 hexanal, 2-heptenal, 2-octenal, 2,4-decadienal, and 4,5-epoxyde-2-enal. 2,4-decadienal is a major decomposition product from linoleic acid and at lower levels can be partially responsible for fried food flavor. At our laboratory, we have monitored 2,4-decadienal in fresh and aged potato chips that were fried in oils with a range of high to low amounts of linoleic acid (Warner et al., 1997). Results showed that potato chips fried in cottonseed oil with 55% linoleic acid had significantly greater amounts of 2,4-decadienal and higher intensities of fried food flavor than potato chips fried in high oleic sunflower oil with only 12% linoleic acid.

Nonvolatile degradation products in used frying oils can include polymeric triacylglycerols, oxidized triacylglycerol derivatives, cyclic substances and breakdown products (Perkins, 1996). Rojo and Perkins (1987) classified the degradation products as polar and

Table 4. Polar compounds (mg/g oil) in high oleic sunflower oils used for frying

Oil	Total polar compounds	Oligomers	Dimers	Oxidized monomers	Diglyceride	Fatty acids
Triglyceride A	17.4	2.1	5.7	6.9	2.0	0.7
Triglyceride B	27.2	5.8	8.6	9.6	2.2	1.0
Triglyceride C	41.5	13.3	12.1	13.0	2.3	0.8

nonpolar polymeric fatty acid methyl esters and monomeric fatty acid methyl esters with unchanged, changed (oxidized, cyclized, isomerized, etc.) and fragmented fatty acid esters. Clark and Serbia (1991) found that large declines in iodine values were needed for a significant amount of polymer formation. Dobarganes and Marquez-Ruiz (1996) reported on the type and quantity of nonvolatile compounds formed in high oleic sunflower oil as it deteriorated during frying (Table 4). The total polar compounds ranged from a moderate level of 17.4% to 41.5% (highly deteriorated). Oligomers, dimers and oxidized monomers increased with increasing polar compounds, whereas the diglycerides and fatty acids remained constant. The type of oil also has a significant effect on the quantities of degradation products produced. Marquez-Ruiz et al. (1995) compared the compounds formed in a polyunsaturated sunflower oil and in a high oleic sunflower oil after 5 hours of frying (Ta-

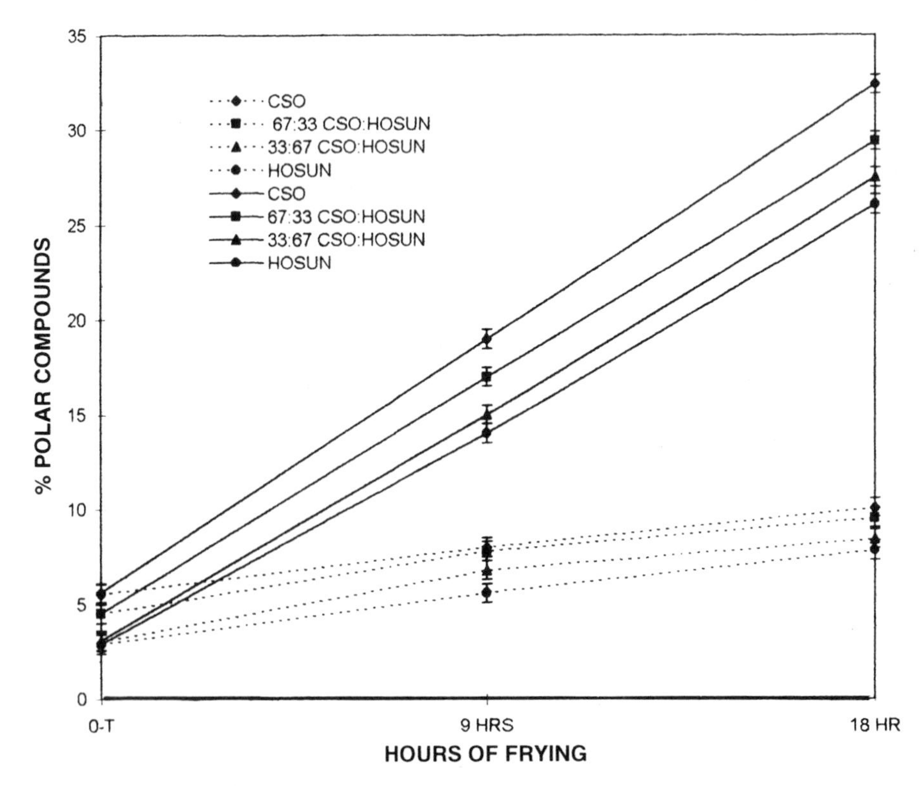

Figure 6. Total polar compound (%) in cottonseed oil (CSO), high oleic sunflower (HOSUN) and blends after 0, 9 and 18 hours of frying french fried potatoes (——)for potato chips (----).

Table 5. Total polar compounds (wt % oil) and polar compound distribution (mg/g oil) of laboratory-used frying oils

		Polar compounds (mg/g)				
		Triglyceride		Oxidized triglyceride		Free fatty
Oil	Total (%)	Polymer	Dimer	monomer	Diglyceride	acid
Sunflower	28.9	50.0	125.1	98.0	11.8	4.1
High oleic sunflower	23.0	33.4	82.3	91.3	19.3	3.7

ble 5). As expected the sunflower oil had higher percentages of total polar compounds and of triglyceride polymers, dimers and oxidized triglyceride monomers. Polar compound formation can be altered by frying conditions. In our laboratory, we used the same oils—cottonseed, high oleic sunflower and blends of these two oils—for two types of frying operations (Figure 6). In oils used for potato chips, the polar compound level were at a low level, ranging from 6–8% in oils used for 18 hours primarily because makeup oil was frequently added. On the other hand, oils used for french fried potatoes had much higher polar compound levels. The effect of fatty acid composition was apparent in these oils more than in the potato chip oil because of a lower rate of oil replenishment for the french fried potatoes. Sebedio and Grandgirard (1989) published a review on the minimum and maximum levels of cyclic acids, another type of compound found in frying oils (Table 6). Maximum values ranged widely from 0.16 to 0.66%. Different frying conditions and other variables that affect degradation of oil contributed to this extensive range.

5.2. Feeding Studies

Animal feeding studies have produced a wide range of results depending on the variables used. A review paper by Clark and Serbia (1991) cited a study by Kantorowitz and Yannai (1974) in which soybean oil and hydrogenated soybean oil heated at 200°C were fed to rats (Table 7). Feeding soybean oil heated more than 10 hours retarded growth and had a toxic effect at 43 hours. On the other hand, hydrogenated soybean oil had no adverse effects. Commercially, soybean oil is rarely used for deep fat frying; however, hydrogenated soybean oil is used extensively, so this the use of soybean oil or other polyunsaturated oils in long-term frying tests is mostly of academic interest for comparing with more stable oils. Clark and Serbia (1991) also reported (Table 7) on a 1988 study by Chanin on feeding rats laboratory-heated oil vs. commercial frying oil. The laboratory-heated oils negatively affected weight gain and feed consumption more than the commercial frying oils. As illustrated in previous examples in this chapter, oils from commercial frying op-

Table 6. Cyclic fatty acids in commercial frying

	Amounts (%)			No. of
Authors	Minimum	Maximum	Country	samples
Frankel et al., 1984	0.02	0.50	USA	25
	0.17	0.66	Egypt, Israel	8
Gere et al., 1985	0.02	0.16	Hungary	8
Sebedio et al., 1987	0.01	0.25	France	31
Poumeyrol et al., 1987	0.01	0.09	France	21

Table 7. Laboratory studies of overheated fats and oils

Purpose	Conditions	Results	Reference
Toxicity evaluated in feeding trials of soybean oil (SBO) and hydrogenated SBO (HSBO)	200°C for 10-43hr	SBO with > 10 hr. of heating retarded growth; toxic at 43 hr; HSBO showed no adverse effects; no effects from polymeric fractions	Kantorowitz and Yanni (1974)
Rat feeding of purified diets at 15% for 28 days of lab-heated corn oil and SBO vs double frying of SBO	Thermally oxidized at 200°C vs single and double-fry SBO	Lab heated oils depressed weight gain, feed consumption; commercial SBO comparable to controls	Chanin et al. (1988)

erations usually have much lower degradation than oils abused in laboratory experiments especially when oil is heated without frying.

5.3. Controlling Frying Oil Degradation

What can be done to help provide frying oils and fried foods that are more healthful and with lower levels of deterioration? This can be accomplished to a large extent by controlling the factors (Table 2) that influence frying oil degradation. For example, fresh oil or fat should have good initial quality with no prior oxidation, have low levels of polyunsaturated fatty acids, and have low amounts of catalyzing metals. Metal chelators, antioxidants and anti-foam additives can be added to the oil to help maintain stability and quality (Warner et al., 1985; Frankel et al., 1985). Filtering oils through adsorbents removes carbonized food particles accumulating in the oil along with other oxidation products that limit oil fry life. Controlling frying conditions such as temperature and time, exposure of oil to oxygen, continuous rather than intermittent frying, oil filtration, and turnover of oil will help decrease degradation of the oil. Replenishing with fresh oil is commonly done in frying operations; however, in the snack food industry where more make-up oil is added than in restaurant-style frying, a complete turnover of the oil in the first 8–12 hr of the frying cycle can be achieved (Moreira et al., 1995).

REFERENCES

Arroyo, R.; Cuesta, C.; Garrido-Polonio, C.; Lopez-Varela, S.; Sanchez-Muntz, F.J. High-performance size-exclusion chromatographic studies on polar components formed in sunflower oil used for frying. *J. Amer. Oil Chem. Soc.* **1992**,*69*, 557.

Chanin, B.E.; Valli, V.E.; Alexander, J.C. Clinical and histopatholgical observations with rats fed laboratory heated or deep-fry fats. *Nutr. Res* **1988**, *8*, 921.

Clark, W.L.; Serbia, G.W. Safety aspects of frying fats and oils. *Food Tech.* **1991**, *45*, 84.

Dobarganes, M.C.; Marquez-Ruiz, G. Dimeric and higher oligomeric triglycerides, In "Deep Frying-Chemistry, Nutrition and Practical Applications", E.G. Perkins and M.C. Erickson, eds., AOCS Press, Champaign, IL, **1996**, 89.

Frankel, E.N.; Smith, L.M.; Hamblin, C.L.; Creveling, R.K.; Clifford,A.J. Occurrence of cyclic fatty acid monomers in frying oils used for fast foods. *J. Am. Oil Chem. Soc.* **1984**, *61*, 87.

Frankel, E.N.; Warner, K.; Moulton, K.J. Effects of hydrogenation and additives on cooking oil performance of soybean oil. *J. Am. Oil Chem. Soc.* **1985**, *62*, 1354.

Fritsch, C.W. Measurements of frying fat deterioration: A brief view. *J. Am. Oil Chem. Soc.* **1981**, *58*, 272.

Gere, A.; Sebedio, J. L.; Grandgirard, A. Studies on some Hungarian fats and oils obtained from commercial frying processes. *Fette Seifen Anstr-Mittel* **1985**, *87*, 359.

Kantorowitz, B.; Yannai, S. Comparison of the tendencies of liquid and hardened soybean oils to form physiologically undesirable materials under simulated frying conditions. *Nutr. Rep. Int.* **1974**, *9*, 331.

Marquez-Ruiz, G., Tasioula-Margari, M., Dobarganes, M.C. Quantitation and distribution of altered fatty acids in frying fats. *J. Amer. Oil Chem. Soc.* **1995**, *72*, 1171.

Moreira, R., Palau, J.; Sun, X. Deep fat frying of tortilla chips: An engineering approach. *Food Tech.* **1995**, *49*, 307.

Morton, I. D. Naturally occurring toxins in foods. *Proc. Nutr. Soc.* **1977**, 36, 101.

Perkins, E.G. Formation of non-volatile decomposition products in heated fats and oils. *Food Tech.* **1967**, *21*, 125.

Perkins, E.G. Formation of lipid oxidation products during deep fat frying: Effects on oil quality and their determination, In "Food Lipids and Health" McDonald, R.E.; Min, D.B., eds., Marcel Dekker, Inc., New York, **1996**, 139.

Pokorny, J. Flavor chemistry of deep fat frying in 0il. In "Flavor Chemistry of Lipid Foods", Min, D.B.; Smouse, T.H., eds., American Oil Chemists Society, Champaign, IL, **1989**, 113–115.

Poumeyrol, G. *Rev. Fr. Corps Gras*, **1987**, *34*, 543.

Rojo, J.; Perkins, E. Cyclic fatty acid monomer formation in frying fats. *J. Am. Oil Chem Soc.* **1987**, *64*, 414.

Sebedio, J-L.; Grandgirard, A.; Septier, C.; Prevost, J. *Rev. Fr. Corps Gras*, **1987**, *34*, 15.

Sebedio, J-L.; Grandgirard, A. Physiological effects of *trans* and cyclic fatty acids. *Prog. Lipid Res.* **1989**, 28, 303.

Selke, E.; Rohwedder, W.K.; Dutton, H.J. Volatile components from triolein heated in air. *J. Amer. Oil Chem. Soc.* **1977**, *54*, 62.

Selke, E.; Rohwedder, W.K.; Dutton, H.J. Volatile components from trilinolein in air. *J. Amer. Oil Chem. Soc.* **1980**, *57*, 25.

U.S. Department of Agriculture, Economic Research Service, Food Consumption Tables, 1995.

Warner, K.; Mounts, T.L.; Kwolek, W.F. Effects of antioxidants, methyl silicone and hydrogenation on room odor of soybean cooking oils. *J. Amer. Oil Chem. Soc.* **1985**, *62*, 1483.

Warner, K.; Orr, P.; Glynn, M. Effect of fatty acid composition of oils on flavor and stability of fried food. *J. Am. Oil Chem. Soc.* **1997**, *74*, 374.

Wessels, H. Determination of polar compounds in frying fats. *Pure and Applied Chem.* **1983**, *55*, 84.

6

CHOLESTEROL OXIDATION PRODUCTS

Their Occurrence and Detection in Our Foodstuffs

Pearlly S. Yan

Experiment Station Chemistry Laboratory
University of Missouri-Columbia
Columbia, Missouri 65211

1. ABSTRACT

The structural similarity of cholesterol oxidation products (COP) to native cholesterol and their xenobiotic effects prompt researchers to study the long-term effects of the assimilation of these compounds into our tissues. COP are present in our food system. The level of exposure changes as our food products and our food choices alter. Therefore, the presence of COP in our food system has to be carefully monitored and their presence in processed foods minimized by optimizing processing and storage conditions. This review will briefly discuss the chemistry of some commonly-occurring COP and their biological significance. A more in-depth survey of the literature on the pitfalls of COP determination is included. It is the intention of the author to impress the readers that 'exogenous' COP can easily form during sample preparation. These artifacts will hinder our understanding of factors that promote COP formation in foods. The effects of heating, dehydrating, packaging and the presence of highly unsaturated lipids on the levels of COP in cholesterol-containing foods are evaluated to gauge the levels of exposure to different consumer groups.

2. CHOLESTEROL AUTOXIDATION

Cholesterol, with its double bond between the C-5 and C-6 of the B-ring (Figure 1), readily undergoes oxidation via the free radical mechanism to form some 66 cholesterol oxidation products (COP). Research in this area is explored extensively in a monograph (1981) and in several reviews by Dr. Leland Smith (Smith, 1987; Smith, 1991). Readers are asked to seek out any one of these works for detailed reactions of cholesterol autoxidation.

Impact of Processing on Food Safety, edited by Jackson et al.,
Kluwer Academic / Plenum Publishers, New York, 1999.

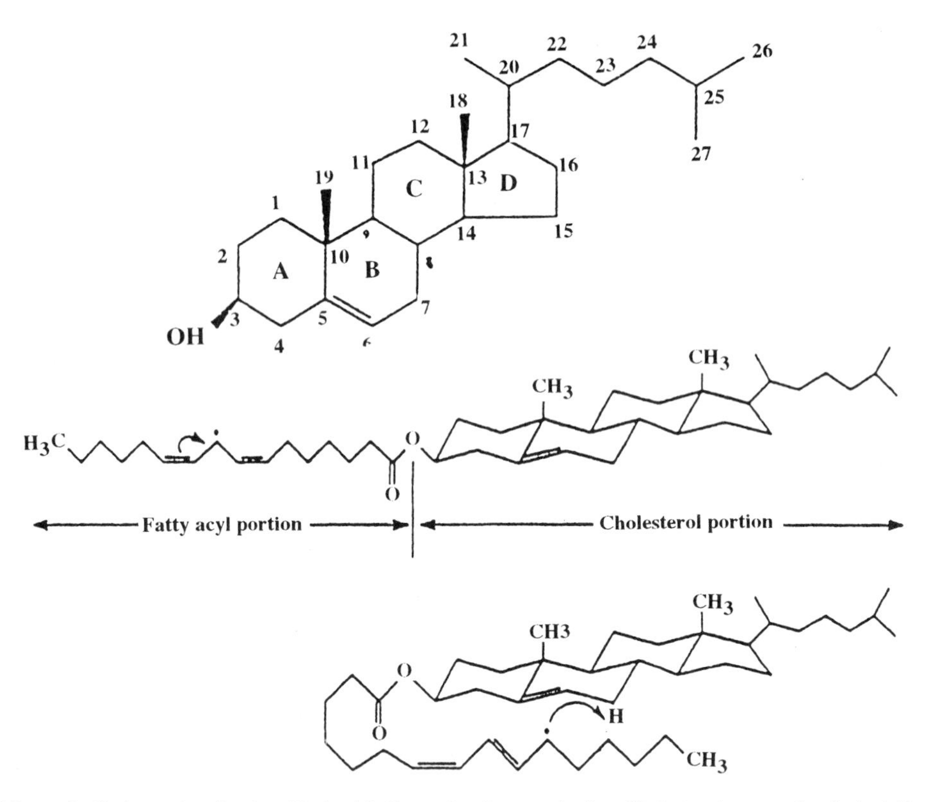

Figure 1. Cholesterol molecule with ring labeling and carbon numbering. Cholesteryl ester molecule depicting the fatty acid portion esterified to the cholesterol portion. From Paniangvait et al. (1995).

At low temperatures, as protons in the allylic C-7 and the tertiary C-25 positions of the cholesterol molecules are abstracted, their respective free radicals are formed. Both of these radicals react with oxygen to give the corresponding peroxyl radicals. However, only the C-7 peroxyl radical survives at room temperature and this becomes the first detectible COP, the epimeric 7-hydroperoxides (Figure 2). These hydroperoxides undergo thermal decomposition to form the epimeric cholest-5-ene-3β-7-diols (7-hydroxycholesterols) and 3β-hydroxycholest-5-en-7-one (7-ketocholesterol). Further decomposition of the latter compound forms cholesta-3,5-dien-7-one. Detection of this compound indicates degradation of 7-ketocholesterol by harsh sample preparation procedures.

Epoxidation of the Δ5-double bond may occur by the attack of 7-hydroperoxides already present and yields the isomeric 5,6-epoxycholestan-3β-ol (epoxycholestanol). The β-isomer usually predominates because of its more sterically hindered epoxide. Both isomers can further degrade into cholestane-3β,5α,6β-triol (cholestantriol) by hydration.

Oxidation of the cholesterol side-chain results in 20-, 24-, 25-, and 26-hydroperoxides and their decomposition products. Cholest-5-ene-3β,25-diol (25-hydroxycholesterol) is among these products. Side-chain oxidation usually takes place in solid cholesterol and not in aqueous dispersions.

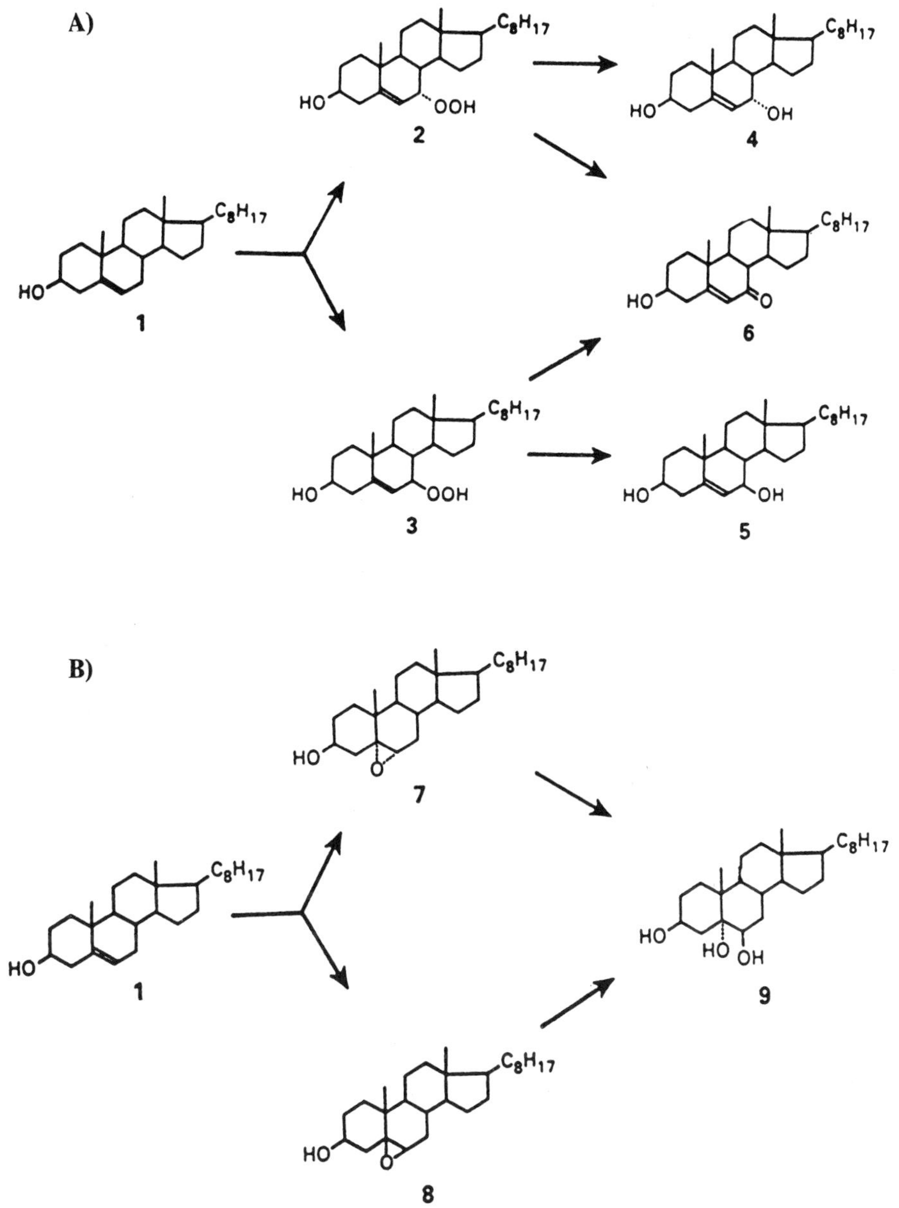

A)

B)

Figure 2. (A) Cholesterol (1) forms the epimeric 7-hydroperoxides (2 and 3) which can be degraded into 7α-hydroxycholesterol (4), 7β-hydroxycholesterol (5) and 7-ketocholesterol (6). (B) Epoxidation of cholesterol (1) to form the isomeric 5,6α-epoxycholesterol (7) and 5,6β-epoxycholesterol (8), both of which can hydrolyze to form cholestanetriol (9). (C) Side chain of cholesterol to form (20S)-cholest-5-ene-3β,20-diol (18), cholest-5-ene-3β,25-diol (19), cholest-5-ene-3β,26-diol (20), and 3β-hydroxycholest-5-en-24-one (21). From Smith (1987).

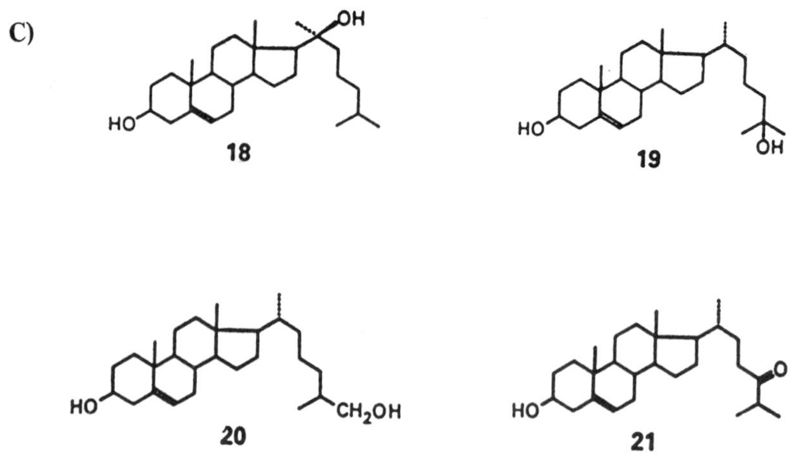

C)

Figure 2. *Continued.*

3. BIOLOGICAL EFFECTS OF CHOLESTEROL OXIDATION PRODUCTS

Cholesterol oxidation products are present in our diet. The important questions to address are if these compounds have any undesirable physiological roles *in vivo* and if they predispose us to debilitating disease states.

Because it is important to establish the residence time of COP and their metabolic fate *in vivo*, research in the area of COP absorption, distribution in the blood stream, and incorporation in various tissues has been conducted. Peng et al. (1986) fed radiolabeled autoxidized cholesterol to rabbits and found that the rate of absorption of COP was not significantly different from that of native cholesterol. Appearance of labeled native- and oxidized cholesterol in the blood stream peaked 24 h after gavaging of such compounds. When humans were given a meal rich in COP (Emanuel et al., 1991), the postprandial increases in concentration of COP peaked 3–4 h after consumption of the test meal. Subjects consuming a fresh egg test meal had very low levels of COP in their plasma. When native or oxidized cholesterol was given to rats via intubation, the appearance of these compounds in the lymph was followed closely by Osada et al. (1994). The proportion of native to oxidized cholesterol absorbed was not as similar as that found in the rabbit (Peng et al, 1986). Rats appeared to absorb less of the oxidized cholesterol present in the feeding mixture. When Bascoul et al. (1986) followed the absorption and the excretion of α-epoxycholesterol in the rat, they noted that COP was cleared from the blood very rapidly and its excretion in the stool continued for several days afterwards, until its disappearance from the blood.

The biological effects of COP are many-fold. They include the induction of atherogenicity, mutagenicity and carcinogenicity. The research studies carried out in these areas are also numerous. Only selected recent work in the area of atherogenicity involving COP will be discussed here, as atherosclerosis is the number one cause of mortality in the United States. Lipid oxidation (occurring *in vivo* or via oxidized lipids in the diet) has been implicated for initiating this disease in humans. Staprans et al. (1996) showed that oxidized lipids from the diet were incorporated into the liver and re-packaged for circulation via the very low density lipoprotein in rats. Nourooz-Zadeh et al. (1996) showed that low-density lipoprotein is the major carrier of lipid hydroperoxides in the plasma. Hodis et al. (1991) established that when rabbits were given a high level of cholesterol, there was a relationship between the level of COP found in circulation to that found in the aorta tissue. These researchers suggested that COP present in dietary cholesterol as well as those formed *in vivo* led to the increased amount found in the blood and in the aorta. These and other findings point to the risk of consuming high-cholesterol foods, which can also be high in COP.

To further pinpoint the deleterious effects of COP, researchers rely on cell culture systems and *ex vivo* studies to accurately define the biological effects of these compounds. It is also through experiments like these that the relative cytotoxic or biological potencies of different COP were determined.

From previous research findings, side-chain 25-hydroxycholesterol and B-ring cholestanetriol were found to be especially cytotoxic. Caboni et al. (1994) substantiated the cytotoxic effect of cholestanetriol by demonstrating its effect on reducing cell proliferation when present at a concentration that did not lead to cell death. The above two COP together with 7-ketocholesterol were shown by Palladini et al. (1996) to affect the barrier function of endothelial cells. They were able to disrupt the organization of actin microfilaments which would eventually lead to cell detachment and cell death by apoptosis. Lizard et al. (1996) also found COP to have the ability to induce apoptosis in endothelial cells, however, the potency of COP observed differed from that of Palladini et al. (1996) in that 7β-hydroxycholesterol > 7-ketocholesterol > 19-hydroxycholesterol > α-epoxycholesterol > 25-hydroxycholesterol. It is important to note that in all these studies, native cholesterol did not exhibit the mentioned cytotoxic effects. These and other studies are pointing to the more commonly occurring COP, i.e., those oxidized at C-7 which are also capable of inducing events that might lead to the onset of human atherosclerosis. As the biological effects of these compounds become established, it will become important that their occurrence in foodstuffs be monitored with accurate and sensitive procedures.

4. ANALYSIS OF CHOLESTEROL OXIDATION PRODUCTS

Analysts who are interested in the determination of COP in food or biological samples are faced with several challenges. These challenges are circumventable as analysts choose the appropriate analytical procedure that has been proven successful in enriching the COP of interest from a specific sample matrix. Possible pitfalls will be briefly discussed and some of the established methods for the determination of COP will be outlined.

4.1. Generation of Exogenous Cholesterol Oxidation Products

Native cholesterol can be as high as 2g/100g edible portion in egg yolk powder in a matrix containing more than 40% lipid material (Sarantinos et al., 1993). Thus the enrichment of COP, which are usually present at low concentrations (0.1 to 50 ppm), without causing the bulk lipid and the native cholesterol to oxidize during the sample preparation steps is highly important to minimize positive errors from artifact formation. Wasilchuk et al. (1992) systematically studied artifact formation during sample preparation by exposing aqueous solutions of multideuterated cholesterol and unlabeled cholesterol to autoxidizing conditions (i.e., aerated, heated at 60–70°C for 2 h, and exposed to UV irradiation) during sample preparation. The aqueous system was spiked with a series of COP as the 'endo-

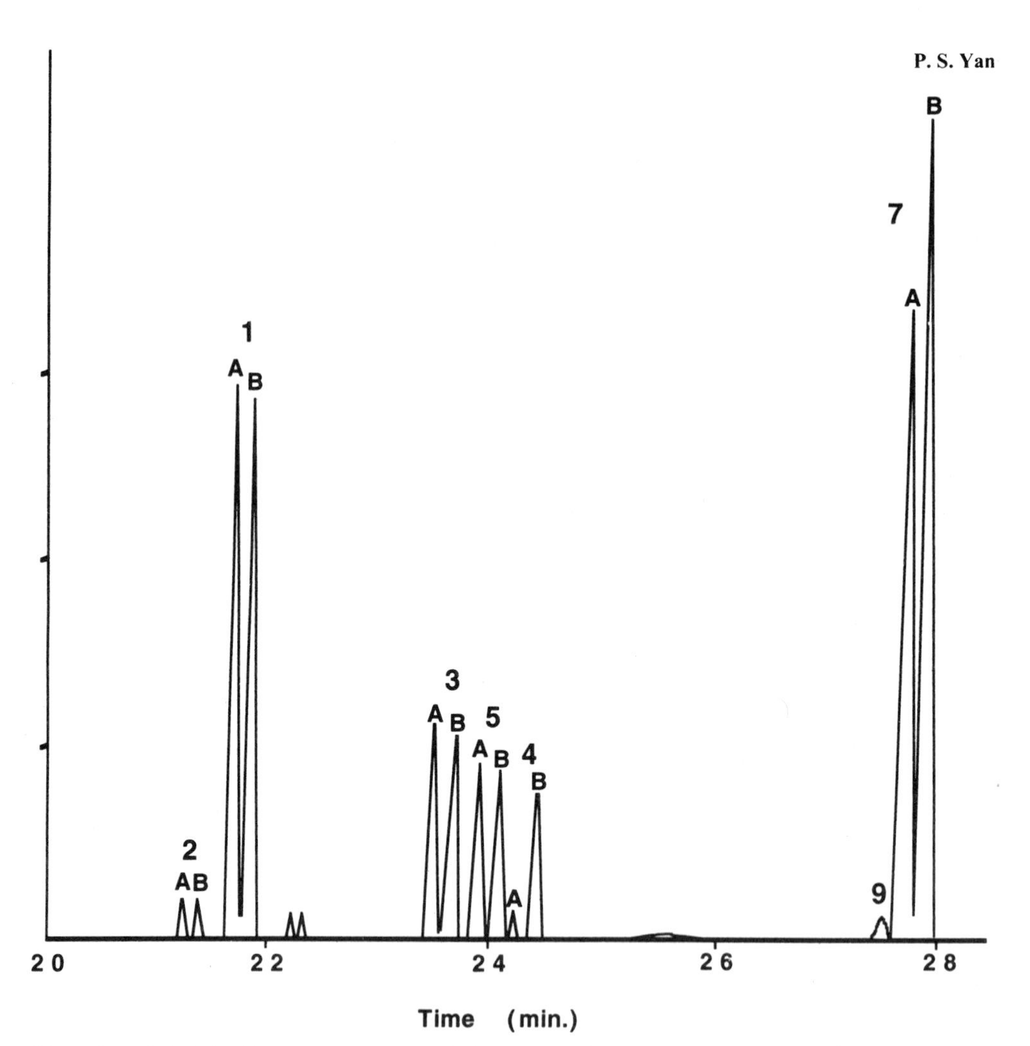

Figure 3. A, Labeled oxide components; B, unlabeled oxide components; 2, 7α-hydroxycholesterol; 1, cholesterol; 3, 7β-hydroxycholesterol; 5, β-epoxycholesterol; 4, α-epoxycholesterol; 7, 7-ketocholesterol. This experiment examined the effectiveness of using multideuterated cholesterol to control for endogenous cholesterol oxidation. Unlabeled α-epoxycholesterol and 7-ketocholesterol were spiked to show the usefulness of the method in their recovery. From Wasilchuk et al. (1992).

genous' COP prior to sample workup. The total ion chromatogram from one of these analyses is presented in Figure 3. In this experiment, the 'endogenous' COP were 7-ketocholesterol and α-epoxycholesterol, and their recoveries were accounted for by the higher abundance of unlabeled 7-ketocholesterol and α-epoxycholesterol. The chromatogram showed that the described autoxidizing conditions formed 7α- and 7β-hydroxycholesterols, α- and β-epoxycholesterols and 7-ketocholesterol with 7-ketocholesterol having the highest and α-epoxycholesterol having the lowest abundance (the labeled peaks) under such conditions. As many studies involving the determination of COP are carried out without the benefit of deuterated cholesterol to aid in determining artifact formation, immense care must be given to sample preparation procedures to minimize such distortions.

The described autoxidizing conditions appear severe, however, there are ample opportunities for autoxidation to occur during the enrichment of COP. Some COP, such as cholestanetriol, are very polar and require polar solvents such as diethyl ether for their extraction. Yet diethyl ether contains ether peroxides upon exposure to light. Dyer et al. (1995) reported that the level of 7-ketocholesterol increased by 400–500% when diethyl ether was used to extract the non-saponifiables after the bulk lipid was removed by saponification. It has long been realized that exposing cholesterol-containing samples to air and light increases their COP levels (VanLier and Smith, 1967). Therefore, modifying the analytical procedure by minimizing exposure to light, distilling solvents used in sample preparation, replacing air with inert gases by purging, reducing the ambient temperature and temperature during solvent removal steps, adding antioxidants and metal chelators to the system, and shortening the analytical procedures have all been described as means to reduce artifact formation. One needs to be mindful that these procedures are effective in lowering exogenous COP levels but may not completely eliminate exogenous COP formation.

The structural similarities between native and oxidized cholesterol also pose another challenge during sample preparation. As mentioned above, native cholesterol needs to be separated from oxidized cholesterol as early as possible during the sample preparation steps. However, oxidized cholesterol may contain 3,5-cholest-dien-7-one or 4,6-cholest-dien-3-one which are more apolar than other commonly occurring COP (Chen & Chen, 1994). If the occurrence of these COP are significant to the system in question, care must be taken so that none of these oxides are eluted with native cholesterol during sample cleanup steps.

As it is important not to create additional COP during sample preparation, it is equally important to avoid incomplete recovery of COP from the sample. Some COP are quite polar and their recoveries are low due to their retention on polar support material such as silica gel. A notable COP that is susceptible to this pitfall is cholest-3β,5α,6β-triol. As this COP is shown to be quite biologically active, it's presence in our food should be carefully monitored.

Poor recoveries of COP can also be attributed to degradation by harsh sample preparation conditions. The most often cited example is the degradation of 7-ketocholesterol as it is exposed to hot saponification (Park & Addis, 1985). This procedure is often included to remove triacylglycerols from the non-saponifiable sterol fraction and to remove the fatty acid moiety of esterified cholesterol. As Dzeletovic et al. (1995) experimented with different saponification conditions, they discovered that 7-ketocholesterol underwent decomposition at temperatures higher than 22°C and that increasing the concentration of KOH from 0.35 M to 0.70 M also resulted in a great reduction in this COP. They also observed that prolonging the exposure to KOH from 1 h to 14 h resulted in 50% loss. These researchers decided on saponifying their plasma samples in 0.35M KOH at 22°C for 2 h. Samples differ in their triacylglycerol and esterified cholesterol contents and it becomes necessary for each analyst to work out the saponification parameters suitable for that sample system. Some researchers employed other means to remove triacylglycerols. If the amount of esterified cholesterol in the sample is low, such as in processed milk (Nourooz-Zadeh and Appelqvist, 1988) where only 10% of the total cholesterol is in the esterified form, researchers may choose to avoid saponification altogether. Procedures other than saponification can be used to free cholesteryl esters in biological samples, which contain far more esterified cholesterol than that present in the free form. Zubillaga and Maerker (1988) as well as Schmarr et al. (1996) described the procedure of transesterification as a means to achieve triglyceride-removal and de-esterification of cholesterol.

If the determination of cholesterol hydroperoxides is part of the objective of the study, analysis by GC or GC-MS should be avoided because hydroperoxides are temperature labile and will be decompose by the high temperatures of these procedures. Hydroperoxides can be determined by TLC (Ansari & Smith, 1994), HPLC (Teng, 1990), and by HPLC-MS with a thermospray or particle beam interface (Sevanian et al, 1994; Caruso et al, 1996).

4.2. Analytical Procedure for the Determination of Cholesterol Oxidation Products

As most analysts are interested in determining the actual levels of COP in their experimental system, the addition of an appropriate internal standard is necessary to achieve this end. Many different compounds were used as internal standards. Criteria used for choosing a suitable compound include the following. First, the internal standard should be structurally similar to the analyte. Second, the internal standard should not be found in the sample. Finally, the detection of the compound should not interfere with the detection of the analytes. Often researchers include a test of response linearity of the internal standard to each of the COP at concentrations encountered in the samples to verify the suitability of the chosen compound. Compounds commonly employed are 5α-cholestane (Park & Addis, 1985; Yan & White, 1990; Sevanian et al., 1994), sitosterol α-epoxide (Dyer et al., 1995), 6-ketocholestanol (Lakritz and Maerker, 1989; Wasilchuk et al., 1992), and 19-hydroxycholesterol (Pie et al., 1990; Rose-Sallin et al., 1995). For researchers who have access to deuterated COP, these compounds are valuable for quantifying COP due to their close structural similarity and the ability to enable discrimination between COP and standards during sample preparation and detection. (Dzeletovic et al., 1995; Wasilchuk et al., 1992; Breuer and Bjorkhem, 1990).

Researchers may also wish to add deuterated cholesterol prior to sample preparation to account for exogenous COP formation during sample preparation as discussed above. Wasilchuk et al. (1992) cautioned about the isotope effect during mass spectral analysis as well as during the oxidation of cholesterol. Fragmentation patterns and the ease of proton abstraction differ between a C-H bond and a C-D bond. The deuterium labeling should therefore be as far away from the oxidation or the cleavage sites as possible to ensure accurate artifact correction and detection.

The first step in sample preparation is usually a total lipid extraction step employing the classic method of Folch et al. (1957). If one is interested in quantifying COP that are associated with the esterified cholesterol fraction, cold saponification or transesterification procedures can precede the lipid fractionation procedure. The cold saponification procedure that is often used was described by Park & Addis (1986) whereby methanolic KOH is mixed with extracted lipid until all the lipid is well dispersed. The atmosphere in the container is flushed with inert gases such as nitrogen or argon and the flask is then held in the dark at room temperature for about 24 h. Neutralization of the medium is necessary prior to the extraction of the unsaponifiables which contain the COP. It can be achieved by extensive washing of the organic phase with deionized water. However, one risks the formation of an emulsion resulting in losses of COP. Neutralization can also be achieved by the addition of an acid. Dzeletovic et al. (1995) cautioned against the use of strong monobasic mineral acids, such as hydrochloric acid, due to its ability to transiently lower local pH drastically and affect acid-sensitive COP, such as β-epoxycholesterol. These researchers chose to use phosphoric acid with a second pKa at 6.6, thereby reducing the risk of overtitration. The transesterification procedure was well described by Zubillaga and Maerker (1988). They reported on the transesterification of various cholesteryl esters to the fatty acid methyl ester and free cholesterol for 2 h at room temperature in 1N NaOH in methanol:benzene (60:40, v/v). 7-Ketocholesterol was found to be stable in this procedure. A slightly different procedure was described by Schmarr et al. (1996).

Because esterified cholesterol is not a major component in most food lipids, and because it is prudent to remove native cholesterol as early as possible to minimize the chance of forming exogenous COP, total lipid from food samples is often fractionated into subclasses, bypassing the saponification/transesterification procedure either by thin-layer chromatography or solid-phase extraction with the latter technique being the one of choice. Aminopropyl solid-phase extraction was used by Schmarr et al. (1996) and John (1996). Schmarr et al. (1996) experimented with both silica gel and aminopropyl bonded-phase columns for the separation and removal of bulk lipid. The more polar COP such as cholest-3β,5α,6β-triol necessitates a polar solvent such as methanol as an eluant. Polar solvents often elute/dissolve silica gel particles which are therefore, less suitable as packing material. Other researchers did not find this to be a problem and silica gel was used in the fractionation of egg lipids (Guardiola et al., 1995; Lai et al., 1995) and in model lipids (Osada et al., 1993; John, 1996).

The analysis of COP can be successfully carried out by gas-liquid chromatography (GC), high-performance liquid chromatography (HPLC), TLC, and a GC or HPLC mass spectrometry (GC-MS or HPLC-MS, respectively). The TLC procedure is sensitive but is only semiquantitative if the intensity of the resolved COP is determined by a densitometer. Ansari and Smith (1994) and Teng (1990) described the color reactions of various COP with chemical reagents. As this procedure does not require heat to volatilize the analytes, cholesteryl hydroperoxides are successfully detected.

The COP can be analyzed by HPLC with both normal phase (Csallany et al., 1989) and reversed-phase columns (Chen and Chen, 1994). The most common detector for lipids is an ultraviolet (UV) detector which relies on the lipid material having π electrons that absorb at 212 nm and sometimes at 234 and 280 nm as well. Among the commonly-occurring COP, cholest-3β,5α,6β-triol, cholest-5α,6α-epoxide and cholest-5β,6β-epoxide do not have π electrons and thus are not detected by UV. Dzeletovic et al. (1995) commented that classical detection techniques such as UV and refractive index are not sensitive enough for determination of COP in human tissues. The employment of a laser light-scattering detector in an HPLC procedure greatly increases the flexibility of the system because a gradient elution system can be used without affecting the baseline of the chromatogram. In addition, this detector is capable of detecting COP without π electrons (Kermasha et al., 1994). Cholesterol hydroperoxides are not degraded by the HPLC procedures, and their detection is drastically improved by using a mercury drop electrochemical detector described by Korytowski et al. (1993). Another method that detects cholesterol hydroperoxides is the HPLC-postcolumn chemiluminescence procedure described byYamamoto et al. (1987).

The GC can readily separate a large number of trimethylsilylated COP and is used extensively for their analysis. Park and Addis (1986) reported COP are sensitive to the high temperature necessary for their volatilization during a GC injection. This resulted in the elution of compounds with trailing peaks. However, trimethylsilyled (TMS) derivatives of COP are stable at GC temperatures. GC procedures were used to analyze COP in dried egg powders (Wahle et al., 1993; Lai et al., 1995), in raw meat and chicken (Zubillaga and Maerker, 1991) and in a model powder system (Granelli et al., 1996). To use this procedure successfully, it is important to determine that all the COP of interest are completely derivatized, and this is especially important for COP that have more than one hydroxyl group such as 7-hydroxycholesterols, the side chain hydroxycholesterols, and cholest-3β,5α,6β-triol. Otherwise these COP could appear as more than one peak and their quantification will be incorrect.

As it is important to positively identify the trace amounts of COP present in complex food and biological matrices, the coupling of mass spectrometry to either GC or HPLC became the detection system of choice. Sevanian et al. (1994) and Caruso et al. (1996) described the types of interfaces used in HPLC/MS systems and Sevanian et al. (1994) evaluated the unique capabilities of the different interfaces as compared to the more established procedure of GC/MS. GC/MS with selected ion monitoring is used more often in food systems (Nielsen et al., 1995) and its detection sensitivity far exceeds that of GC with flame ionization detection. As the MS becomes more affordable, these detection methods shall gain more prominence in the arena of COP analysis.

5. FORMATION OF CHOLESTEROL OXIDATION PRODUCTS DURING PROCESSING AND STORAGE

Over the last ten years, interest in cholesterol oxidation has been on the rise and many excellent reviews were published in this area. A recent review by Paniangvait et al. (1995) included an extensive list of COP found in a variety of foods and their respective treatment conditions. The biological significance of COP was examined thoroughly in a review by Guardiola et al. (1996). The chemical and physical properties of COP were discussed in the monograph (Smith, 1981) and a review article (1987) by the same author. Readers are encouraged to seek out these reviews to explore each area at greater depth. The review by Paniangvait et al. (1995) also discussed factors affecting cholesterol oxidation during food processing. To avoid repeating information presented by these authors, this review will focus on more recent research findings or information that was not explored.

5.1. Heating

High temperature increases the formation as well as the decomposition of lipid hydroperoxides. As such, Kim and Nawar (1993) illustrated with their cholesterol model system that a temperature beyond 100°C resulted in a sudden increase in COP formation. Because COP themselves are heat labile and decompose into more polar compounds or polymerize into high molecular weight compounds, their levels at any point in time are an equilibrium between COP formation and degradation. In Figure 4, work by Kim and Nawar (1993) and Osada et al. (1994) points to the need for studying processing conditions systematically. In their model systems, cholesterol was exposed to a series of increasing temperatures. Both groups reported that with sufficiently high heat (140 and 150°C), COP levels increased drastically very early on, followed by a comparable sharp drop in their levels. Under less harsh conditions, the maximum COP levels were lower and were reached at a later time. The levels also decreased after reaching a maximum. With the least harsh condition, COP accumulated very slowly in the medium, and never reached a maximum within the observed time frame. Osada et al. (1993) observed that with very high temperatures (i.e., 200°C), little COP was accumulated in the medium because they were degraded faster than they were formed. Consequently, if random samples were analyzed for COP for the purpose of studying the heat treatment on COP formation, the levels seen in different samples might not mean a great deal in that a low level may actually represent excessive COP degradation due to high processing temperatures.

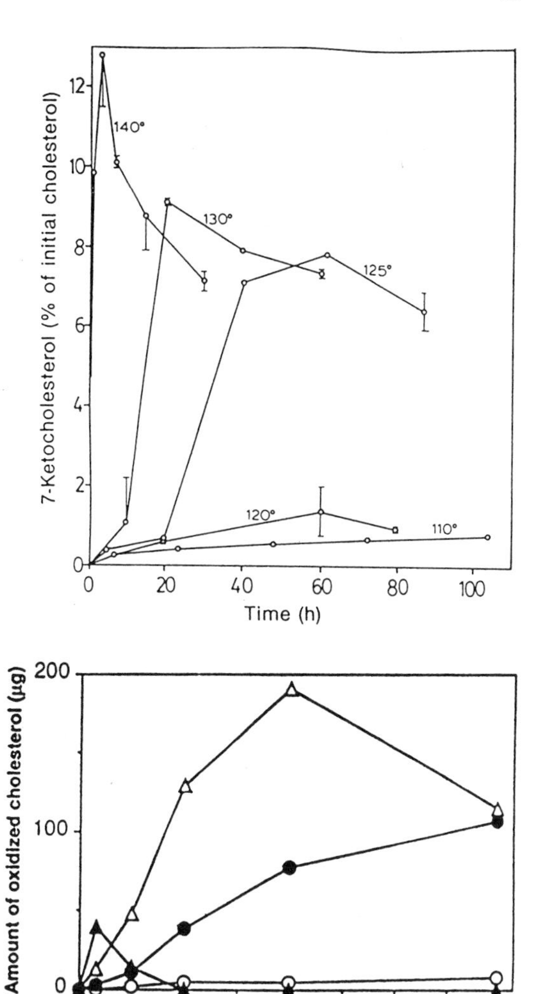

Figure 4. Formation of 7-ketocholesterol when pure cholesterol was heated at 100–200°C. From Kima and Nawar (1993). Figure on the bottom illustrates the time course of the production of oxidized cholesterol by heating at the following temperatures: ○, 100°C; ●, 120°C; △ 150°C; ▲, 200°C. From Osada et al. (1993).

Cholesterol is a minor component in food lipid, the bulk of the lipid being triacylglycerols followed by phospholipids. However, both cholesterol and unsaturated fatty acids undergo oxidation via the free radical mechanism (Smith, 1981). The number of double bonds present in the very-long-chain polyunsaturated fatty acids (vlc-PUFA) makes them highly susceptible to oxidation. The presence of such lipid can lead to extensive cholesterol oxidation because vlc-PUFA peroxyl radicals, once formed, can oxidize nearby cholesterol molecules by abstracting allylic protons (C-7 on the B-ring of the cholesterol molecule) and the tertiary proton (C-25 of side chain of the cholesterol molecule), forming hydroperoxides and other secondary COP. The content of vlc-PUFA and cholesterol in seafoods vary greatly (Shozen et al., 1995; Osada et al., 1993). As we encourage the public to increase their fish intake (especially fatty fish that contains high levels of vlc-PUFA) and since seafood products are in many traditional diets (Chen and Yen, 1994; Yankah et al., 1996; Ohshima et al., 1996), it is no surprise that increasing research emphasis is placed on processed seafood and cholesterol oxidation. Ohshima et al. (1996) demonstrated that grilling boiled and dried anchovies for short periods (220°C for up to

15 min) can lead to high levels of COP during the first 6 min. The accumulated COP were later degraded upon further grilling. Both cholestanetriol and 25-hydroxycholesterol were formed under those conditions. Yankah et al. (1996) looked at the effect of refined salt and rock salt on the quality of a fermented fish product. Rock salt rather than refined salt is traditionally used in the preparation of this product. However, it contains higher moisture, more impurities, and even trace metals. Yankah et al. (1996) found that use of refined salt produced a higher quality product with lower levels of COP after drying and storage. The COP level found in products prepared with the rock salt was very high (total COP were 363 ppm after 2 months storage), almost approaching levels detected in unprotected spray-dried whole egg powder aged for 12 months (7-ketocholesterol present at 500 ppm) (Fontana et al., 1993). Other processed food items contain much less COP. Dried egg pasta contains about 15 ppm 7-ketocholesterol (Zunin et al., 1996) and infant formula powders can have up to 86 ppm total COP (Rose-Sallin et al., 1995).

As prepared food products are ever so popular with busy consumers, the findings of Pie et al. (1991) are particularly noteworthy. These researchers previously noticed that butter that was heated formed more COP during frozen storage at -20°C in than unheated butter. They proceeded to study the effect of pre-cooking on cholesterol oxidation in frozen meat patties. Their data showed that cooking after frozen storage only resulted in slightly higher COP whereas pre-cooked frozen patties had much more COP. In order to study similar phenomenon in consumer items, these researchers analyzed the COP content in two identical frozen meals, one of which was stored for an additional 3 months. The latter sample showed much higher levels of 7-ketocholesterol and epoxycholesterols in comparison to the sample frozen for shorter duration. In view of these results, only the freshest ingredients should be used in the preparation of frozen entrees due to the lengthy expiration date carried by these items.

5.2. Dehydration Procedures

Porous cholesterol-rich products such as dried milk powder, dried egg powder, and freeze-dried meat products can be important contributors of COP to our diet. With the development of an electron spectrometry technique to study the surface coverage of food powder with dispersed lipid, Granelli et al. (1996) discovered that the amount of COP found in the model food powder correlated well with the surface-covering ability of the tested food lipids as shown in Figure 5. Technical grade tristearin was found to cover around 70% of the spray-dried powder and thus had the highest level of COP. Highly purified tristearin covered the least surface area and thus had the lowest level of COP. The coverage and COP values of triolein were intermediate between the other two fats. The authors theorized that lipids having less tendency to spread are probably protected from the atmosphere by the matrix itself thus leading to lower cholesterol oxidation. Model systems such as these bring about important understanding in the area of cholesterol oxidation in foods.

Another model system reported by Lai et al. (1995) further identified oxides of nitrogen (NO_x) as the agent that induces more COP in food powder produced in a direct gas-fired spray-dryer. In their experiment, NO_x was added to an indirect gas-fired spray dryer in levels ranging from 0.5 to 50 ppm (the normal level of NO_x found in gas-fired spray-dryer is about 8 ppm). The effect of another oxidant, cumene hydroperoxide, was also tested in the indirect gas-fired spray-dryer. Cumene hydroperoxide undergoes decomposition by heat to generate alkoxyl or peroxyl radicals. These radicals are highly reactive to unsaturated lipids similar to those generated by the decomposition of NO_x (forming a mix-

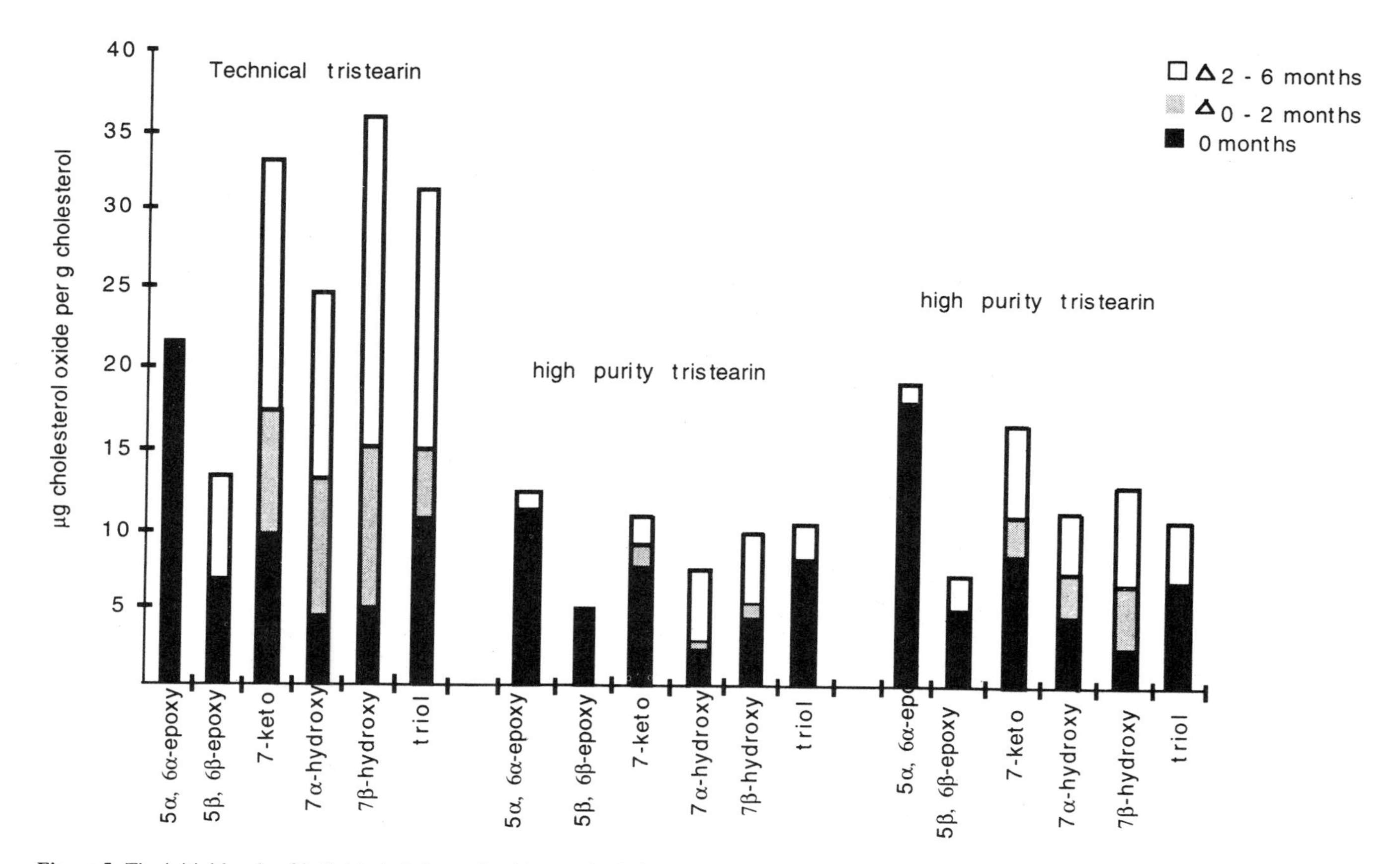

Figure 5. The initial levels of individual cholesterol oxides (µg/g cholesterol) and increments for 0–2 and for 2–6 months storage for model powders containing different oil phases. From Granelli et al. (1996).

ture of oxidizing nitrogen oxide gases) and hydrogen peroxide (forming hydroxyl radical). Lai et al (1995) found that direct gas-fired drying produced higher levels of COP thus confirming previous findings by other researchers (Missler et al., 1985; Morgan and Armstrong, 1987). They reported that egg powders exposed to NO_x during processing (gas-fired or NO_x-added indirect dryer) are characterized by great abundance of β-epoxycholesterol, and a ratio of β to α-epoxycholesterol as high as 4.9:1. This COP pattern was also observed in samples prepared by the cumene hydroperoxide-added indirect gas-fired spray-dryer. Because adding this organic hydroperoxide resulted in the epoxidation of cholesterol not seen with indirect gas-fired spray drying alone, these researchers were confident that highly-reactive oxidizing species present in the direct gas-fired dryer induced a greater degree of cholesterol oxidation when spray-drying cholesterol-containing systems. Experiments such as these help to persuade food processors not to use direct-gas spray-dryer.

Researchers have also documented that the incorporation of spray-dried ingredients into processed products also increase their COP levels in the final products. Zunin et al. (1995) evaluated baked goods prepared from either fresh or powdered eggs. In order to single out the effect of powdered eggs in a baked product, a simple formulation without other cholesterol-containing ingredients was used. A biscuit recipe was chosen. Prepared biscuit was baked at 185°C for 20 min. The fresh eggs used in this research did not contain detectable amount of COP whereas the powdered eggs contained 4.7 ppm in lipid fraction. After baking, the biscuits made with fresh eggs or powdered eggs had 9.3 and 13.0 ppm total COP in lipid, respectively. Upon storage, far more COP were formed in the biscuits made with powdered eggs than those make with fresh eggs (9.3 vs 57.0 ppm in lipid, respectively).

In a later study, Zunin et al. (1996) examined cholesterol oxidation in dried egg pasta. Their data offered yet another critical point in the processing of cholesterol-containing foods materials. In this experiment, ten batches of commercially-prepared egg pasta were selected as reference samples because the researchers knew these pastas were prepared with four eggs/kg semolina flour (as specified by the product of identity in Italy) and that the drying conditions were well-controlled (75°C for 20 min and then at 65°C for 8 h). Other dried egg pastas prepared with both fresh or powdered eggs were purchased from local markets. Commercially-prepared egg pastas containing powdered eggs tend to have a wide range of COP concentrations. In this study, the researchers quantified both native and oxidized cholesterol. This additional information helped to evaluate pasta samples containing low to medium levels of COP and low levels of native cholesterol (in comparison to cholesterol level estimated from the product identity). This type of sample could have undergone extensive cholesterol oxidation (which explained the low levels of native cholesterol). The absence of much higher levels of COP signified that the commonly-occurring COP were further degraded or polymerized and thus not detected. Among the thirty-two dried egg pastas examined, no correlation between native cholesterol and 7-ketocholesterol (the major COP found) was seen. This confirms that, within a reasonable range, the initial cholesterol level has no effect on the COP level of the finished product. The manufacturing protocols, on the other hand, have a significant impact on the extent of cholesterol oxidation in the product. As we are striving to produce less COP in our foodstuffs, drying and heating conditions need to be carefully evaluated.

The population that needs the most safeguard from the ingestion of COP is probably our young. Infant formulas are usually high in fat. Some are supplemented with iron. The low water activity in powdered formulas rendered them more susceptible to lipid oxidation. As such, powdered infant formulas need to be monitored with great care. Rose-Sallin

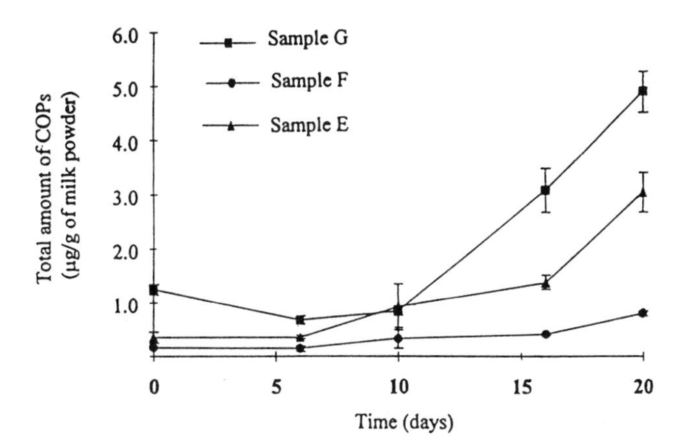

Figure 6. Formation of COP in infant formulas used in conditions corresponding to those normally applied at home (room temperature and opened packages). Three different samples (G, F, E) were opened (day 0), and then aliquots of powder were taken at intervals up to day 20. From Rose-Sallin et al. (1995).

et al. (1995) examined the formation of COP in three locally purchased infant formula powders. All of them contained around 260 mg fat/g formula. Among the three infant formulas tested, two of them had an initial COP level of <350 ng/g whereas one had about 1200 ng/g. Prior to correcting for artifact formation, 7-ketocholesterol was the major COP present. However, after correcting for the amount of deuterated 7-ketocholesterol, the highest COP in the infant formulas were 7β-or 7α-hydroxycholesterols, and there was little endogenous 7-ketocholesterol. Because of the correction for 'exogenous' 7-ketocholesterol, the amount of COP found in these formulas was lower than levels reported previously (MuCluskey and Devery, 1993). As shown in Figure 6, little increase in COP was observed in all three formulas during the first 10 days of storage. However by day 20 of storage, the COP levels increased greatly in two of the formulas. With this information, it is important for the manufacturers to establish the level of cholesterol oxidation in their products that are opened and stored so as to offer consumers clear guidelines on handling powdered infant formulas.

5.3. Additives and Packaging Materials in Easily Oxidized Products

Consumers desire to reduce their saturated fat intake yet would like to retain in their diet items that are high in saturated fat and cholesterol, such as eggs, red meat, and dairy spreads. This facet of consumer demands prompted the development of new products with fatty acid profiles modified to become more unsaturated. Concomitant with the increase in unsaturation is the increased risk of lipid oxidation, leading to the oxidation of co-existing cholesterol. Food scientists thus need to come up with solutions for these new challenges.

Eggs and poultry are two important consumer items and modification of their fatty acid profiles can lead to significant changes in the dietary fatty acids consumed. The fatty acid composition of laying hens were modified by including fish oil, flax oil, palm oil, and sunflower oil (Li et al., 1996a) in their diet. With the exception of palm oil, all the other food lipids were high in either omega-3 or omega-6 fatty acids which are susceptible to lipid oxidation. These researchers examined the effect of adding 0.07% of mixed tocopherols to the diets on storage stability of freeze-dried breast meat from these laying hens.

The storage conditions were deliberately made harsh by storing the meat in open bags exposed to normal daylight for up to 4 months. The fatty acid profiles as well as the tocopherol levels of the breast meat were significantly altered by the respective diets. Tocopherol supplementation lowered thiobarbituric acid reactive substances in freeze-dried breast meat right after processing, but not after 4 months storage. The protection exerted by tocopherol on cholesterol oxidation was different in that the tocopherol supplemented products exhibited similar levels of COP after processing but had lower total COP when stored for 4 months. Among the four dietary lipids, breast meat from fish oil-fed hens was consistently less stable while meat from the palm-oil fed hens was the most stable. As much as 18.4% of the cholesterol in these stored products was oxidized. Since freeze-dried meat powder is often incorporated into convenience food products, meats that have more healthful fatty acid profiles need to be adequately protected.

Li et al. (1996b) looked at the stability of egg yolk powder from laying hens given fish , flax, palm, or sunflower oils with and without tocopherol supplementation. The fatty acid profiles of the egg powders reflected those of the dietary lipids. The tocopherol content of the egg from hens supplemented with dietary tocopherol increased by 3- to 4-fold. Like that of the breast meat, the eggs from fish oil-fed hens had the highest COP levels. Tocopherol was effective in lowering COP in all diets except the sunflower oil diet. The cytotoxic COP, 25-hydroxycholesterol, was detected in the egg powders from fish oil- and flaxseed oil-hens. When stored unprotected for 4 months, cholesterol losses were up to 50%. Such losses were not affected by dietary lipids of the laying hens.

A similar protective effect of dietary tocopherol was observed when Buckley et al. (1995) studied the oxidative stability and quality of pork by supplementing the pig diet with vitamin E. These researchers felt that disrupting meat muscle membranes by processes such as mechanical deboning, mincing, restructuring, or cooking changes the cellular compartmentalization. This leads to the migration of prooxidants such as iron to move from a small 'transit pool' to membrane lipids. Transition metals are capable of bringing on lipid oxidation by abstracting a proton from unsaturated fatty acids or by catalyzing the breakdown of lipid hydroperoxides, thereby propagating lipid oxidation reactions. The supplementation of tocopherols in the animal's diet can increase the level of antioxidant in meat membranes counteracting the damaging effect of prooxidative meat processing techniques mentioned above.

Huber et al. (1995) studied the effect of a tocopherol blend, ascorbyl palmitate, and BHA on cholesterol oxidation in spray-dried egg yolk. The egg yolk powders were stored at 60°C for up to 28 d. Their findings pointed to the need for examining the whole spectrum of COP formed during spray-drying and during accelerated storage. The tocopherol blend and BHA were found to be equally effective in reducing the levels of COP generated from the C-7 position on the cholesterol molecule. The levels of epoxycholestanols and cholestanetriol were not affected by either of the tested antioxidants. Samples protected with ascorbyl palmitate had less 7-ketocholesterol and 7β-hydroxycholesterol than the control. Therefore, more information is gained if more of the commonly-occurring COP can be quantified following processing and storage of food products.

As air and light both accelerate the lipid oxidation process, reducing their access by modifying the package atmosphere, including of oxygen absorbers, or blocking with light-, oxygen-, and moisture-barrier wraps are potential means to reduce cholesterol oxidation in foodstuffs. Shozen et al. (1997) showed that when boiled and dried anchovy was vacuum-packaged with a metal based oxygen absorber, the levels of COP found after 165 d storage were similar to those in the control stored in gas-tight plastic bags laminated with ethylenevinyl acetate (EVA)/polyvinylidene chloride/EVA for 14 d. Fontana et al. (1993) reported that when light was blocked by light-barrier wrappers, prepared cookies did not accumulate COP during the 12-month storage period. If the cookies were exposed to daylight, β-epoxycholestanol increased in the samples but not 7-ketocholesterol. This indicates that daylight is capable of bringing about epoxidation of cholesterol in a manner similar to γ-irradiation as observed by Maerker and Jones (1992). The effectiveness of packaging on the reduction of cholesterol oxidation was also reported by Rose-Sallin et al. (1995). They observed that by sealing powdered milk in inert gas in a container, only 250 ng COP/g powder was formed after storing for one year. If the powder milk was left opened for the same period of time, a level of 1895 ng/g powder was found.

As consumers are shying away from butter, new products such as dairy spreads are replacing butter in our diets. Nielsen et al. (1996) reported that the cholesterol present in the spreads tends to be less stable than that found in butter. These researchers noted that dairy spreads are given a shelf life of 10 wk at 4 °C, yet the time course of COP formation indicated that by 8 wk of storage the total COP as well as epoxycholestanols had already reached a maximum. This signifies that from the standpoint of cholesterol oxidation, better packaging or protection of these products needs to be instigated.

5.4. Food Irradiation

Food irradiation is gaining importance as a method for preserving food and can affect food constituents including lipids and cholesterol. Maerker and Jones (1992) studied the effects of γ-irradiation on cholesterol oxidation. This subject has also been thoroughly reviewed by Paniangvait et al. (1995) and little data have been generated since then. Readers are referred to the above review for the effects of irradiation on cholesterol oxidation.

6. SUMMARY

Cholesterol oxidation products are shown to be present in the food we consume. Little COP are found in fresh products, but they can be present in high amounts if the processing conditions are not well controlled. These include: high processing temperatures, presence of prooxidants, improper or prolonged storage, inadequate packaging, and presence of other oxidation sensitive lipids. Some of these conditions are discussed here. As we are mindful of the pitfalls of producing exogenous COP (or artifacts) during the quantification, we are closer to estimating the levels of these compounds in our diet. This information coupled with recent findings on the possible roles of COP on the onset of atherosclerosis shall help to increase public awareness and to steer the food industry around the world to re-examine processing conditions to not only produce organoleptically-superior products but also products with low levels of COP as well.

REFERENCES

Ansari, G.A.S.; Smith, L.L. Assay of cholesterol autoxidation. *Methods In Enzymol.* **1994**, 233, 332–338.

Bascoul, J.; Domergue, N.; Mourot, J.; Debry, G.; Crastes de Paulet, A. Intestinal absorption and fecal excretion of 5,6 α-epoxy-5α-cholesta-3β-ol by the male Wistar rat. *Lipids.* **1986**, 21, 744–747.

Breuer, P.; Bjorkhem, I. Simultaneous quantification of several cholesterol autoxidation and monohydroxylation products by isotope-dilution mass spectrometry. *Steroids.* **1990**, 55, 185–192.

Buckley, D.J.; Morrissey, P.A.; Gray, J.I. Influence of dietary vitamin E on the oxidative stability and quality of pig meat. *J. Anim. Sci.* **1995**, 73, 3122–3130.

Caboni, M.F.; Hrelia, S.; Bordoni, A.; Lercker, G.; Capella, P.; Turchetto, E.; Biagi, P.L. *In vitro* effects of 5α-cholestane-3β,5,6β-triol on cultured rat cardiomyocytes. *J. Agric. Food Chem.* **1994**, 42, 2367–2371.

Caruso, D.; Rasetti, M.F.; De Angelis, L.; Galli, G. Identification of 3β-hydroxy-5α-cholest-6-ene-5-hydroperoxide in human oxidized LDL. *Chem. Phys. Lipids* **1996**, 79, 181–186.

Chen, B.H.; Chen, Y.C. Evaluation of the analysis of cholesterol oxides by liquid chromatography. *J. Chromatogr.* A **1994**, 661, 127–136.

Chen, J.S.; Yen, G.C. Cholesterol oxidation products in small sun-dried fish. *Food Chem.* **1994**, 50, 167–170.

Csallany, A.S.; Kindom, S.E.; Addis, P.B.; Lee, J.H. HPLC method for quantitation of cholesterol and four of its major oxidation products in muscle and liver tissues. *Lipids*. **1989**, 21, 645–651.

Dyer, R.G.; Hetherington, C.S.; Alberti, K.G.; Laker, M.F. Simultaneous measurement of phytosterols (campesterol and β-sitosterol) and 7-ketocholesterol in human lipoproteins by capillary column gas chromatography. *J. Chromatogr. B: Biomed. Applications*. **1995**, 663, 1–7.

Dzeletovic, S.; Breuer, O.; Lund, E.; Diczfalusy, U. Determination of cholesterol oxidation products in human plasma by isotope dilution-mass spectrometry. *Anal. Biochem.* **1995**, 225, 73–80.

Emanuel, H.A.; Hassel, C.A.; Addis, P.B.; Bergmann, S.D.; Zavoral, J.H. Plasma cholesterol oxidation products (oxysterols) in human subjects fed a meal rich in oxysterols. *J. Food Sci.* **1991**, 56, 843–847.

Fontana, A.; Antoniazzi, F.; Ciavatta, M.L.; Trivellone, E.; Cimino, G. 1H-NMR study of cholesterol autooxidation in egg powder and cookies exposed to adverse storage. *J. Food Sci.* **1993**, 58, 1286–1290.

Folch, J.; Lees, M.; Stanley, G.H.S. A simple method for the isolation and purification of total lipids from animal tissues. *J. Biol. Chem.* **1957**, 726, 497–509.

Granelli, K.; Faldt, P.; Appelqvist, L.A.; Bergentstahl, B. Influence of surface structure on cholesterol oxidation in model food powders. *J. Sci. Food Agric.* **1996**, 71, 75–82.

Guardiola, F.L.; Codony, R.; Miskin, D.; Rafecas, M.; Boatella, J. Oxysterol formation in egg powder and relationship with other quality parameters. *J. Agric. Food Chem.* **1995**, 43, 1903–1907.

Guardiola, F.; Condony, R.; Addis, P.B.; Rafecas, M.; Boatella, J. Biological effects of oxysterol: current status. *Food Chem. Toxic.* **1996**, 34, 193–211.

Hodis, H.N.; Crawford, D.W.; Sevanian, A. Cholesterol feeding increases plasma and aortic tissue cholesterol oxide levels in parallel: Further evidence for the role of cholesterol oxidation in atherosclerosis. *Atherosclerosis*. **1991**, 89, 117–126.

Huber, K.C.; Pike, O.A.; Huber, C.S. Antioxidant inhibition of cholesterol oxidation in a spray-dried food system during accelerated storage. *J. Food Sci.* **1995**, 60, 909–912, 916.

John, C.B. Isolation of cholesterol oxidation products from animal fat using aminopropyl solid-phase extraction. *J. Chromatogr. A*. **1996**, 736, 205–210.

Kermasha, S.; Kubow, S.; Goetghebeur, M. Comparative high-performance liquid chromatographic analyses of cholesterol and its oxidation products using diode-array ultraviolet and laser light-scattering detection. *J. Chromatogr. A*. **1994**, 685, 229–235.

Kim, S.K.; Nawar, W.W. Parameters influencing cholesterol oxidation. *Lipids*. **1993**, 28, 917–922.

Korytowski, W.; Bachowski, G.J.; Girotti,A.W. Analysis of cholesterol and phospholipid hydroperoxides by high-performance liquid chromatography with mercury drop electrochemical detection. *Anal. Biochem.* **1993**, 213, 111–119.

Lai, S.M.; Gray, J.I.; Buckley, D.J.; Kelly, P.M. Influence of free radicals and other factors on formation of cholesterol oxidation products in spray-dried whole egg. *J. Agric. Food Chem.* **1995**, 43, 1127–1131.

Lakritz, L.; Maerker, G. Effect of ionizing radiation on cholesterol inaqueous dispersion. *J . Food Sci.* **1989**, 54, 1569–1572.

Li, S.X.; Ahn, D.U.; Cherian, G.; Chung, T.Y.; Sim, J.S. Dietary Oils and tocopherol supplementation on cholesterol oxide formation in freeze-dried chicken meat durıng storage. *J. Food Lipids* **1996a**, 3, 27–42.

Li, S.X.; Cherian, G.; Ahn, D.U.; Hardin, R.T.; Sim, J.S. Storage, heating, and tocopherols affect cholesterol oxide formation in food oils. *J. Agric. Food Chem.* **1996b**, 44, 3830–3834.

Li, S.X.; Cherian, G.; Sim, J.S. Cholesterol oxidation in egg yolk powder during storage and heating as affected by dietary oils and tocopherol. *J. Food Sci.* **1996c**, 61, 721–725.

Lizard, G.; Deckert, V.; Dubrez, L.; Moisant, M.; Gambert, P.; Lagrost, L. Induction of apoptosis in endothelial cells treated with cholesterol oxides. *Am. J. Path.* **1996**, 148, 1625–1638.

Maerker, G.; Jones, K.C. Gamma-irradiation of individual choelsterol oxidation products. *J. Am. Oil Chem. Soc.* **1992**, 69, 451–455.

McCluskey, S.; Devery, R. Validation of chromatographic analysis of cholesterol oxides in dried foods. *Trends Food Sci. Technol.* **1993**, 4, 175–178.

Misseler, S.R.; Wasilchuk, B.A.; Merritt, C. Separation and identification of cholesterol oxidation products in dried egg preparations. *J. Food Sci.* **1985**, 50, 595–598.

Morgan, J.N.; Armstrong, D.J. Formation of cholesterol 5,6-epoxides during spray-drying egg yolk. *J. Food Sci.* **1987**, 52, 1224–1227.

Nielsen, J.H.; Olsen, C.E.; Jensen, C.; Skibsted, L.H. Cholesterol oxidation in butter and dairy spread during storage. *J. Dairy Res.* **1996**, 63, 159–167.

Nielsen, J.H.; Olsen, C.E.; Duedahl, C.; Skibsted, L.H. Isolation and quantification of cholesterol oxides in dairy products by selected ion monitoring mass spectrometry. *J. Dairy Res.* **1995**, 62, 101–113.

Nourooz-Zadeh, J.; Appelqvist, L. Cholesterol oxides in Swedish foods and food ingredients: milk powder products. *J. Food Sci.* **1988**, 53, 74–79.

Nourooz-Zadeh, J.; Tajaddini-Sarmadi, J.; Ling, K.L.E.; Wolff, S.P. Low-density lipoprotein is the major carrier of lipid hydroperoxides in plasma. Relevance to determination of total plasma lipid hydroperoxide concentrations. *Biochem. J.* **1996**, 313, 781–786.

Ohshima, T.; Shozen, K.I.; Ushio, H.; Koizumi, C. Effects of grilling on formation of cholesterol oxides in seafood products rich in polyunsaturated fatty acids. Food Sci. & Technol. *Lebensm. Wiss. U. Technol.* **1996**, 29, 94–99.

Osada, K.; Kodama, T.; Yamada, K.; Sugano, M. Oxidation of cholesterol by heating. *J. Agric. Food Chem.* **1993**, 41, 1198–1202.

Park, S.W.; Addis, P.B. Capillary column gas-liquid chromatographic resolution of oxidized cholesterol derivatives. *Anal. Biochem.* **1985**, 149, 275–283.

Park, S.W.; Addis, P.B. Identification and quantitation estimation of oxidized cholesterol derivatives in heated tallow. *J. Agric. Food Chem.* **1986**, 34, 653–659.

Palladini, G.; Finardi, G.; Bellomo, G. Disruption of actin microfilament organization by cholesterol oxides in 73/73 endothelial cells. *Expt. Cell Res.* **1996**, 223, 72–82.

Paniangvait, P.; King, A.J.; Jones, A.D.; German, B.G. Cholesterol oxides in foods of animal origin. *J. Food Sci.* **1995**, 60, 1159–1174.

Peng, S.K.; Phillips, G.A.; Xia, G.Z.; Morin, R.J. Transport of cholesterol autoxidation products in rabbits lipoproteins. *Atherosclerosis.* **1986**, 64, 1–6.

Pie, J.E.; Spahis, K.; Seillan, C. Cholesterol oxidation in meat products during cooking and frozen storage. *J. Agric. Food Chem.* **1991**, 39, 250–254.

Rose-Sallin, C.; Huggett, A.C.; Bosset, J.O.; Tabacchi, R.; Fay, L.B. Quantification of cholesterol oxidation products in milk powders using [2H7]cholesterol to monitor cholesterol autoxidation. *J. Agric. Food Chem.* **1995**, 43, 935–941.

Sarantinos, J.; O'Dea, K.; Sinclair, A.J. Cholesterol oxides in Australian foods. Indentification and quantification. *Food Australia.* **1993**, 45, 485–491.

Schmarr, H.G.; Gross, H.B.; Shibamoto, T. Analysis of polar cholesterol oxidation products: Evaluation of new method involving transesterification, solid phase extraction and gas chromatography. *J. Agric. Food Chem.* **1996**, 44, 512–517.

Sevanian, A.; Seraglia, R.; Traldi, P.; Rossato, P.; Ursini, F.; Hodis, H. Analysis of plasma cholesterol oxidation products using gas- and high-performance liquid chromatography/mass spectrometry. *Free Rad. Biol. Med.* **1994**, 17, 397–409.

Shozen, K.I.; Ohshima, T.; Ushio, H.; Koizumi, C. Formation of cholesterol oxides in marine fish products induced by grilling. *Fisheries Sci.* **1995**, 61, 817–821.

Shozen, K.I.; Ohshima, T.; Ushio, H.; Takiguchi, A.; Koizumi, C. Effects of antioxidants and packing on cholesterol oxidation in processed anchovy during storage. Food Sci. & Technol. *Lebensm. Wiss. U. Technol.* **1997**, 30, 2–8.

Smith, L.L. Cholesterol autoxidation. New York: Plenum Press, 1981.

Smith, L.L. Cholesterol autoxidation 1981–1986. *Chem. Phys. Lipids.* **1987**, 44, 87–125.

Smith, L.L. Another cholesterol hypothesis: Cholesterol as antioxidant. *Free Rad. Biol. Med.* **1991**, 11, 47–61.

Straprans, I.; Rapp, J.H.; Pan, X.M.; Feingold, K.R. Oxidized lipids in the diet are incorporated by the liver into very low density lipoprotein in rats. *J. Lipid Res.* **1996**, 37, 420–430.

Teng, J.I. Oxysterol separation by HPLC in combination with thin layer chromatography. *Chromatogram.* **1990**, 8–10.

Van Lier, J.E.; Smith, L.L. Sterol metabolism. I. 26-hydroxycholesterol in the human aorta. *Biochemistry* **1967**, 6, 3269–3278.

Wahle, K.W.J.; Hoppe, P.P.; McIntosh, G. Effects of storage and various intrinsic vitamin E concentrations on lipid oxidation in dried egg powders. *J. Sci. Food Agric.* **1993**, 61, 463–469.

Wasilchuk, B.A.; Le Quesne, P.W.; Vouross, P. Monitoring cholesterol autoxidation processes using multideuterated cholesterol. *Anal. Chem.* **1992**, 64, 1077–1098.

Yamamoto, Y.; Brodsky, M.H.; Baker, J.C.; Ames, B.N. Detection and characterization of lipid hydroperoxides at picomole levels by high-performance liquid chromatography. *Anal. Biochem.* **1987**, 160, 7–13.

Yan, P.S.; White, P.J. Cholesterol oxidation in heated lard enriched with two levels of cholesterol. *J. Am. Oil Chem. Soc.* **1990**, 67, 927–931.

Yankah, V.V.; Ohshima, T.; Ushio, H.; Fujii, T.; Koizumi, C. Study of the differences between two salt qualities on microbiology, lipid and water-extractable components of momoni, a Ghanaian fermented fish products. *J. Sci. Food Agric.* **1996**, 71, 33–40.

Zubillaga, M.P.; Maerker, G. Quantification of three cholesterol oxidation products in raw meat and chicken. *J. Food Sci.* **1991**, 56, 1194–1196, 1202.

Zubillaga, M.P.; Maerker, G. Transesterification of cholesteryl esters. *J. Am. Oil Chem. Soc.* **1988**, 65, 780–782.

Zunin, P.; Evangelisti, F.; Caboni, M.F.; Penazzi, G.; Lercker, G.; Tiscornia, E. Cholesterol oxidation in baked foods containing fresh and powdered eggs. *J. Food Sci.* **1995**, 60, 913–916.

Zunin, P.; Evanelisti, F.; Calcagno, C.; Tiscornia, E. Cholesterol oxidation in dried egg pasta: Detecting 7-keto-cholesterol content. *Cereal Chem.* **1996**, 73, 691–694.

7

THE IMPACT OF FOOD PROCESSING ON THE NUTRITIONAL QUALITY OF VITAMINS AND MINERALS

Manju B. Reddy and Mark Love

Department of Food Science and Human Nutrition
Iowa State University, Ames, Iowa 50011

1. ABSTRACT

Processing (including preparation) makes food healthier, safer, tastier and more shelf-stable. While the benefits are numerous, processing can also be detrimental, affecting the nutritional quality of foods. Blanching, for example, results in leaching losses of vitamins and minerals. Also, milling and extrusion can cause the physical removal of minerals during processing. The nutritional quality of minerals in food depends on their quantity as well as their bioavailability. The bioavailability of key minerals such as iron, zinc and calcium is known to be significantly affected by the fiber, phytic acid, and tannin content of foods. Concentrations of these constituents are altered by various processing methods including milling, fermentation, germination (sprouting), extrusion, and thermal processing. Vitamins, especially ascorbic acid, thiamin and folic acid, are highly sensitive to the same processing methods. The time and temperature of processing, product composition and storage are all factors that substantially impact the vitamin status of our foods.

2. INTRODUCTION

The vitamin and mineral content of foods subjected to processing is influenced by several factors. The first determinant factor is the chemical stability of the food vitamin or mineral. In addition, the extent of processing, environmental factors, and the form in which foods are delivered can also impact their stability. This short treatment of the topic cannot cover all of the components associated with these factors. However, there are numerous reviews and monographs that can fill in the missing detail (Harris and Von Loesecke, 1960; Karmas and Harris, 1975; Karmas and Harris, 1988; Muller and Tobin, 1980; Bender, 1978 and Tannenbaum, 1979). A cursory survey of the literature in this area might

Impact of Processing on Food Safety, edited by Jackson et al.,
Kluwer Academic / Plenum Publishers, New York, 1999.

seem to suggest that ascorbic acid and thiamin are the only vitamins studied in this area; but a review by Gregory (1996) contains a broad and detailed information on known chemical changes in vitamins during processing, handling and storage.

Gauging the magnitude of vitamin loss or inter-conversion is rather difficult largely due to the variability of the data base as it has been accumulated historically (Murphy et al., 1973). Other factors mentioned above significantly change the vitamin and mineral content of foods. Among these factors are the inherent variability of vitamins due to the nature of the food as a biological material and the variable distribution within the anatomy of the plant or animal tissue. Depending on how a particular food is processed or the extent to which it is refined, as dictated by cultural preference or desired end use, there can be significant and unavoidable losses of nutrients. The processing of grain into refined fractions results in losses of the vitamins with respect to the whole grain. These degree of loss depends on the location of the nutrients in grain which are removed during cereal refining.

An important factor to consider when conducting or evaluating processing studies is how nutrient losses are calculated. Many published studies report apparent rather than true nutrient losses. Apparent losses are calculations based on nutrient content of moisture-free unprocessed and processed foods (Murphy et al., 1975). True losses of nutrients, defined as calculations based on nutrient content of known weights of food before and after processing. True losses are more accurate calculations since they take into account changes in the moisture and solid content of the food during processing. Murphy et al (1975) underscored the need for studies that measure the true nutrient losses during processing. Recently, there has been an increasing number of studies completed which adhere to these criteria. Whenever possible, only studies employing the true loss analyses will be cited in this review.

3. EFFECT OF PROCESSING ON VITAMINS

The chemical nature and chemical stability are key factors in determining the vitamin content of food. A brief summary of this material can be found in the chapter by Harris (1977) on nutrient stability which includes a tabular summary for the vitamins. More extensive treatment of the chemical changes experienced by nutrients can be found in reviews by Wong (1989) and Gregory (1996) and to a lesser extent in the *Handbook of Vitamins* (Machlin, 1991).

3.1. Fat Soluble Vitamins

The chemical properties of vitamins dictate the mechanism and extent of losses during processing. Fat soluble vitamins are degraded by a distinctly different set of chemical processes than water soluble vitamins. The fat soluble vitamins and vitamin principles (carotenoids and tocotrienes) are destroyed by autocatalytic processes similar to those experienced by unsaturated fatty acids. Potent catalysts of these processes are light, air, transition metal elements (particularly Fe and Cu), and radicals from co-oxidizing olefinic long-chain fatty acids. Many food processes do not have a significant impact on the fat soluble vitamin content unless large volumes of air are introduced into the food. Processes which do not limit contamination by transition metal ions from equipment or water supplies used in processing, and storage conditions which do not block light and limit exposure to air (by packaging under nitrogen) promote significant vitamin losses due to the catalytic effects of these elements.

Certain fat soluble vitamins (particularly, vitamin A and the carotenoids) experience geometric isomerization upon thermal processing with losses of vitamin value (Wong, 1989). All of the fat soluble vitamins are lost to a varying degree during thermal processing with the exception of vitamin K. The moisture content or water activity (aw) of foods during processing and storage further influences the stability of the fat soluble vitamins. Fat soluble vitamins are most stable when water exists as a monolayer in food (D'Arcy and Watt, 1981; Labuza, 1984). Degradation increases at hydration rates below and above this value (Gregory, 1996).

3.2. Water Soluble Vitamins

Chemical and physical factors determining the retention of water soluble vitamins are similar to those for the fat soluble vitamins. While certain water soluble vitamins are susceptible to oxidation (thiamin and cobalamin), the processes are different from those for the fat soluble vitamins. Processing medium or the environment is a critical factor in influencing the stability or retention of water soluble vitamins. Being water-soluble components, any processing operation which increases the exposure of the vitamin to aqueous media will potentially lead to leaching of the vitamin (Adams and Erdman, 1988; Lachance and Fisher, 1988).

Vitamins stable at acidic pHs include ascorbic acid, niacin, free folacin, and thiamin. Biotin, thiamin, free folic acid, pantothenic acid, and ascorbic acid are lost more readily at alkaline pHs. Biotin and pantothenic acid are most stable at pHs near 7.0. Acid or alkaline treatment of cereals is sometimes necessary to release niacin from it protein (niacytin) or carbohydrate (niacyanogen) bound forms. Treatment with lye ($Ca[OH]_2$) or sodium hydroxide is the basis of the nutritional improvement in the vitamin value of corn flour when it is processed into nixtamal or masa flour for tortilla making in Mexico and Central and Latin America.

Other chemical processing agents will contribute to the destruction of some vitamin principles. Biotin is readily oxidized in the presence of H_2O_2. Bisulfite (or SO_2) attacks the methylene bridge of thiamin and accounts for FDA's prohibition against bisulfite or SO_2 use in foods which are significant sources of thiamin (Code of Fed. Reg., Title 21, 1997). The presence of transition elements such as Cu^{+2} and Fe^{+3} in processing water catalyzes the oxidation of ascorbic acid to dehydro-ascorbic acid without loss of vitamin potency and further to diketoglulonic acid with loss of bio-potency.

Physical factors also contribute to the loss of vitamins during processing and storage. Electromagnetic radiation in the visible and near ultra-violet region is one such factor. Riboflavin and pyridoxine are photochemically degraded with attendant loss of vitamin potency. Temperature is another factor. Some vitamins are stable to the effects of thermal processing including niacin (although there is inter-conversion of nicatinamide to nicotinic acid when heated in the presence of acid or alkali), biotin, riboflavin, and vitamin K. Others lost during heating including pantothenic acid, ascorbic acid, thiamin at pHs > 7.0, folate, and cobalamin. Under heating temperatures necessary to produce ready-to-eat cereals, as much as 17 % of the initial cobalamin content is lost and another 17 % is lost after storage for one year. During pasteurization losses are lower: 4 % by high temperature short time (HTST) processing and 10 % by ultra-high temperature (UHT) processing (Burton, 1984). Processing and storage losses of cobalamin under these conditions are accelerated by the presence of ascorbic acid (Wong, 1989) Methods utilized for ground beef preparation had little effect on the amount of cobalamin available for consumption. Cooking crumpled ground beef of two initial fat contents (4.7 and 24.5 %) by pan frying, pan broiling, or microwave heating showed equal retention of cobalamin. Rinsing the cooked meat samples with hot water to lower their fat content had no dramatic effect on losses of cobalamin (Love and Prusa, 1992).

4. EFFECT OF PROCESSING ON MINERALS

Minerals, unlike vitamins, are not destroyed by heat, light, oxidizing agents or pH. However, minerals can either be removed from foods during processing (leaching, physical separation) or can be added from the instruments used to process foods (Ummadi et al., 1995). The bioavailability of minerals is mostly affected by the processes of milling, soaking, cooking, germination, fermentation, and heat processing. All of the above processes influence mineral bioavailability either directly by affecting their solubility or indirectly by destroying the inhibitory effect of phytic acid or tannins. Phytic acid, a phosphorus-containing compound normally present in large amounts in cereals, is suggested to be a major factor in causing impaired absorption of several essential elements such as zinc, iron, magnesium and calcium.

4.1. Milling

Grains generally have a high concentration of minerals in the bran and germ fractions, and their removal by milling leaves behind a pure endosperm with a low mineral content. Conversion of whole wheat to white flour results in 16–86% loss of iron, zinc, copper, magnesium and selenium (Miller, 1996). Although losses of minerals are substantial during milling, mineral bioavailability can improve due to the reduction in the phytic acid/bran content of the grain. Iron absorption from the bread made with white flour was 23% compared to 3% absorption from the same bread made with bran, suggesting that either the fiber or phytic acid in bran was responsible for the reduction in iron absorption (Hallberg et al., 1987). The inhibitory effect of bran was primarily attributed to phytic acid in the later studies. A 10-fold reduction of iron absorption in humans was found even when a small amount of phytate (50 mg) was added to a semi-synthetic meal indicating the inhibiting potency of phytic acid (Reddy et al., 1996). The phosphorus content of phytic acid greatly dictates the amounts of minerals absorbed, especially iron and zinc (Navert et al., 1985; Sandberg, 1991). The rice obtained from various rice mills in Thailand had phytic phosphorus concentrations ranging from 30 to 175 mg. Tuntawiroon et al (1990) found that iron absorption was three-fold higher at the lower range than at the higher range of phytic phosphorus concentrations. Pearling of sorghum also increases iron absorption due to the reduction in polyphenol and phytate content. Latunde-Dada (1991) reported that dehulling soy beans reduced iron absorption since the iron in soy hulls was similar to that of $FeSO_4$, a highly available form (Latunde-Dada, 1991).

4.2. Cooking

Mineral losses occur by means of leaching out into the cooking water and are less when foods are steamed rather than boiled. Zinc and iron losses by conventional cooking of broccoli, spinach, sweet potato and collards varied from 10–27% (Lane et al., 1986) and even a 40% loss of iron was reported from Tanzanian foods due to cooking (Lyimo et al., 1991). Although significant losses occur by cooking, mineral bioavailability generally increases with cooking (Kapandis and Lee, 1995). Cooking might improve mineral bioavailability by increasing solubility due to cell wall disruption, protein denaturation and release of organic acids. For example, iron bioavailability increased by at least 200% when vegetables such as broccoli, kale and cabbage were cooked (Kapandis and Lee, 1995). Hydrochloric acid extractability, an indicator of mineral availability, was greatly enhanced for calcium and zinc by cooking and blanching of spinach and amaranth leaves (Yadav and Sehgal, 1995).

4.3. Soaking, Germination, and Fermentation

The bioavailability of minerals is affected by many complex, often interrelated factors. Mineral availability from cereal grains can be improved by hydrolyzing phytates during processing. Phytate content can be lowered by the activation of the normally occurring phytase, which hydrolyzes phytate phosphorus, thereby increasing mineral availability. Myoinositol hexaphosphates are known to have a stronger inhibitory effect on iron bioavailability than lower inositol phosphates and can easily be hydrolyzed to mono to penta-phosphates by soaking, germination, fermentation or treating with the enzyme, phytase (Brune et al., 1992; Sandberg et al., 1996). Phytate hydrolysis in oats, wheat, barley and rye has been shown to be dependent on time and temperature during fermentation. However, phytate in oats is more resistant to hydrolysis than in other cereals (Sandberg, 1991). Calcium, zinc, iron, manganese and copper availability increased when pearl millet, a staple food of Asia and Africa, was fermented (Mahajan and Chauhan, 1988; Khetarpaul and Chauhan, 1989). Reduction of phytate by germination and fermentation was shown to improve iron availability from soy beans and wheat products (Latunde-Dada, 1991; Sandberg, 1991). Iron absorption was two-fold higher when human subjects were fed a yeast-fermented bread rather than an unfermented flat bread made with the same flour (unpublished results). Sorghum, due to its high content of phytate and tannins, has minerals of poor availability. The high tannin content of cereals was reported to interfere with phytate hydrolysis during fermentation (Svanberg et al., 1993). However, tannin levels can be reduced by soaking and germination, both of which improve iron and zinc availability from sorghum products (Stuart et al., 1987; Indumadavi and Agte, 1992; Agarwal and Chitnis, 1995). Malting and roasting of weaning foods (wheat, barley and green gram) increased iron bioavailability by 16–32% (Gahlawat and Sehgal, 1995). Iron and zinc absorption in humans were greatly improved by reducing phytate levels by soaking and malting breakfast cereal made from oats (Larsson and Sandberg, 1993; Larsson et al., 1996).

Fermentation improves the bioavailability of minerals not only by reducing the phytate content but also by producing lactic acid which improves mineral solubility. Fermentation of milk with *Staphylococcus thermophilus* and *Lactobacillus bulgaricus* increased zinc availability from 6.3% to 12.5%. The increase in zinc solubility was attributed to the fermentation of lactose to lactic acid which either increased zinc solubility or decreased the binding of zinc to casein (Van Dael et al., 1993). Fermentation of soy bean meal by lactic acid bacteria increased zinc availability in rats both by destroying phytate and by producing zinc binding ligands (Moeljopawiro et al., 1988).

4.4. Storage

Very little information is available on the effect of storage on mineral bioavailability. Freezing cooked vegetables for six months had no effect on iron or zinc availability (Lane et al., 1986). Nine to twelve months of storage produced no effect on the bioavailability of iron compounds added to canned milk products as determined in rats by the hemoglobin repletion test (Clemens, 1981). One of the factors limiting the expanding consumption of beans is the development of a textural defect when beans are stored under relative humidities and high temperatures prevalent in tropical countries. The defects (hard to cook and hard shells) are linked to the structure of the seed and are related to the polyphenol, phytate and fiber content. Rat studies have shown that bioavailability of iron increases when beans were irradiated with a ^{60}Co source. The radiation dose, which was shown to decrease the phytate, tannin and insoluble fiber content, was positively correlated with iron bioavailability (Pinn et al., 1993).

4.5. Fortification

Many iron compounds are used to fortify foods. Iron bioavailability depends on the type of iron added and the chemical environment in the food. It is a common practice in food industry to add the most available iron salt at the final processing step, with the hope of maintaining good iron availability without sacrificing product quality. Some iron compounds are not compatible with certain foods because of the associated organoleptic problems. Hurrell (1989) tabulated the relative biological values (RBV) of iron compounds in humans and reported that highly soluble compounds such as $FeSO_4$ have RBVs of 100%, but cause rapid fat oxidation. The less reactive and more compatible compounds unfortunately have low iron bioavailability. For example, the insoluble iron compounds such as ferric pyrophosphate and elemental iron cause a few organoleptic problems but have a RBV of only 40% that of $FeSO_4$. Iron bioavailability from infant cereals can be improved by adding ascorbic acid, a well known enhancer of iron absorption. The effectiveness of ascorbic acid in increasing iron absorption depends on the type of food and the amount of inhibiting factors present in the food. Fifty mg of ascorbic acid increased iron absorption from infant cereals, maize, rice and wheat (Cook et al., 1997). Ascorbic acid was less effective in enhancing iron absorption from quinoa because of its high phytate and polyphenol content.

4.6. Heat Processing

Heat processing can affect bioavailability by changing mineral solubility and by destroying food constituents that either increase or decrease availability. Cooking and baking can destroy ascorbic acid and its effect on iron availability (Hallberg, 1981). *In vitro* studies have shown that Maillard reaction products, produced during browning, bind with zinc. The degree of binding is related to the extent of browning and the nature of the proteins found in the food (Johnson, 1991).

Extrusion processing of cereals can cause an increase in iron content due to contamination from the extruder. The process can also increase mineral bioavailability by reducing the phytate content of food. Extrusion cooking reduced the phytic acid content of cereals from 66–79% to 20–50% of the total inositol phosphates, resulting in increased iron bioavailability (Ummadi et al., 1995). Studies by Hurrell et al. (1991) have shown that heat processing has differing effects on different forms of iron. Iron absorption in humans from chocolate milk powder fortified with ferrous fumarate was two-fold higher than for ferrous sulfate when the ferrous fumarate was added to the milk before it was dried (under vacuum for 3 h at 95°C). When ferrous fumarate was added to the milk after drying, absorption of the iron compound was only 1.2-fold higher than that of ferrous sulfate. In contrast, iron absorption from ferric pyrophosphate was reduced by 72% when it was added to the milk before processing (Hurrell et al., 1991).

5. CONCLUSIONS

All foods that processed are subjected to nutrient losses. However, processing can increase nutrient bioavailability due to inactivation of antinutritive factors. In conclusion, food processing practices can generally be beneficial in terms of increasing mineral availability but sometimes they can impose detrimental effects especially on vitamins. We discussed in this paper the major factors affecting the vitamin and mineral availability, but many other factors such as additives and packaging may also have an impact on the nutritional quality of foods.

REFERENCES

Adams, C.E.; Erdman, J.W. Effects of home food preparation practices on nutrient content of foods, In *Nutritional Evaluation of Food Processing;* Karmas, E., Harris, R., Eds.; Van Nostrand Reinhold: New York, NY, **1988**.

Agrawal, P.; Chitnis, U. Effect of treatments on phytate phosphorus, iron bioavailability, tannins and in vitro protein digestibility of grain sorghum. *J. Food Sci. Technol.* **1995**, *32 (6)*, 453–458.

Bender, A.E. *Food Processing and Nutrition;* Academic Press, London, **1978**.

Brune, M.; Rossander-Hultén, L.; Hallberg, L.; Gleerup, A.; Sandberg, A. Iron absorption from bread in humans: Inhibiting effects of cereal fiber, phytate and inositol phosphates with different numbers of phosphate groups. *J. Nutr.* **1992**, *122*, 442–449.

Burton, H. Reviews of the progress of Dairy Science: The bacteriological, chemical, biochemical, and physical changes that occur in milk at temperatures of 100 to 150°C. *J. Dairy Res.* **1984**, *51*, 341–363.

Clemens, R. A. Effects of storage on the bioavailability and chemistry of iron powders in a heat-processed liquid milk-based product. *J. Food Sci.* **1981**, *47*, 228–230.

Code of Federal Regulations, Title 21; Government Printing Office, Washington, D.C.; 182.3798, **1997**.

Cook, J. D.; Reddy, M. B.; Burri, J.; Juillerat, M. A.; Hurrell, R. F. The influence of different cereal grains on iron absorption from infant cereal foods. *Am. J. Clin. Nutr.* **1997**, *65*, 964–969.

D'Arcy, R.I.; Watt, I.C. Water vapor sorption isotherms on macromolecular substrates. In *Water Activity: Influences on Food Quality;* Rockland, L., Stewart, G., Eds.; Academic Press: New York, NY, **1981**.

Gahlawat, P.; Sehgal, S. In vitro starch and protein digestibility and iron availability in weaning foods as affected by processing methods. *Plant Foods for Human Nutrition.* **1995**, 47, 173–179.

Gregory, J. Vitamins. In *Food chemistry*; Fennema, O.R., Ed.; Marcel Dekker: New York, NY, **1996**.

Hallberg, L.; Rossander, L.; Skanberg, A.B. Phytates and inhibitory effect of bran on iron absorption in man. *Am J Clin Nutr.* **1987**, *45*, 988–996.

Hallberg, L. Bioavailability of dietary iron in man. *Ann Rev. Nutr.* **1981**, *1*, 123–146.

Harris, R.S; Von Loescke, H.W., Eds.; *Nutritional Evaluation of Food Processing;* John Wiley & Sons: New York, NY, **1960**.

Harris, R.S. General discussion on stability of nutrients. In *Nutritional Evaluation of Food Processing;* Harris, R., Karmas, E., Eds.; AVI: Westport, CT, **1975**.

Hurrell, R.F. Food manufacturing processes and their influence on the nutritional quality of foods. In *Nutritional Impact of Processing;* Muller, H.R, Somogyi, J.C., Eds.; Bibl. Nutr. Dieta: Basel, Karger, **1989**.

Hurrell, R.F.; Reddy, M.B.; Dassenko, S.A.; Cook, J.A.; Shepherd, D. Ferrous fumarate fortification of a chocolate drink powder. *Brit. J. Nutr.* **1991**, *65*, 271–283.

Indumadhavi, M.; Agte, V. Effect of fermentation on ionizable iron in cereal-pulse combinations. *Int. J. Food Sci. Tech.* **1992**, *27*, 221–228.

Johnson, P.E. Effect of food processing and preparation on mineral utilization. In *Nutritional & Toxicological Consequences of Food Processing.* Friedman, M., Ed.; Plenum Press: New York, NY, **1991**.

Kapanidis, A.N.; Lee, T. Heating cruciferous vegetables increases in vitro dialyzability of intrinsic and extrinsic iron. *J. Food Sci.* **1995**, *60 (1)*, 128- 141.

Karmas, E.; Harris, R., Eds.; *Nutritional Evaluation of Food Processing;* AVI: Westport, CT, **1975**.

Karmas, E.; Harris, R., Eds.; *Nutritional Evaluation of Food Processing;* Van Nostrand Reinhold: New York, NY, **1988**.

Khetarpaul, N.; Chauhan, B.M. Effect of germination and pure culture fermentation on HCl-extractability of minerals of pearl millet (Pennisetum typhoideum). *Int. J. Food. Sci. and Tech.* **1989**, *24*, 327–331.

Lachance, P.A.; Fisher, M.C. Effects of food preparation procedures in nutrient retention with emphasis on food service practices. In *Nutritional Evaluation of Food Processing;* Karmas, E., Harris, R., Eds.; Van Nostrand Reinhold: New York, NY, **1988**.

Labuza, T.P. *Moisture sorption: practical aspects of isotherm measurement and use*; The American Association of Cereal Chemists: St. Paul, MN, **1984**.

Lane, R.H.; Neggers, Y.B.; Bonner, J.L.; Stitt, K.R. Nutrient quality of selected vegetables prepared by conventional and cook-freeze methods. *J. Food Qual.* **1986**, *9*, 407- 412.

Larsson, M.; Sandberg, A.S. Phytate reduction in oats during malting. In *Bioavailability '93 - Nutritional, Chemical and Processing Implications of Nutrient Availability;* Schlemmer, U., Ed.; Karlsruhe: Bundesforschungsanstalt fur Ernahrung, **1993**.

Larsson, M.; Rossander-Hultén, L.; Sandström, B.; Sandberg, A. Improved zinc and iron absorption from breakfast meals containing malted oats with reduced phytate content. *Brit. J. Nutr.* **1996**, *76*, 677–688.

Latunde-Dada, G.O. Some physical properties of ten soy bean varieties and effects of processing on iron levels and availability. *Food Chem.* **1991**, *42*, 89–98.

Love, J.A.; Prusa, K.J., Nutrient composition and sensory attributes of cooked ground beef: effects of fat content, cooking method, and water rinsing. *J. Am. Diet. Assoc.* **1992**, *92*, 1367–1371.

Lyimo, M.H.; Nyagwegwe, S.; Mnkeni, A.P. Investigations on the effect of traditional food processing, preservation and storage methods on vegetable nutrients: a case study in Tanzania. *Plant Foods for Hum. Nutr.* **1991**, *41*, 53–57.

Machlin, L.J., Ed.; *Handbook of Vitamins;* Marcel Dekker: New York, NY, **1991**.

Mahajan, S.; Chauhan, B.M. Effect of natural fermentation on the extractability of minerals from pearl millet flour. *J. Food Sci.* **1988**, *53 (5)*, 1576–1577.

Miller, D. In *Food Chemistry*; Fennema, O.R., Ed.; Marcel Dekker, Inc: New York, NY, **1996**.

Moeljopawiro, S.; Fields, M.L.; Gordon, D.D. Bioavailability of zinc in fermented soybeans. *J Food Sci.* **1988**, *53*, 1546–1573.

Muller, H.G.; Tobin, G. *Nutrition and food processing;* AVI: Westport, CT, **1980**.

Murphy, E.W.; Criner,; P.E.; Gray, B.C. Comparisons of Methods for calculating retentions of nutrients in cooked foods. *J. Agri. Food Chem.* **1975**, *23* , 1153–1157.

Murphy, E.W.; Watt, B.K.; Rizek, R.L. Tables of food composition: availability, uses, and limitations. *Food Technology.* **1973**, 40–51.

Nävert, B.; Sandström, B.; Cederblad. A. Reduction of the phytate content of bran by leavening in bread and its effect on zinc absorption in man. *Brit. J. Nutr.* **1985**, *53*, 47–53.

Pinn, A.B.O.; Colli, C.; Mancini-Filho, J. Beans (Phaseolus vulgaris L.) irradiation - I-iron bioavailability. In *Bioavailability '93 - Nutritional, Chemical and Processing Implications of Nutrient Availability.* Schlemmer, U., Ed.; Karlsruhe: Bundesforschungsanstalt fur Ernahrung, **1993**.

Reddy, M.B.; Hurrell, R.F.; Juillerat, M.A.; Cook, J.D. The influence of different protein sources on phytate inhibition of nonheme-iron absorption in humans. *Am. J. Clin. Nutr.* **1996**, *63*, 203–207.

Sandberg, A. The effect of food processing on phytate hydrolysis and availability of iron and zinc. In *Nutritional & Toxicological Consequences of Food Processing;* Friedman, M., Ed.; Plenum Press: New York, NY, **1991**.

Sandberg, A.; Rossander, H.; Turk, M. Dietary Aspergillus niger phytase increases iron absorption in humans. *J. Nutr*, **1996**, *126*, 476–480.

Svanberg, U.; Lorri, W.; Sandberg, A. Lactic fermentation of non-tannin and high-tannin cereals: Effects on *in vitro* estimation of iron availability and phytate hydrolysis. *J. Food Sci.* **1993**, *58 (2)*, 408–412.

Stuart, M.A.; Johnson, P.E.; Hamaker, B.; Kirleis, A. Absorption of zinc and iron by rats fed meals containing sorghum food products. *J. Cereal Sci.* **1987**, *6*, 81–90.

Tannenbaum, S.R.. *Nutritional and Safety Aspects of Food Processing*; Marcel Dekker: New York, NY, **1979**.

Tuntawiroon, M.; Sritongkul, N.; Rossander-Hultén, L.; Pleehachinda, R.; Suwanik, R.; Brune, M.; Hallberg, L. Rice and iron absorption in man. *Eur. J Clin. Nutr.* **1990**, *44*, 489–497.

Ummadi, P.; Chenoweth, W.L.; Uebersax, M.A. The influence of extrusion processing on iron dialyzability, phytates and tannins in legumes. *J Food Process and Preserv.* **1995**, *19*, 119–131.

Van Dael, P.; Shen, L.H.; Deelstra, H. Influence of milk processing on the *in vitro* availability of zinc and selenium from milk. In *Bioavailability '93 - Nutritional, Chemical and Processing Implications of Nutrient Availability;* Schlemmer, U., Ed.; Karlsruhe: Bundesforschungsanstalt fur Ernahrung, **1993**.

Wong, D.W.S. *Mechanisms and Theory in Food Chemistry*; Van Nostrand Reinhold: New York, NY, **1989**.

Yadav, S.K.; Sehgal, S. Effect of home processing on ascorbic acid and β-carotene content of spinach (Spinacia oleracia) and amaranth (Amaranthus tricolor) leaves. *Plant Foods for Human Nutrition.* **1995**, *47*, 125–131.

8

IMPACT OF PROCESSING ON FOOD ALLERGENS

Susan L. Hefle

Food Allergy Research and Resource Program, University of Nebraska
Department of Food Science and Technology
351 Food Industry Building, Lincoln, Nebraska 68583-0919

1. ABSTRACT

In general, allergenic foods are resistant to processes commonly used in food manufacturing. Nearly all the causative proteins (allergens) retain their allergenicity after treatment by heat and/or proteolysis. Notable exceptions exist; for example, the allergenicity of many fresh fruits and vegetables is decreased or removed by relatively mild processes such as gentle heating or mashing. The use of proteolytic enzymes to remove allergenicity is successfully used in the production of hypoallergenic infant formulas, but this approach with other allergenic foods has resulted in only limited success. Processing effects can result in decreased or complete removal of allergenic qualities of a food, such as the removal of proteins in oilseed processing, which renders the oils hypoallergenic and safe for consumption by allergic individuals. This discussion will address the different allergenic foods and processes which can affect or decrease their allergenicity.

2. ADVERSE REACTIONS TO FOODS

An adverse food reaction is defined as any untoward reaction following the ingestion of food (Lifshitz, 1988). These reactions generally fall into two categories; food intolerance and food hypersensitivity. Food intolerances are nonimmunologic in nature (Sampson and Cooke, 1990) and are responsible for most adverse food reactions. Food intolerances may be idiosyncratic, due to metabolic disorders, or caused by pharmacological substances such as toxins or drugs present in food. Food additives may cause respiratory and gastrointestinal complaints in some individuals (Lifshitz, 1988). With the exception of sulfite-induced asthma, these complaints are mild and transient, not life-threatening.

Impact of Processing on Food Safety, edited by Jackson et al.,
Kluwer Academic / Plenum Publishers, New York, 1999.

Food allergy (or hypersensitivity), is an adverse reaction to food involving the body's immune system. In contrast to most food intolerance symptoms, the symptoms of a true food-allergic reaction may be severe and life-threatening.

3. FOOD ALLERGY

Food allergies are initiated by the body's production of specific antibodies, known as immunoglobulins, in reaction to food components. The body manufactures antibodies as part of its regular defense system against foreign invaders such as viruses and bacteria. In certain individuals, the immune system is triggered to elicit a specific antibody, called immunoglobulin E (IgE), against various environmental representatives such as pet dander, pollens, insect venoms, or foods. The common immune mechanisms involved cause food-allergic reactions to resemble allergic reactions to honeybee stings or penicillin.

3.1. Allergic Mechanism

In food-allergic individuals, IgE is produced against naturally-occurring food components, primarily protein. After ingestion, the food components are subject to digestion, then make their way through the intestinal barrier and get into the circulatory system. Through the circulatory highway, they are presented by sentinels of the immune system to specialized cells called white blood cells. White blood cells produce IgE in response to the protein intruder. The IgE is released from the white blood cells, and travels in the circulatory system until it comes into contact with certain cells known as mast cells (in the tissues) or basophils (in the blood), which have a unique property in that they fix IgE to their cell surfaces. When the mast cells/basophils become armed with IgE, they are said to be "sensitized". Upon additional exposure, the responsible food protein, or "allergen", again is put through the digestive paces, then circulates in the blood, coming in contact with sensitized mast cells or basophils. The fixed IgE recognizes the food allergen specifically, and the allergen becomes bound to it - this contact causes a complex chain of events to occur in the sensitized mast cells or basophils, leading to release of granules containing certain substances that are responsible for the symptoms of the allergic reaction. The substances released from the cells include histamine and serotonin, but many other mediators are also released (Barrett and Metcalfe, 1988). These mediators cause effects such as vasodilation, smooth muscle contraction, and other responses of the body that are associated with food-allergic reactions (discussed below). A very small amount of allergen can be responsible for the release of large amounts of these cell mediators.

Food allergy can only develop if the allergen crosses the gastrointestinal barrier partially intact. The symptoms of a food-allergic reaction depend on the transport of allergens across the barrier. Local allergic reactions can occur, or if the allergen reaches the systemic circulation in an intact form, it can give rise to systemic responses. Penetration of the gastrointestinal mucosa depends on size and structure of the food allergen, changes in the allergen occurring as a result of digestion, gut permeability, and interaction with other factors (i.e. IgA or protein-binding fiber components) located in the gut.

3.2. Symptoms of a Food-Allergic Reaction

Symptoms of food-allergic reactions are dependent on which part of the body the mediators are released. Table 1 lists symptoms associated with true food allergy. The most

Table 1. Symptoms of food allergy

Gastrointestinal	Respiratory	Cutaneous
Abdominal cramps	Asthma	Angioedema
Diarrhea	Laryngeal edema	Atopic dermatitis
Nausea	Rhinitis	Urticaria
Vomiting	Wheezing	

common manifestations of food-allergic reactions are gastrointestinal, cutaneous, and respiratory (Sampson and Cooke, 1990), and they represent contact of allergen with populations of sensitized mast cells present in the affected tissues. Gastrointestinal symptoms are common, especially in infants and young children. These include nausea and vomiting, cramping, and diarrhea (Barrett and Metcalfe, 1988). Cutaneous reactions to food allergens in sensitive individuals can include itching and edema of the lips, tongue, gums, oral mucosa, and pharynx. Urticaria (hives) is the most common skin manifestation, and can be of a general or localized nature. Atopic dermatitis, a chronic inflammatory skin disease, is characterized by dry, easily irritated, intensely pruritic skin. True food allergy may contribute to the pathogenesis of atopic dermatitis (Sampson and McCaskill, 1985; Burks et al.,1988). Respiratory symptoms can be divided into two categories: upper airway distress, which in food-allergic reactions are usually caused by laryngeal edema, and middle airway distress, produced as a consequence of bronchoconstriction (Collin-Williams and Levy, 1984). Respiratory symptoms are somewhat rare with food allergies, but asthma has been associated with allergies to cow's milk, soybeans, and peanuts (Minford et al., 1982; Chiaramonte and Rao, 1988). Food-allergic reactions are very individualistic and diverse (Collin-Williams and Levy, 1984); for example, while some individuals may initially experience immediate reactions in their mouth, others do not experience symptoms until the offending food has moved farther down the gastrointestinal tract.

Anaphylactic shock is a rare, acute, and severe food-allergic response which can be life-threatening. Anaphylactic shock is a generalized form of shock reaction triggered by significant mast cell degranulation, usually involving a number of organ systems. In addition to some or many of the other symptoms of food-allergic reactions discussed above, the cardiovascular system can be affected. Anaphylactic reactions may advance rapidly, beginning with mild symptoms, but then can progress to cardiorespiratory arrest and shock over 1–3 hours. For example, an individual experiencing an anaphylactic food-allergic reaction may notice tongue itching and swelling, or palatal itching at first, then throat tightening, perhaps followed by wheezing and cyanosis. Chest pain and urticaria may be noted, and the individual may have gastrointestinal symptoms such as abdominal pain, vomiting, or diarrhea. A progression of symptoms can lead to potentially life-threatening hypotension and shock.

3.3. Incidence and Natural History

The incidence of true food allergy is less than the general population perceives. While studies have shown that at least one in four adults with allergies believe that they have experienced adverse reactions following ingestion or handling of foods (Sampson and Metcalfe, 1992), it is estimated that 2–3 percent (Bock, 1987; Sampson and Cooke, 1990) of the pediatric population and 1–2 percent of the adult population are afflicted (Sampson and Cooke, 1990). The true prevalence is unknown, however, and other estimates range from 0.3 to 10 percent of the population on the whole (Taylor, 1980;

Johnstone, 1981; Taylor, 1985; Barrett and Metcalfe, 1988; Schreiber and Walker, 1989). Food allergy also is influenced by cultural eating habits. For example, allergies to fish are more common in Japan and Scandanavia than elsewhere because consumption of fish is higher in those countries (Aas, 1966).

Frequency of food allergy is highest in infancy, and decreases with increasing age (Collin-Williams and Levy, 1984). It is most prevalent between 1.5 - 3 years of age (Kjellman, 1991). Avoiding the offending food can result in loss of sensitivity, as investigations have shown that one-third of children and adults lose their clinical reactivity after 1–2 years of allergen avoidance (Sampson and Scanlon, 1989). While cow's milk and egg allergies tend to be outgrown, allergies to nuts, legumes, fish and shellfish tend to persist (Bock, 1982; Collin-Williams and Levy, 1984).

3.4. Allergenic Foods

3.4.1. Commonly-Allergenic Foods. The most common allergenic foods are listed in Table 2. The substances which elicit allergic reactions are usually proteins (Aas, 1978). While adults tend to be allergic to shellfish, legumes (especially peanuts), crustacea, tree nuts, and wheat (Bock and Atkins, 1990; Sampson, 1990a; Sampson and Cooke, 1990), children tend to be allergic to milk and egg more frequently. Any food, however, has the potential to cause an allergic reaction. Very severe reactions are most often seen with peanuts, eggs, fish, and nuts (Collin-Williams and Levy, 1984). Allergic reactions to peanuts are often acute and severe, and life-threatening reactions to peanuts are more common than to other foods, including tree nuts and seafood (Sampson, 1990b).

Other factors may influence prevalence rates. The relatively recent introduction of soybean to the diet in France has resulted in an increase in the incidence of soybean allergy (Moneret-Vautrin, 1986), and soy has become the third most common food allergy in that country. Another example is kiwi fruit, which is not indigenous to the U.S. and became available as a result of importing and distribution in the 1980s. After the introduction of kiwi to the marketplace, literature reports of allergic reactions to kiwi fruit began to appear in the literature (Fine, 1981; Fallier, 1983).

3.4.2. Cross-Reactivity. When a food-allergic individual produces IgE directed against a certain food allergen, and then encounters another food with similar proteins, an allergic response may occur. Structural similarities may exist within families of biologically-related foods. Since dietary elimination of the offending food is the only method of avoiding an allergic reaction, cross-allergenicity can be of concern. The most common food families associated with cross-reactions are fish, legumes, and crustacea (Chiaramonte and Rao, 1988). Certain protein structures are also apparently common to both foods and pollens. Common allergens have been reported in melon, banana, and ragweed pollen (Anderson et al., 1970), celery and mugwort pollen (Pauli et al., 1985), and apple and birch pollen (Lahti et al., 1980). Reports in the literature seem to indicate that the oc-

Table 2. Common allergenic foods

Cow's milk	Soybeans
Eggs	Wheat
Peanuts	Crustacea
Tree nuts	Fish

currence of clinical cross-reactions are infrequent (Bock, 1991). Extensive in vitro "allergenic cross-reactivity" (binding of IgE antibody that is specific for a different food allergen) has been documented, but clinical manifestations are apparently rare, and being allergic to one food does not necessarily rule out a diet including botanically-related foods.

3.4.3. Avoidance of Food Allergens. The only real preventative mechanism for food allergic reactions is to avoid the offending food. Food-allergic individuals must read food ingredient labels diligently, since they usually reveal the presence of the offending ingredient or food. This can be difficult, as particular terms used by food processors can disguise the presence of allergens. "Natural flavorings" could contain soybean and/or milk proteins, and "caramel flavoring" could contain milk proteins. In addition, it can difficult to identify and avoid some types of allergenic foods. An example is deflavored peanuts, which are peanuts that are pressed and deflavored, then reflavored and sold as other types of nuts, such as almonds. Though they smell, taste, and look like tree nuts, these deflavored peanuts have been found to retain their allergenic qualities (Nordlee et al., 1981), and can pose a serious threat to unsuspecting peanut-allergic people.

Food-allergic individuals may also be inadvertently exposed to foods contaminated with allergenic proteins during processing, from carryover due to inadequate cleaning of processing equipment, or in re-work of allergen-containing products in making other products. For example, in one documented case, due to inadequate cleaning of common equipment, sunflower butter became contaminated with peanut butter and elicited an allergic reaction in a peanut-sensitive patient (Yunginger et al., 1983). Also, cases of allergic reactions have occurred due to milk protein contamination of non-milk and "pareve"-labeled foods (Gern et al., 1991; Jones et al.,1992). The amounts needed to trigger a serious reaction in a sensitive individual can be very small; for example, in one case described by Yunginger et al.(1988), a fish-allergic individual died from ingesting french fries that had been fried in oil previously used to fry fish.

3.5. Food Allergens

3.5.1. General Properties of Food Allergens. Food allergens are defined as those substances in foods that initiate and provoke the immunological reactions of food allergy. While almost all allergens are proteins, the vast majority of proteins are not allergens. They are constrained in molecular dimensions, as the food allergens isolated and described to date are all approximately 10–70 kD in size (Aas, 1976; King, 1976; Chiaramonte and Rao, 1988). These values reflect the usual method of allergen characterization, sodium dodecyl sulfate-polyacrylamide electrophoresis, which is run under denaturing conditions. In the native state, some allergens such as the peanut allergens *Ara h* 1 (63.5 kD) and *Ara h* 2 (17 kD)(Burks et al., 1991a; Burks et al., 1992a) exist in native form as proteins of 200 to 300 kD size. In terms of size, the allergen must be of adequate molecular intricacy to interact with the elements of the immune system. However, quite low limits of molecular size exist; for example, small fragments of the codfish allergen, 6500 and 8500 daltons in size, possess pronounced allergenic activity (Elsayad et al., 1972).

3.5.2. Allergen Nomenclature. In response to the rapid progress in recombinant technology and the use of this technique in the study of allergens, an allergen nomenclature system has been adopted (King et al., 1994). Allergens are designated according to the taxonomy of their source. The first three letters of the genus name are used, followed by the first letter of the species name, and then an Arabic number. The numbers are assigned in the order in which the allergens were discovered and isolated. Table 3 gives some examples of food allergens named using this nomenclature system.

3.5.3 Biochemical and Physicochemical Properties of Food Allergens. Most food allergens are glycoproteins possessing acidic isoelectric points. However, this is a general property of most antigens, and thus is not a unique property. All allergens are proteins but most proteins are not allergens. Many allergens contain post-translational modifications such as oligosaccharide addition. Allergens are often the major proteins in the food, with some exceptions. Most allergenic foods contain multiple allergens. For example, egg white is a complex mixture of at least twenty proteins, only 5 - 6 of which are allergenic (Langeland, 1982). The existence of multiple allergens in cow's milk (Goldman et al., 1963; Bleumink and Young, 1968) and peanuts (Barnett et al., 1983) is well-documented. Common food allergens that have been fully or partially purified or characterized include codfish (Elsayad and Aas, 1971), cow's milk (Goldman et al., 1963; Bleumink and young, 1968), eggs (Anet et al., 1985), peanuts (Barnett and Howden, 1986; Burks et al., 1991a; Burks et al., 1992a), soybeans (Shibaski et al., 1980; Herian et al., 1990), and shrimp (Hoffman et al., 1981; Daul et al., 1992) (Table 3).

Most common allergenic food proteins are heat-stable and resistant to proteolytic processes (Astwood et al., 1996). They are resistant to pH extremes; however, for example, fresh fruits and vegetable allergens are susceptible to digestion, cooking, and proteolytic processes (Aas, 1984). Individuals allergic to fresh fruits and vegetables can often tolerate these foods when they are cooked, canned, or frozen (Hannuksela and Lahti, 1977; Eriksson, 1978). Therefore, the allergenicity of a food may be influenced by the way in which the food is prepared, processed, or stored.

Amino acid sequencing has not elucidated a unique or typical pattern for allergens in general. There have been no tertiary structure patterns or biological function patterns (Table 3) elucidated that would shed light on why certain proteins are allergens, while most are not. Food allergens have similarities to many other proteins in the environment, and in some cases, share a great deal of homology with other non-allergenic substances; for example, an IgE-binding section of *Pen a* 1, the major shrimp allergen and a tropomyosin,

Table 3. Identified food allergens

Name	Source	Molecular weight (kD)	Identity
Ara h 1	peanut	63.5	vicilin
Ara h 2	peanut	17	
Ber e 1	brazil nut	12	2S albumin
Bra j 1	oriental mustard	14	2S albumin
Gad c 1	codfish	12	parvalbumin
Gal d 1	egg	28	ovomucoid
Gal d 2	egg	44	ovalbumin
Gal d 3	egg	78	ovotransferrin
Gal d 4	egg	14	lysozyme
Gly m 1	soybean	30	globulin
Met e 1	shrimp	34	tropomyosin
Pen a 1	shrimp	36	tropomyosin
Pen i 1	shrimp	34	tropomyosin
Sin a 1	yellow mustard	14	2S albumin

shares 60–85% homology with tropomyosins from various non-allergenic species (Daul et al., 1994).

4. EFFECT OF PROCESSING ON ALLERGENS

4.1. Thermal Processing

Food allergens are generally resistant to heat (Taylor and Lehrer, 1996), and therefore, would not be affected appreciably by the heat treatment received in food processing. Heat treatment promotes denaturation, loss of tertiary structure, and aggregation of allergens, suggesting that the immune system would respond to the linear amino acid sequence of the allergen instead of conformational structures. However, some exceptions exist. The allergenicity of fresh fruits and vegetables is particularly susceptible to heating (Dreborg and Foucard, 1983; Ortolani et al., 1988). Microwaving destroys the allergenicity of apples (Oei et al., 1995), and Binkley (1994) described an anaphylactic reaction in a tree nut- and tree pollen-allergic subject to raw maple sap, but the finished (cooked) maple syrup could be ingested without problem. Canned tuna or salmon was less allergenic than raw in one study (Bernhisel-Broadbent et al., 1992), although this is not true of all fish. The codfish allergen, *Gad c* 1, is resistant to heat treatment.

Cow's milk retains its allergenicity after intense heat treatment (Baldo, 1984), and also retains allergenicity through the condensation, drying, and evaporation process (Moneret-Vautrin et al., 1992) but isolated cow's milk allergens are susceptible to different degrees to heat (Bahna and Gandi, 1983). Caseins have been reported to retain their allergenicity after heat treatments of 100°C (Kohno et al., 1994), while the allergenicity of the whey proteins can be reduced at 80–90°C for 30 min. (Baldo, 1984); serum albumin and milk immunoglobulins, both minor allergens, are heat-labile, but α-lactalbumin is somewhat resistant to heat (Baldo, 1984). The susceptibility of the whey protein bovine serum albumin and the immunoglobulins to heat has been theorized to be the reason why individuals allergic to beef can tolerate well-cooked beef, but not less-cooked beef (Fiocchi et al., 1995; Werfel et al., 1997). The selective resistance of cow's milk allergens to heat treatment explains the problems in using it as a hypoallergenic process in the infant formula industry.

Ovalbumin and ovomucoid are the major allergens of the egg (Hoffman, 1983). Debate flourishes over the heat resistance of the allergenicity of ovalbumin. In one study, ovalbumin treated for 100°C for 3 min showed a 90% reduction in allergenicity (Honma et al., 1994), but in another report (Elsayed et al., 1986), the allergenicity of ovalbumin was resistant to heating (80°C for 10 min). Ovomucoid retains allergenicity after prolonged heating at 100°C (Gu et al., 1986).

Legume allergens are generally quite heat stable. The allergenicity of the major peanut allergens is stable to heat (100°C) (Barnett and Howden, 1986; Burks et al., 1991b; Burks, et al.1992b), although a few minor peanut allergens are heat-labile (Barnett et al., 1983). Commercially processed peanut products, including peanut butter and various flours, retain their allergenicity (Nordlee et al., 1981). The heat resistance of soybean allergens can be influenced in a variable manner according to the conditions encountered during processing. Shibasaki et al., 1980, in studies of the soybean globuin fractions 11S, 7S, and 2S, found that specific IgE reactivity was decreased in the 11S and 7S fractions to 39–75% of the native globulin when heated to 80°C for 30 minutes, while the allergenicity of the 2S fraction was enhanced. While Burks et al. (1991b) found that the allergenicities of the 11S and 7S fractions were substantially decreased after 80°C for 60 min, and 120°C at 60 min, in later experiments, they found that the allergenicity of the three major soy protein fractions were only minimally affected by heating at 37°C for 60 min, 56°C for 60 min, 100°C for 5 min, 100°C for 20 min, or 100°C for 60 min (Burks et al., 1992b).

Heat can increase the allergenicity of certain foods; for example, in one study, an individual was allergic to roasted pecans, but not raw ones (Malanin et al., 1995). One investigator hypothesized that the allergens in the heated pecan nuts might be products of Maillard-type degradation (Berrens, 1996). Maillard reaction products ("browning") are produced during heating and involve the conjugation of free sugars and amino groups or sidechains. Maillard reaction products have been proposed to be highly allergenic, although human evidence is lacking (Bleumink et al., 1966).

4.2. Chemical Treatment

As discussed previously, most food allergens are resistant to pH extremes; they must survive the harsh acidic environment of the stomach in order to enact their allergenic influences. For example, *Ara* h 1, the major peanut allergen, is stable at pH 2.8 and 11.0 (Burks et al., 1992b), and ovalbumin is stable at pH 3.0 (Honma, 1994). However, fresh fruits and vegetable allergens are acid-labile, and cease to exert their allergenic influence after encountering the stomach environment (Hannuksela and Lahti, 1977).

Various chemical treatments have been explored in trying to reduce the allergenicity of food proteins. Cyanogen bromide was evaluated to try to destroy the allergenic activity of ovomucoid and ovalbumin. Ovomucoid allergenicity was not affected (Kurisaki et al., 1981), while that of ovalbumin was decreased (Elsayed et al., 1986). Treatment of ovalbumin with urea does not affect allergenicity (Honma et al., 1994). The production of soy protein isolates utilizes an acid and alkali extraction of defatted soybean, or an extraction of soy flour with hot aqueous ethanol. Studies have shown that these commercial isolates have diminished IgE-binding capability compared to whole soybean (Pedersen, 1988; Herian et al., 1990), while soy products such as soy flours and soy protein concentrates retain most of their allergenicity (Herian et al.,1990).

4.3. Proteolysis/Hydrolysis

Food allergens are generally resistant to proteolysis or hydrolysis. For example, *Gad c* 1, the major codfish allergen, was found to be quite resistant to proteolysis, as a combination of four proteases was necessary to destroy IgE-binding (Aas and Elsayed, 1969). The nature and cost of this intense treatment is not economically feasible. The allergens of eggs (Elsayed et al., 1986), peanuts (Burks et al., 1992b), and soybeans (Burks et al., 1992b) are resistant to proteolytic processes. In a study by Herian et al. (1993), commercial- and acid-hydrolyzed soy proteins were found to retain their allergenicity, as did fermented soy products such as soy sauce, tempeh, miso, and tofu.

Proteolytic or hydrolytic cleavage of allergens denatures the conformational IgE-binding epitopes that may be present, as well as destroying the sequential IgE-binding epitopes of the protein. While these processes can eliminate IgE-binding activity, they can also result in bitter taste from the presence of small peptides. The infant formula industry has struggled for years with proteolytic processes for cow's milk and soybean proteins to attempt to produce palatable hypoallergenic formulas for the food-allergic infant. Extensive hydrolysis of casein does diminish allergenicity to a large extent (Wahn et al., 1992); one commercial infant formula is based on a casein hydrolysate that contains 70% free amino acids and peptides with chain lengths of 5–8 amino acid residues (Siemensma et al., 1993). While most hypoallergenic infant formulas in the market are based on extensively-hydrolyzed casein, residual allergenicity is occasionally demonstrated by allergic reactions to them in certain milk-sensitive infants (Plebani et al., 1990). Whey protein hydrolysates have also been shown to produce reactions in certain milk-allergic infants (Ellis et al., 1991), except for one preparation in which the hydrolysate was ultrafiltered after hydrolysis (van Beresteijn et al., 1994), thereby removing the immunoreactive peptides.

Other "hypoallergenic" foods have been produced using enzymatic proteolytic processes. "Hypoallergenic" wheat was produced by treating wheat flour with various proteases such as bromelain, actinase, transglutaminase, or collagenase (Watanabe et al., 1994; Tanabe et al., 1996). Similarly, "hypoallergenic" rice was produced by treatment with proteolytic enzymes (Watanabe et al., 1994) or using the enzyme actinase followed by exposure to a reduced pressure for degassing (Watanabe et al., 1990).

4.4. Seed Oil Extraction

Solvent-extracted, highly-refined seed oils pose no threat to allergic individuals, as the protein has been removed. Oral challenge studies in allergic subjects have borne this out (Taylor et al. 1981; Bush et al., 1985). However, cold-pressed oils and other minimally-processed oils pose risks (Hoffman and Collins-Williams, 1994; Brown et al., 1996). For example, in one study, Porras et al. (1985) found soy protein in some samples of European soy oil and margarine.

4.5. Physical Treatment

Physical treatment, can, in some cases, influence allergenicity. A soybean allergen, *Gly m* 1, can be removed by ultracentrifugation (Samoto et al., 1994), although this has limited usefulness, as *Gly m* 1 is not an allergen for most soy-allergic individuals. Ultrafiltration of proteolytic or hydrolytic preparations of cow's milk resulting in peptides of less than 8,000 daltons in molecular weight, can reduce the allergenicity of the preparation substantially (Halken et al., 1993). Homogenization of cow's milk theoretically should expose more allergen on the surface of the micelles, but no increased allergenicity was observed in one study (Host and Samuelsson, 1988).

In another case, differences in the extent of milling influenced allergenicity. Psyllium husk, a much-used ingredient in bulk laxatives, was incorporated into a cereal by the Kellogg Company, because of its ability to lower serum cholesterol levels. After a short time on the market, Kellogg received reports of allergic reactions to Heartwise™ cereal among consumers who were health-care providers with histories of being involved in dispensing bulk laxatives in powder form. The individuals in question had become sensitized to psyllium through the inhalation route, and were now experiencing reactions to psyllium proteins after ingestion. Kellogg's found that more extensive milling of the psyllium would reduce the allergenicity of the preparation used in Heartwise™. The patented milling process removes pieces of the seed coat which contain the allergens (Simmons, 1993). After the more extensive milling procedure was used, no future allergic complaints were reported.

4.6. Combination of Processes

Often, a combination of proteolysis or hydrolysis with other processes such as heat treatment, ultrafiltration, or centrifugation is used to produce a "hypoallergenic" infant formula. Combining processes holds promise, but should be approached with caution; in one study, β-lactoglobulin was selectively removed after digestion with thermolysin under high hydrostatic pressure (100–300 kg.cm2). While the product lacked b-lactoglobulin, it still contained α-lactalbumin, another major cow's milk allergen (Okamoto et al., 1991). Proteolytic digestion of whey followed by heat treatment has proven promising in hypoallergenic infant formula development (Asselin et al., 1989). As discussed above, proteolysis of whey followed by ultrafiltration can produce a hydrolysate devoid of IgE-binding (van Beresteijn et al., 1994). Twin screw extrusion cooking was effective at reducing antigenicity of soybean meal, as it reduced the molecular weights of soy proteins, but no allergenicity studies were done (Ohishi et al., 1994).

5. SUMMARY

Food allergens are proteins that are usually very resistant to heat, digestion, acid, and alkali. Some food allergens have remarkable tenacity, and most food processing treatments do nothing to reduce their allergenicity. Food processing methods are mild in general, do not reduce the IgE-binding capability of allergens appreciably in most cases, and, in fact, may actually increase the allergenicity of some foods, although fresh fruits and vegetables are the exception. As more food allergen identification and information on the responsible protein structures becomes available, perhaps better ways to use processing methods to reduce or remove allergenicity may become apparent and feasible.

REFERENCES

Aas, K. Studies of hypersensitivity to fish. *Int. Arch. Allergy* **1966**, 29, 346–363.

Aas, K. What makes an allergen an allergen. *Allergy* **1978**, 33, 3–14.

Aas, K. Antigens in food. *Nutr. Rev.* **1984**, 42, 85–91.

Aas, K.; Elsayed, S. M.; Characterization of a major alleren (cod): Effect of enzymic hydrolysis on the allergenic activity. *J. Allergy* **1969**, 44, 333–343.

Anderson, L. B. Jr.; Dreyfuss, E. M.; Logan, J.; Johnston, D. E.; Glaser, J.. Melon and banana sensitivity coincident with ragweed pollenosis. *J. Allergy* **1970**, 45, 310–319.

Anet, J.; Back, J. F.; Baker, R. S.; Barnett, D.; Burley, R. W.; Howden, M. E. H. Allergens in the white and yolk of hen's egg. A study of the IgE binding by egg proteins. *Int. Arch. Allergy App. Immunol.* **1985**, 77, 364–371.

Asselin, J.; Hebert, J.; Amiot, J. Effects of *in vitro* proteolysis on the allergenicity of major whey proteins. *J. Food Science* **1989**, 54, 1037–1039.

Astwood, J.D.; Leach, J. N.; Fuchs, R. L. Stability of food allergens to digestion in vitro. *Nature Biotech.* **1996**, 14, 1269–1273.

Bahna, S. L.; M. D. Gandhi, M.D. Milk hypersensitivity. I. Pathogenesis and symptomatology. *Ann. Allergy* **1983**, 50, 218–223.

Baldo, B.A. Milk allergies. *Aust. J. Dairy Technol.* **1984**, 39, 120–128

Barnett, D.; M. E. H. Howden, M. E. H. Partial characterization of an allergenic glycoprotein from peanut (Arachis hypogaea L.). *Biochim. Biophys. Acta* **1986**, 882, 97–105.

Barnett, D.; Baldo, B. A.; Howden, M. E. H. Multiplicity of allergens in peanuts. *J. Allergy Clin. Immunol.* **1983**, 72, 61–68.

Barrett, K. E.; Metcalfe, D. D. Immunologic mechanisms in food allergy. In *Food Allergy*, ed. Chiaramonte, L. T.; Schneider, A. T.; Lifshitz, F. 1988, 23–43, Marcell Dekker, New York.

Bernhisel-Broadbent, J; Strause, D; Sampson, H.A. fish hypersensitivity. II: clinical relevance of altered fish allergenicity caused by various preparation methods. *J. Allergy Clin. Immunol.* **1992**, 90, 622–629.

Berrens, L.; Neoallergens in heated pecan nut: products of Maillard-type degradation? *Allergy* **1996**, 51, 277–278.

Binkley, K.E. Making maple syrup: hazardous avocational ingestion of raw sap in a patient with tree nut and tree pollen sensitivity. *J. Allergy Clin. Immunol.* **1994**, 94, 267–268.

Bleumink, E.; Berrens, L. Synthetic approaches to the biological activity of b-lactoglobulin in human allergy to cow's milk. *Nature* **1966**, 212, 541–543.

Bleumink, E.; Young, E. Identification of the atopic allergen in cow's milk. *Int. Arch. Allergy* **1968**, 34, 521–543.

Bock, S. A. Natural history of food sensitivity. *J. Allergy Clin. Immunol.* **1982**, 69, 173–177.

Bock, S. A. Prospective appraisal of complaints of adverse reaction to foods in children during the first three years of life. *Pediatrics* **1987**, 79, 683–688.

Bock, S. A. Oral challenge procedures. In *Food Allergy*; Metcalfe, D.D., Sampson, H.A., Simon, R. A., Ed.; Blackwell Scientific Publishers: Cambridge, England, 1991; pp. 81–95.

Bock, S. A.; Atkins, F. M. Patterns of food hypersensitivity during sixteen years of double-blind, placebo-controlled food challenges. *J. Pediatrics* **1990**, 117, 561–567.

Burks, A. W.; Mallory, S. A.; Williams, L. W.; Shirrell, M. A. Atopic dermatitis: Clinical relevance of food hypersensitivity reactions. *J. Pediatrics* **1988**, 113, 447–451.

Burks, A. W.; Williams, L. W.; Helm, R. M.; Connaughton, C.; Cockrell, G.; O'Brien, T. Identification of a major peanut allergen, *Ara h* 1, in patients with atopic dermatitis and positive peanut challenges. *J. Allergy Clin. Immunol.* **1991a**, 88, 172–179.

Burks, A. W.; Williams, L. W.; Helm, R. M.; Thresher, W.; Brooks, J. R.; Sampson, H. A.; Identification of soy protein allergens in patients with atopic dermatitis and positive soy challenges: determination of change in allergenicity after heating or enzyme digestion. In *Nutritional and Toxicological Consequences of Food Processing*; Friedman, M., Ed.; Plenum Press: New York, NY, 1991b, pp. 295–307.

Burks, A. W.; Williams, L. W.; Connaughton, C.; Cockrell, G.; O'Brien, T. J.; Helm, R. M. Identification and characterization of a second major peanut allergen, *Ara h* II, with use of the sera of patients with atopic dermatitis and positive peanut challenge. *J. Allergy Clin. Immunol.* **1992a**, 900, 962–969.

Burks, A.W.; Williams, L.W.; Thresher, W.; Connaughton, C.; Cockrell, G.; Helm, R.M. Allergenicity of peanut and soybean extracts altered by chemical or thermal denaturation in patients with atopic dermatitis and positive food challenges. *J. Allergy Clin. Immunol.* **1992b**, 90, 889–897.

Bush R. K.; Taylor S. L.; Nordlee, J. A.; Busse, W. W. Soybean oil is not allergenic to soybean-sensitive individuals. *J. Allergy Clin. Immunol.* **1985**, 76, 242–245.

Chiaramonte, L. T.; Rao, Y.A. Common food allergens. In *Food Allergy*; Chiaramonte, L. T., Schneider, T. A., Lifshitz, F., Ed.; Marcel Dekker: New York, NY, 1988, pp. 89–106.

Collin-Williams, C.; Levy, L. D. Allergy to food other than milk. In *Food Intolerance*, Chandra, R. K., Ed.; Elsevier, New York, NY, 1984, pp. 137–186.

Daul C. B.; Slattery, M.; Morgan, J. E.; Lehrer, S. B. Identification of a common major crustacea allergen. *J. Allergy Clin. Immunol.* **1992**, 89, 194(abstract).

Daul, C. B.; Slattery, M.; Reese, G.; Lehrer, S.B. Identification of the major brown shrimp (*Penaeus aztecus*) allergen (*Pen a* 1) as the muscle protein tropomyosin. *Int. Arch. Allergy Appl. Immunol.* **1994**, 105, 49–52.

Dreborg, S.; Foucard, T.; Allergy to apple, carrot, and potato in children with birch pollen allergy. *Allergy* **1983**, 38, 167–172.

Ellis, M. H.; Short, J. A.; Heiner, D. C.; Anaphylaxis after ingestion of a recently introduced hydrolyzed whey protein formula. *J. Pediatrics* **1991**, 118, 74–77.

Elsayad, S.; Aas, K. Characterization of a major allergen (cod): observations on effect of denaturation on the allergenic activity. *J. Allergy* **1971**, 47, 283–291.

Elsayad, S.; Aas, K.; Sletten, K.; Johansson, S. G. O. Tryptic cleavage of a homogenous cod fish allergen and isolation of two active polypeptide fragments. *Immunochemistry* **1972**, 9, 647–661.

Elsayed, S.; Hammer, A. S. E.; Kalvenes, M. B.; Flovagg, E.; Apold, J.; Vik, H.; Antigenic and allergenic determinants of ovalbumin. I. Peptide mapping, cleavage at the methionyl peptide bonds and enzymic hydrolysis of native and carboxymethyl OA. *Int. Arch Allergy. Appl. Immunol.* **1986**, 79, 101–107.

Eriksson, N. E. Food sensitivity reported by patients with asthma and hay fever. *Allergy* **1978**, 33, 189–196.

Fallier, C. J. Anaphylaxis to kiwi fruit and related "exotic" items. *J. Asthma* **1983**, 20, 193–196.

Fine, A. J. Hypersensitivity reaction to kiwi fruit (Chinese gooseberry, Actinidia chinensis). *J. Allergy Clin. Immunol.* **1981**, 68, 235.

Fiocchi, A.; Restani, P.; Riva, E.; Restelli, A. R.; Biasucci, G.; Galli, C. L.; Giovanni, M.; Meat allergy: II - Effects of food processing and enzymatic digestion on the allergenicity of bovine and ovine meats. *J. Am. College Nutrition* **1995**, 14, 245–250.

Gern, J.E.; Yang, E.; Evrard, H. M.; Sampson H. A.. Allergic reaction to milk-contaminated "nondairy" products. *N. Eng. J. Med.* **1991,** 324, 976–979.

Goldman, A. S.; Anderson, D. W.; Sellers, W. A.; Saperstein, S.; Kniker, W. T.; Halpern, S. R. Milk allergy. I. Oral challenge with milk and isolated milk proteins in allergic children. *Pediatrics* **1963**, 32, 425–443.

Gu, J.; Matsuda, T.; Nakamura, R.; Antigenicity of ovomucoid remaining in boiled shelled eggs. *J. Food Science* **1986**, 51, 1448–1450.

Halken, S.; Host, A.; Hansen, L. G.; Osterballe, O.; Safeety of a new, ultrafiltrated whey hydrolysate formula in children with cow milk allergy: a clinical investigation. *Pediatric Allergy Immunol.* **1993**, 4, 53–59.

Hannuksela, M.; Lahti, A. Immediate reaction to fruits and vegetables. *Contact Derm.* **1977**, 3, 79–84.

Herian, A.; Taylor, S. L.; Bush, R. K. Identification of soybean allergens by immunoblotting with sera from soy-allergic adults. *Int. Arch. Allergy Appl. Immunol.* **1990**, 92, 192–198.

Herian, A. M.; Taylor, S. L.; Bush, R. K. Allergenic reactivity of various soybean products as determined by RAST inhibition. *J. Food Science* **1993**, 58, 385–388.

Hoffman, D. Immunochemical identification of allergens in egg white. *J. Allergy Clin. Immunol.* **1983**, 71, 481–486.

Hoffman, D. R.; Day, E. D.; Miller, J. S. The major heat stable allergen of shrimp. *Ann. Allergy* **1981**, 47, 17–22.

Hoffman, D. R.; Collins-Williams, C.; Cold-pressed peanut oils may contain peanut allergen. *J. Allergy Clin. Immunol.* **1994**, 93, 801–802.

Honma, K.; Kohno, Y.; Saito, K.; Shimojo, N.; Tsunoo, H.; Niimi, H. Specificities of IgE, IgG and IgA antibodies to ovalbumin. *Int. Arch. Allergy Immunol.* **1994,** 103, 28–35.

Host, A.; Samuelsson, E. G. Allergic reactions to raw, pasteurized, and homogenized/pasteurized cow milk: a comparison. *Allergy* **1988**, 43, 113–118.

Jones, R. T.; Squillace, D. L., Yunginger, J. W. Anaphylaxis in a milk-allergic child after ingestion of milk-contaminated kosher-pareve-labeled "dairy-free" dessert. *Ann. Allergy* **1992**, 68, 223–227.

King, T. P. Chemical and biological properties of some atopic allergens. *Adv. Immunol.* **1976**, 23, 77–105.

King, T. P.; Hoffman, D.; Lowenstein, H.; Marsh, D.G.; Platts-Mills, T.A.; Thomas, W. Allergen nomenclature. *Int. Arch. Allergy Immunol.* **1994**, 10, 224–227.

Kjellman, N. M. Natural history and prevention of food hypersensitivity. In *Food Allergy*; Metcalfe, D. D., Sampson, H. A., Simon, R. A., Ed.; Blackwell Scientific Publishers: Cambridge England, 1991, pp. 319–331.

Kohno, Y.; Honma, K.; Saito, K.; Shimojo, N.; Tsunoo, H.; Kaminogawa, S.; Niimi, H.; Preferential recognition of primary protein structures of a-casein by IgG and IgE antibodies of patients with milk allergy. *Annals Allergy* **1994**, 73, 419–422.

Kurisaki, J.; Konishi, Y.; Kaminogawa, S.; Yamauchi, K.; Studies on the allergenic structure of hen ovomucoid by chemical and enzymic fragmentation. *Agr. Biol. Chem.* **1981**, 45, 879–886.

Lahti, A.; Bjorksten, F.; Hannuksela, M. Allergy to birch pollen and apple, and cross-reactivity of the allergens studies with the RAST. *Allergy* **1980**, 35, 297–300.

Langeland, T. A clinical and immunological study of allergy to hen's egg white. III. Allergens in hen's egg white studied by crossed radioelectrophoresis (CRIE). *Allergy* **1982**, 37, 521–530.

Lifshitz, F. Food intolerance. In *Food Allergy*, Chiaramonte, L. T., Schneider, A. T., Lifshitz, F., Ed.; Marcel Dekker: New York, NY, 1988, pp. 3–21.

Malanin, K.; Lundberg, M.; Johansson, S. G. O. Anaphylactic reaction caused by neoallergens in heated pecan nut. *Allergy* **1995**, 50, 988–991.

Minford, A. M. B.; MacDonald, A.; Littlewood, J. M. Food intolerance and food allergy in children: a review of 68 cases. *Arch. Dis.Child.* **1982**, 57, 742–747.

Moneret-Vautrin, D. A. Food antigens and additives. *J. Allergy Clin. Immunol.* **1986**, 78, 1039–1045.

Moneret-Vautrin, A.; Humbert, G.; Alais, C.; Grilliat, J. P. Donnees recentes sur les proprietes immunoallergologiques des proteins laitieres. *Le Lait* **1992**, 62, 396–399.

Nordlee, J. A.; Taylor, S. L.; Jones, R. T.; Yunginger, J. W. Allergenicity of various peanut products as determined by RAST inhibition. *J. Allergy Clin. Immunol.* **1981**, 81, 376–382.

Oei, H. D.; Tjiook, S. B.; de Haas, R.; Does the allergenicity of apple disappear after microwave treatment? *J. Allergy Clin. Immunol.* **1995**, 95, 329 (abstract).

Ohishi, A; Watanabe, k.; Urushibata, M.; Utsuno, K.; Ikuta, K.; Sugimoto, K.; Harada, H. Detection of soybean antigenicity and reduction by twin-screw extrusion. *J. Assoc. Official Analy. Chem.* **1994**, 71, 1391–1396.

Okamoto, M.; Hayashi, R.; Enomoto, A.; Kaminogawa, S.; Yamauchi, K. High-pressure proteolytic digestion of food proteins: selective elimination of b-lactoglobulin in bovine milk whey concentrate. *Agric. Biol. Chem.* **1991**, 55, 1253–1257.

Ortolani, C.; Ispano, M.; Pastorello, E.; Bigi, A.; Ansaloni, R. The oral allergy syndrome. *Ann. Allergy* **1988**, 67, 47–52.

Pauli, G.; Bessot, J. C.; Dietemann-Molard, A.; Braun, P. A.; Thierry, R. Celery sensitivity: clinical and immunological correlations with pollen allergy. *Clin. Allergy* **1985**, 15, 273–279.

Pedersen H. E.; Allergenicity of soy proteins. In *Vegetable Protein Utilization in Human Foods and Animal Feedstuffs*; Applewhite, T, H, Ed.; American Oil Chemists Society: Champaign, IL, 1988, p. 204–212.

Plebani, A.; Albertini, A.; Scotta, S.; Ugazio, A.G.; IgE antibodies to hydrolysates of cow milk proteins in children with cow milk allergy. *Annals Allergy* **1990**, 64, 279–280.

Porras, O.; Carlsson, B.; Fallstrom, S. P.; Hanson, L. A. Detection of soy protein in soy lecithin, margarine, and, occasionally, soy oil. *Int. Arch. Allergy Appl. Immunol.* **1985**, 78, 30–32.

Samoto, M.; Akasaka, T.; Mori, H.; Manabe, M.; Ookura, T.; Kawamura, Y. Simple and efficient procedure for removing the 34kDa allergenic soybean protein *Gly m* 1, from defatted soy milk. *Bioscience Biotech. Biochem.* **1994**, 58, 2123–2125.

Sampson, H. A. Food allergy. *Curr. Opinion Immunol.* **1990a**, 2, 542–547.

Sampson, H. A. Peanut anaphylaxis. *J. Allergy Clin. Immunol.* **1990b**, 86, 1–3.

Sampson, H. A.; Cooke, S.K. Food allergy and the potential allergenicity-antigenicity of microparticulated egg and cow's milk proteins. *J. Am. Coll. Nutr.* **1990**, 9, 410–417.

Sampson, H. A.; McCaskill, C. C. Food hypersensitivity and atopic dermatitis: evaluation of 113 patients. *J. Pediatrics* **1985**, 1071, 669–675.

Sampson, H. A.; Metcalfe, D. D. Food allergies. *J. Am. Med. Assoc.* **1992**, 268, 2840–2844.

Sampson, H. A.; Scanlon, S. M. Natural history of food hypersensitivity in children with atopic dermatitis. *J. Pediatrics* **1989**, 115, 23–27.

Schreiber, R. A.; Walker, W. A. Food allergy: facts and fiction. *Mayo Clinic Proc.* **1989**, 64, 1381–1391.

Shibaski, M.; Suzuki, S.; Nemob, H.; Kurome, T. Allergenicity of major component protein of soybean. *Int. Arch. Allergy Appl. Immunol.* **1980**, 61, 441–448.

Siemensma, A. D.; Weijer, W. J.; Bak, H. J. The importance of peptide lengths in hypoallergenic infant formulas. *Trends Food Science Tech.* **1993**, 4, 16–21.

Simmons, C. T. Method of decreasing the allergenicity of psyllium seed husk. United States Patent Number 5, 273,764, 1993.

Tanabe, S.; Arai, S.; Watanabe, M.. Modification of wheat flour with bromelain and baking hypoallergenic bread with added ingredients. *Bioscience Biotech. Biochem.* **1996**, 60, 1269–1272.

Taylor, S. L. Food allergy. *J. Food Prot.* **1980**, 43, 300–306.

Taylor, S. Food allergies. *Food Technol.* **1985**, 39, 98–105.

Taylor, S; Lehrer; S.B. Principles and characteristics of food allergens. *Crit. Rev. Food Sci. Nutr.* **1996**, 36(S), S91-S118.

Taylor, S. L.; Busse, W. W.; Sachs, M.I.; Parker, J. L.; Yunginger, J. W.. Peanut oil is not allergenic to peanut-sensitive individuals. *J. Allergy Clin. Immunol.* **1981**,68,372–375.

Teuber, S.D.; Brown, R.L., Haapanen, L. A. D. S. Allergenicity of gourmet nut oils processed by different methods. *J. Allergy Clin. Immunol.* **1997**, 99, 502–507.

Van Beresteijn, E. C. H.; Peeters, R. A.; Kaper, J.; Meijer, R. J. G. M.; Robben, A. J. P. M., Schmidt, D. G.. Molecular mass distribution, immunological properties and nutritive value of whey protein hydrolysates. *J. Food Science* **1994**, 57, 619–625.

Wahn, U.; Wahl, R.; Rugo, E. Comparison of the residual allergenic activity of six difference hydrolyzed protein formulas. *J. Pediatrics* **1992**, 21, 80S-84S.

Watanabe, M.; Miyakawa, J.; Ikezawa, Z.; Suzuki, Y.; Hirao, T.; Yoshizawa, T.; Arai, S. Production of hypoallergenic rice by enzymic decomposition of constituent proteins. *J. Food Science* **1990**, 55, 781–783.

Watanabe, M.; Suzuki, Y.; Ikezawa, Z.; Arai, S. Controlled enzymatic treatment of wheat proteins for production of hypoallergenic flour. *Bioscience Biotech. Biochem.* **1994**, 58, 388–390.

Werfel, S. J.; Cooke, S. K.; Sampson, H. A.; Clinical reactivity to beef in children allergic to cow's milk. *J. Allergy Clin. Immunol.* **1997**, 99, 293–300.

Yunginger, J. W.; Gaurerke, M. B.; Jones, R. T.; Dahlberg, M. E.; Ackerman, S. J. Use of radioimmunoassay to determine the nature, quantity, and source of allergenic contamination of sunflower butter. *J. Food Prot* **1983**, 46, 625–629.

Yunginger, J. W.; Sweeney, K. G.; Sturner, W. Q.; Giannandrea, L. A.; Teigland, J. D.; Bray, M.; Benson, P. A.; York, J. A.; Biedrzycki, L.; Squallace, D. L., Helm, R. M. Fatal food-induced anaphylaxis. *J. Am. Med. Assoc.* **1988**, 260, 1450–1452.

9

POSTHARVEST CHANGES IN GLYCOALKALOID CONTENT OF POTATOES

Mendel Friedman and Gary M. McDonald

Western Regional Research Center
Agricultural Research Service, U.S. Department of Agriculture
800 Buchanan Street, Albany, California 94710

1. ABSTRACT

Potatoes contain antinutritional and potentially toxic compounds including inhibitors of digestive enzymes, hemagglutinins, and glycoalkaloids. Solanum glycoalkaloids are reported to inhibit cholinesterase, disrupt cell membranes, and induce teratogenicity. In this overview, we describe the role of potatoes in the human diet, reported changes in glycoalkaloid content of fresh and processed potatoes during storage, under the influence of light and radiation, following mechanical damage, and as a result of food processing. Also covered are safety aspects and suggested research needs to develop a protocol that can be adopted by the potato producers and processors to minimize post-harvest synthesis of glycoalkaloids in potatoes. Reducing the glycoalkaloid content of potatoes will provide a variety of benefits extending from the farm to processing, shipping, marketing, and consumption of potatoes and potato products. A commercially available ELISA kit is described which permits rapid assay of glycoalkaloid content of parts of the potato plant including leaves, tubers, and peel, as well as processed potato products including french fries, chips, and skins. Understanding the multiple overlapping aspects of glycoalkaloids in the plant and in the diet will permit controlling postharvest glycoalkaloid production for the benefit of the producer and consumer.

2. INTRODUCTION

The main objectives of this overview based largely on our own studies are (a) to review safety aspects of glycoalkaloids, so as to better define the post-harvest fate of the potato glycoalkaloids α-chaconine and α-solanine in tubers and processed products; (b) to provide a data base that will permit a realistic assessment of risks associated with glycoalkaloid consumption; and (c) to recommend procedures for post-harvest handling and sam-

Impact of Processing on Food Safety, edited by Jackson et al.,
Kluwer Academic / Plenum Publishers, New York, 1999.

pling of potatoes to minimize glycoalkaloid formation. Other compositional changes which accompany formation of glycoalkaloids which impact the quality of potatoes and recent efforts to improve analysis of glycoalkaloids will also be mentioned.

2.1. Structures of Glycoalkaloids

For the purpose of this paper, we define the following terms:

glycoalkloids naturally-occurring, nitrogen-containing steroidal glycosides with a carbohydrate side chain attached to the 3-OH position; e.g.α-chaconine and α-solanine from potatoes, α-tomatine and dehydrotomatine from tomatoes, and solamargine and solasonine from eggplants.

glycone the steroidal part of the glycoalkaloid lacking the carbohydrate side chain; e.g. solanidine from α-chaconine and α-solanine; solasodine from solamargine and solasonine; and tomatidine from α-tomatine and dehydrotomatine.

alkaloids glycoalkaloids and aglycones.

Figure 1 illustrates the structures of the common potato, eggplant, and tomato glycoalkaloids; Figures 2 depicts the hydrolysis pathways of the carbohydrate side chains of a potato glycoalkaloids; Figures 3 and 4 show HPLC chromatograms of potato glycoalkaloids and hydrolysis products. Tables 1–2 summarize the distribution of glycoalkaloids in fresh and processed potatoes reported in the literature.

3. POTATOES IN THE HUMAN DIET

3.1. Composition and Nutrition

Potatoes are an excellent source of carbohydrates (starch and free sugars), free amino acids, and good quality proteins (Friedman, 1996a; Rodriguez-Saona and Wrolstad, 1997). They also contain biologically active compounds including inhibitors of digestive enzymes, hemagglutinins, polyphenols, and glycoalkaloids (Friedman, 1992, 1997; Friedman and McDonald, 1997). Human consumption varies by country. For example, the average daily per capita intake in the United States in 1996 was about 142 g, a more than 50% increase from 1952 (Friedman, 1996a; Jones, 1998); in the United Kingdom, 140 g (Hopkins, 1995); and in Sweden, 300 g (Slanina, 1990). The cited amount for the United Kingdom is estimated to contain 14 mg of glycoalkaloids. Although the glycoalkaloid content of most commercial potato varieties is usually below a suggested guideline of 200 mg/kg fresh potatoes (which some investigators consider to be too high), the content can increase significantly during storage, on exposure to light, and as a result of mechanical injury such as peeling or slicing. Potatoes are processed both commercially and in the home (Willard, 1993). After processing, further accumulation of glycoalkaloids is halted as the enzymes necessary for their biosynthesis have been deactivated. However, since glycoalkaloids are largely unaffected by home processing conditions such as baking, boiling, frying, and microwaving, any glycoalkaloids present in the tubers before cooking will still remain afterwards (see below).

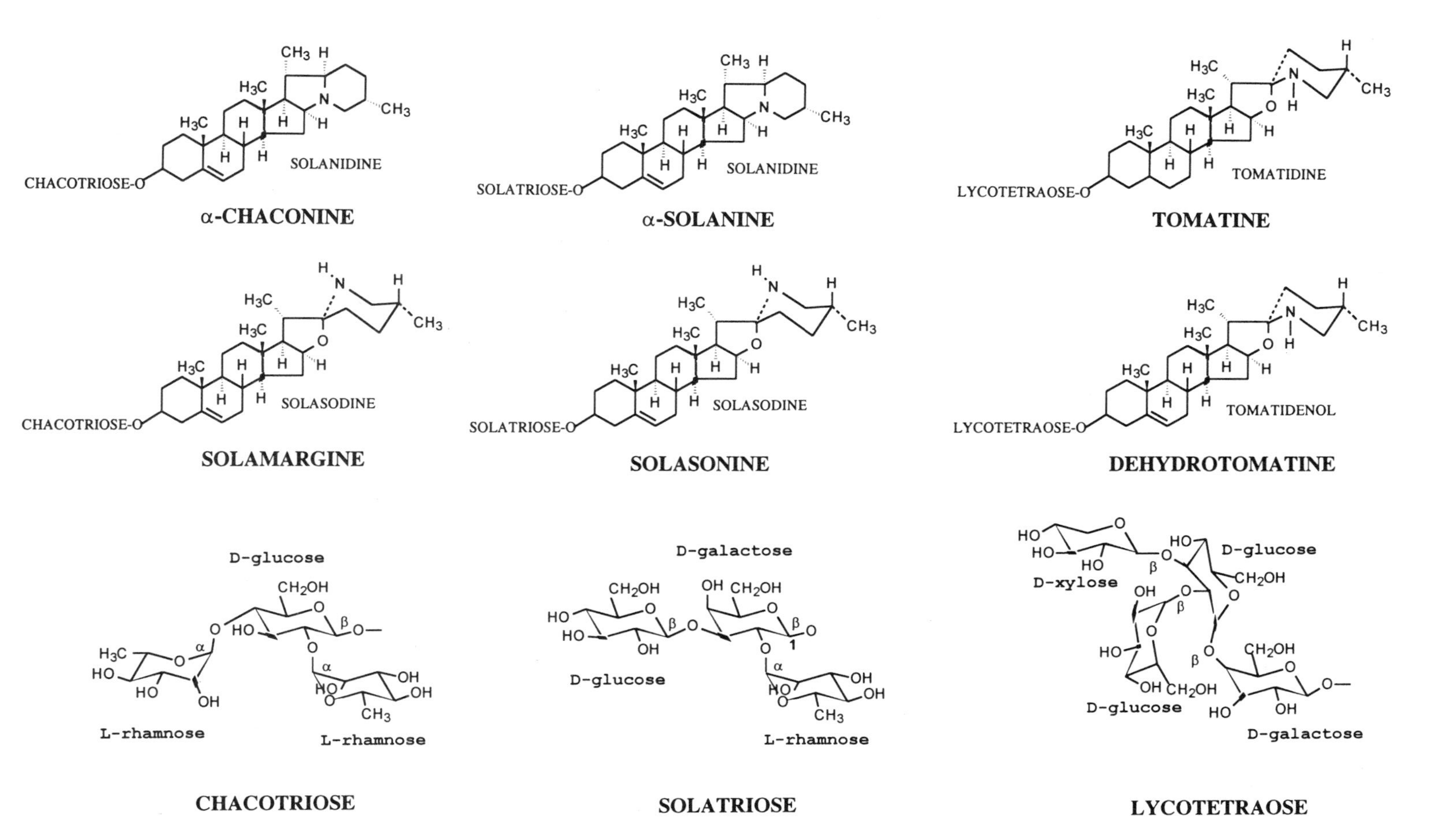

Figure 1. Structures of potato glycoalkaloids α-solanine and α-chaconine, eggplant glycoalkaloids solasonine and solamargine, the tomato glycoalkaloids α-tomatine and dehydrotomatine and the three carbohydrate side chains chacotriose, solatriose, and lycotetraose.

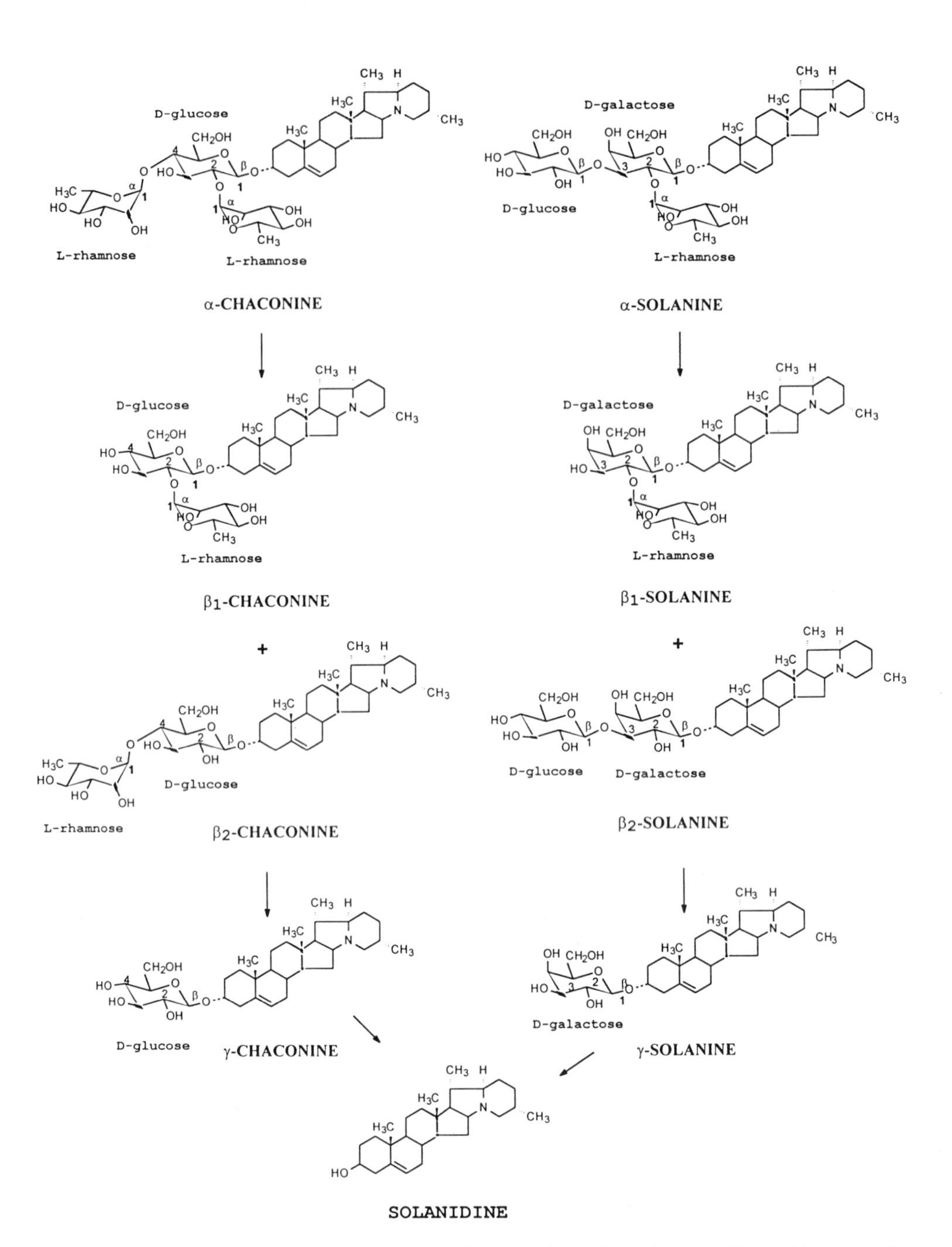

Figure 2. Hydrolysis of the trisaccharide side chains of α-chaconine and α-solanine to diglycosides, monoglycosides, and the aglycone solanidine.

Table 1. Total glycoalkaloid content of parts of the potato plant and tuber

Plant part	Friedman and Dao (1992)	Kozukue et al. (1987)	Coxon (1981)
Roots	860[a]	—	
Stems	320–450[a]	3071	
Leaves	1450[c]	230–1000	
Flowers	—	3000–5000	
Berries	380	—	255–1355
Sprouts	2750–10000[a]	—	
Peel	850[b]	13–400	
Flesh	60100[b]	—	

[a] NDA 17251, a cultivar known to be high in glycoalkaloids.
[b] Lenape, a cultivar known to be high in glycoalkaloids.

Consumers often ask whether the green potatoes are safe to eat. The green color merely suggests that the potatoes exposed to light produced the green pigment chlorophyll. Although the synthesis of chlorophyll and glycoalkaloids may not be related biosynthetic processes (Dao and Friedman, 1994; Griffiths et al., 1994), stress conditions such as light and bruising also induce the formation of glycoalkaloids. Greening is therefore often accompanied by increased concentrations of glycoalkaloids.

3.2. Potato Peel

Potato peel is also a good source of antioxidative compounds. For example, polyphenolic compounds in peel prevented soybean and sunflower oil oxidation *in vitro* (Onyeneho and Hettiaachchy, 1993; Rodriguez de Sotillo et al., 1994). In related studies, Camire et al. (1995) and Zhao et al. (1994) found that potato peel bound more of the carcinogen benzpyrene than did wheat bran, cellulose, or arabinogalactan. Extrusion of the peel at 110°C reduced the affinity of the carcinogen for the peel. This result suggests that heat may inactivate or destroy compounds responsible for binding carcinogens.

Lazarov and Werman (1996) found that consumption of potato peel induced a lowering of cholesterol in rats. They suggested that the fiber component of the peel is responsible for the observed cholesterol-lowering effect. This is unlikely, in view of the fact that

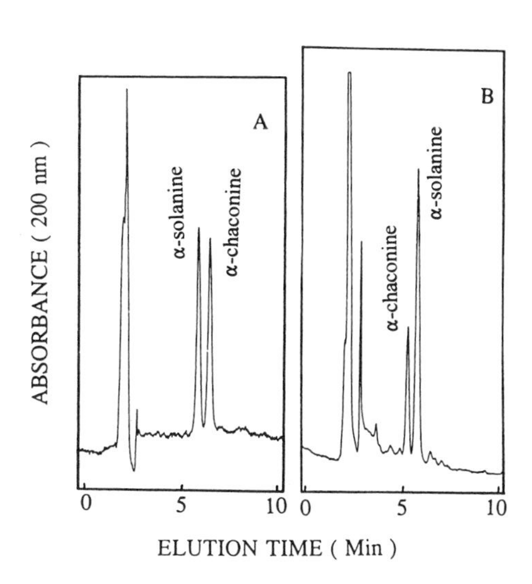

Figure 3. HPLC chromatograms of a mixture of α-chaconine and α-solanine (A) and a potato leaf extract (B). (Adapted from Dao and Friedman, 1996).

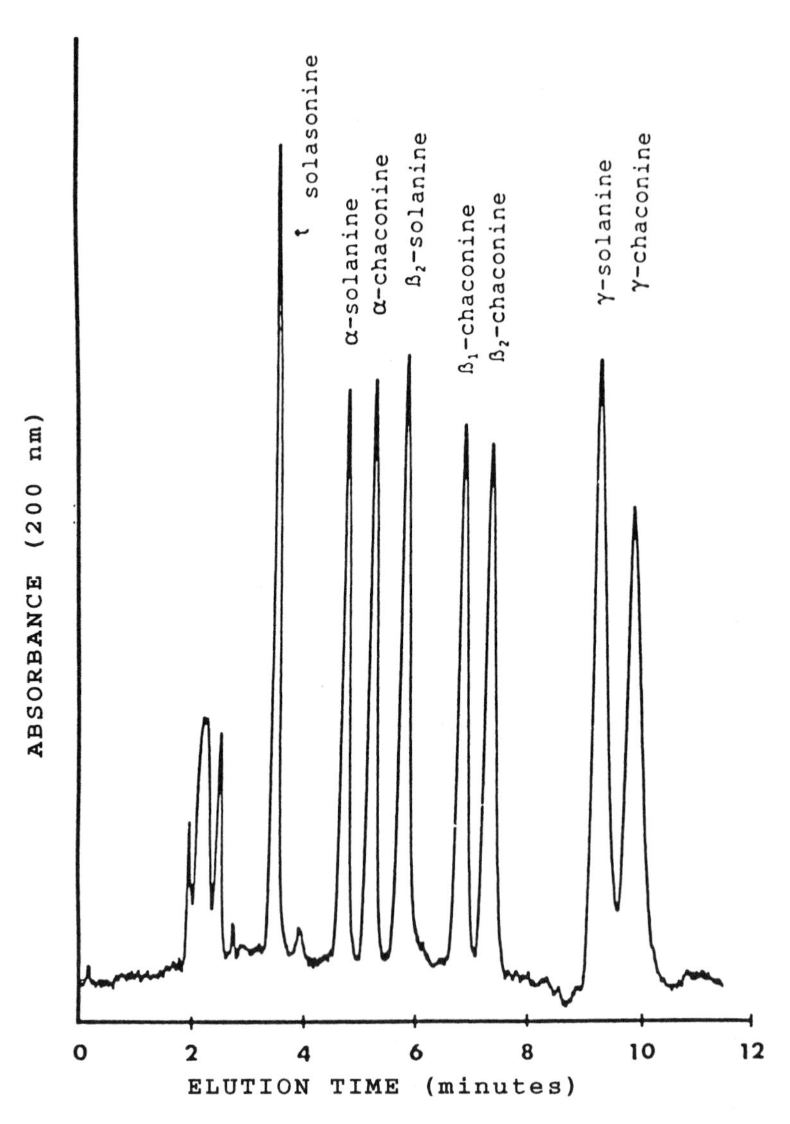

Figure 4. HPLC chromatogram of α-solanine and α-chaconine and their respective hydrolysis products whose structures are depicted in Figure 2. (Adapted from Friedman and Levin, 1992).

insoluble dietary fiber does not induce a reduction in cholesterol (Kritchevsky, 1988) and our finding that of the total dietary fiber of 20 g per 100 g freeze-dried peel in red Lasoda potatoes, more than 80% fiber of this peel is insoluble fiber (unpublished results). Other components of the peel including protein, free amino acids, free organic acids, phenolic compounds, and glycoalkaloids may contribute to the beneficial effect of potato peel on plasma cholesterol. These findings imply that potatoes are an excellent source of nutrients and health-promoting compounds.

The distribution of glycoalkaloids in the peeled part of tubers and in the peel deserves additional comment. Although potato peel is generally reported to contain 80 to 90% of the total amount present in whole tubers (Bushway et al., 1983; Kozukue et al.,

Table 2. Glycoalkaloid content of various potato products

Product	Total glycoalkaloids (mg/kg)	Reference
Commercial french fries, fresh	0.8–8.4	Friedman and Dao (1992)
	19–58	Davies and Blincow (1984)
Partially cooked fries, frozen	23–55	Jones and Fenwick (1981)
Pre-cooked fries, frozen	19–35	Jones and Fenwich (1981)
Commercial wedges, fresh	44	Friedman and Dao (1992)
Commercial skins, baked	31	Friedman and Dao (1992)
	52–63	Bushway et al. (1983)
Commercial skins, fried	55–203	Friedman and Dao (1992)
	120–242	Bushway et al. (1983)
Commercial potato chips	24–109	Friedman and Dao (1992)
	95–720	Sizer et al. (1980)
	32–184	Davies and Blincow (1984)
	59–70	Jones and Fenwick (1981)
Potato pancake powder	45	Friedman and Dao (1992)
Peel wedges, frozen	76–120	Bushway et al. (1983)
Peel slices, frozen	66–71	Bushway et al.(1983)
Canned potatoes	29–99	Davies and Blincow (1984)
	24–34	Jones and Fenwick (1981)

1987; Kubo and Fukuhara, 1996; Table 3), Panovska et al. (1997) found that for seven varieties grown in Czechia, the glycoalkaloid concentration in peeled tubers (flesh) in relation to whole tubers varied between 28 to 59%. Possible reasons for this surprising observation are not immediately apparent. Both this study and a related one by Hellenas et al. (1994) found that unpeeled tubers with a high glycoalkaloid content also had a high content after peeling. This is confirmed by our observations shown in Table 3. The variable partitioning of glycoalkaloids between peel and flesh in different potato cultivars should be taken into consideration when potato peel or flesh are to be used in animal and human nutrition.

3.3. Flavor and Taste

Experiments with human taste panels revealed that potato varieties with glycoalkaloid content exceeding 14 mg/100 g fresh weight tasted bitter (Johns and Keen, 1986; Mondy and Gosselin, 1988; Sinden et al., 1976; Zitnak and Filadelfi, 1985). Those in excess of 22 mg/100 g also induced mild to severe burning sensations in the mouths and throats of panel members. In a related observation, Kaaber (1993) reports that the Norwegian potato variety Kerrs Pink was quite susceptible to greening related glycoalkaloid syn-

Table 3. Glycoalkaloid content of freeze-dried peeled potatoes and of the potato peel determined by HPLC[a]

	Glycoalkaloid levels (mg/kg)		
Cultivar	Peeled tubers (flesh)	Peel	Ratio
Russet Norkota	94	996	1 : 10.5
Red Lasoda	95	965	1 : 10.2
Ranger Russet	170	1694	1 : 10.0
Russet Burbank	290	1570	1 : 5.0

[a] Sum of α-chaconine plus α-solanine determined by HPLC.

thesis and accompanying increases in bitterness and burning sensations, whereas the Bintje variety was not.

Zitnak and Filadelfi-Keszi (1988) describe the isolation of the diglycoside β_2-chaconine, a so-called potato bitterness compound. β_2-Chaconine and other glycoalkaloid hydrolysis products (Figure 2) are readily formed on exposure of the glycoalkaloids in pure form or in potatoes to enzymes and to acid conditions (Filadelfi and Zitnak, 1982; Friedman and McDonald, 1995; Friedman et al., 1993). It is also formed in sprouts during storage of potatoes (unpublished results). As far as we know, the taste of the other hydrolysis products shown in Figure 2 has not been evaluated.

In addition to glycoalkaloids, phenolic compounds also influence the net organoleptic properties of potatoes (Friedman, 1996b). Since potatoes contain both glycoalkaloids and phenolic compounds in various amounts depending on variety, the net effect on taste and flavor could be the result of combined effects of both components.

4. SAFETY ASPECTS

4.1. Symptomology

Here we offer a brief synopsis of the literature on safety-related aspects of glycoalkaloids, which was comprehensively evaluated elsewhere (Friedman and McDonald, 1997). Steroidal glycoalkaloids have been found in potatoes, green tomatoes, and eggplants. Symptoms of glycoalkaloid toxicity experienced by animals and humans include colic pain in the abdomen and stomach, gastroenteritis, diarrhea, vomiting, burning sensation about the lips and mouth, hot skin, fever, rapid pulse, and headache. These symptoms are similar to those experienced by people exposed to human pathogens such as *E. coli*. It is possible that many patients are misdiagnosed about the etiology of these symptoms in the absence of confirmatory evidence of the presence of the pathogens in tissues of affected individuals.

The estimated highest safe level of total glycoalkaloids for human consumption is about 1 mg/kg body weight, a level that may cause gastrointestinal irritation (Slanina, 1990). The acute toxic does is estimated to be about 1.75 mg/kg body weight. A lethal dose may be as low as 3–6 mg/kg body weight (Cieslik, 1997; Morris and Lee, 1984). Glycoalkaloids appear to be less toxic to laboratory animals than to humans. Their toxicity is also significantly lower when administered orally than by injection. Thus, the LD_{50} (mg/kg body weight needed to kill 50% of test animals) for solanine determined by intraperitoneal injection ranges from 20 for rabbits to 34 for mice and 70 for the rats. The value for rats consuming solanine orally was found to be 590 (Azim et al., 1982; Gonmori and Yoshioka, 1994). Surprisingly, the oral LD_{50} dose of the tomato glycoalkaloid tomatine (900–1000 mg/kg body weight) is quite high, i.e. this compound exhibits low toxicity. This maybe because after consumption very little tomatine is actually absorbed from the digestive tract into the blood stream, presumably because tomatine forms a strong insoluble complex with both dietary and endogenous (bile) cholesterol, which is then eliminated in the feces (Friedman et al., 1998).

Also noteworthy is the finding by Phillips et al. (1996) that consumption of potato leaves (2–5 g/kg body weight/day) by laboratory animals (rats, mice, or hamsters) did not result in any significant toxicity. Leaves from different plants are reported to be a good source of good quality protein and other nutrients (Domek et al., 1995; Friedman, 1996a). Potato leaves are reported to be part of the human diet in Bangladesh (Phillips et al., 1996).

In a relevant study, we found that the analysis of glycoalkaloids in potato leaves was less precise when determined by colorimetry than by HPLC (Dao and Friedman, 1996).

The reported toxicity of the glycoalkaloids may be due to such adverse effects as (a) anticholinesterase effects on the central nervous system (Nigg et al., 1996); (b) disruption of cell membranes affecting the digestive system (Blankemeyer et al., 1992, 1995, 1997, 1998; Gee et al., 1996); (c) induction of ornithine dacarboxylase (Caldwell et al., 1991); and (d) reduction in feed consumption in mice and rabbits (Friedman et al., 1996, 1998). Although toxicity does not seem to occur at the genetic level since we found that potato glycoalkaloids produced negative responses in both the Ames mutagenicity and erythrocyte micronucleus chromosomal damage assays (Friedman and Henika, 1992), one manifestation of these adverse effects may be glycoalkaloid-induced teratogenicity. However, since human teratogenicity appears to be a multifactorial event, the question whether potato glycoalkaloids contribute to neural tube defects and related malformations in humans is unresolved (Morris and Lee, 1984; Friedman and McDonald, 1997).

Moreover, since the two major potato glycoalkaloids α-chaconine and α-solanine differ in biological potency, occur in varying ratios in different cultivars, and may act synergistically, care should be exercised in relating dose-response data for individual glycoalkaloids to the total amount in potatoes. Specifically, since the biological potency of α-chaconine is reported to be three or more times greater that of α-solanine (Friedman et al., 1991, 1992a), it would be better if new potato cultivars could be developed with a low α-chaconine to α-solanine ratio. New varieties may also inherit new glycoalkaloids of unknown structure and function from their progenitors (Vazquez et al., 1997).

4.2. Synergy

With respect to potential toxicity of glycoalkaloids to humans, Hopkins (1995) points out that although glycoalkaloids are present in foods such as potatoes consumed daily by animals and humans, their toxicological status is poorly defined. Moreover, since potatoes contain two glycoalkaloids which may act additively, synergistically, or antagonistically, studies are also needed to address the interactions of glycoalkaloids when consumed as mixtures in varying proportions.

Rayburn et al. (1995a) examined the embryo toxicities of α-chaconine and α-solanine individually and in mixtures. Toxic units (TU's) were calculated to assess possible synergism of several mixtures ranging from 3: 1 to 1: 20 TU's of α-chaconine to α-solanine. Some combinations exhibited strong synergism in both embryo lethality and malformations. These studies suggested that (a) synergism observed for a specific mixture cannot be used to predict possible synergism of other mixtures with different ratios of the two glycoalkaloids; (b) toxicities observed for individual glycoalkaloids may not predict toxicities of mixtures; and (c) specific combinations found in different potato varieties need to be tested to assess the safety of a particular plant variety.

These considerations suggest that predicted safety limits for glycoalkaloid-containing foods based on individual compounds may not be justified. The observed synergism between α-chaconine and α-solanine suggests the need for additional studies on the mechanism of interaction between different glycoalkaloids at the cellular-physiological level. This is a complex and challenging problem since consumption of glycoalkaloid-containing foods can result in the ingestion of at least six different glycoalkaloids - α-chaconine and α-solanine from potatoes, dehydrotomatine and α-tomatine from tomatoes, and solamargine and solasonine from eggplants (Friedman and Levin, 1998; Friedman et al., 1996, 1997a; Blankemeyer et al., 1998). The results obtained from our studies support the

Table 4. Protection against α-chaconine-induced development toxicity in the frog embryo[a]

Treatment	Malformation (%)	Mortality (%)
Controls	4.9	10.3
4 mg/L α-chaconine	100.0	99.4
4 mg/L α-chaconine +G6P+G6PD+NADP+NADPH[b]	10.5	28.8
4 mg/L α-chaconine +G6P+NADP+NADPH	11.1	21.3
4 mg/L α-chaconine +G6PD	NA[c]	100.0
4 mg/L α-chaconine +G6P	26.2	23.8
4 mg/L α-chaconine +NADP	32.5	50.0
4 mg/L α-chaconine +NADPH	NA	100.0

[a] Adapted from Rayburn et al. (1995a).
[b] G6P = glucose-6-phosphate; G6PD = glucose-6-phosphate dehydrogenase; NADP = oxidized nicotinamide adenine dinucleotide; NADPH = reduced form.
[c] NA = not applicable because of 100% mortality.

continuing use of the frog embryo and cell membrane assays for assessing mixture interactions of glycoalkaloids.

4.3. Protective Effect of Nutrients

4.3.1. Glucose-6-Phosphate and Nicotinamide Adenine Dinucleotide. Our studies also revealed that it may be possible to manipulate the diet to minimize adverse effects of glycoalkaloids based on the following observations. Rayburn et al. (1995a) showed that glucose-6-phosphate and nicotinamide adenine dinucleotide phosphate (NADP) protected frog embryos against adverse effects of α-chaconine (Table 4). Glucose-6-phosphate could exert its protective effect by competing with carbohydrate groups for receptor sites of cell membranes in the frog embryos. This is a plausible explanation since we also showed that both the nature and number of sugars in the carbohydrate side chain of glycoalkaloids are important in influencing biological potency (Rayburn et al., 1994).

4.3.2. Folic Acid. In related studies, Friedman et al. (1997b) found that folic acid protected against α-chaconine-induced disruption of frog embryo cell membranes and developmental toxicity (Figures 5–6). These observations suggest that ingredients present in complex diets may protect against adverse manifestations of glycoalkaloids. They also suggest that the simple and inexpensive endpoints used may validate and possibly replace animal studies, thus minimizing the need to use animals in safety evaluations of glycoalkaloids and other membrane-disruptive compounds including bacterial toxins (Louise and Obrig, 1995).

To stimulate further studies in this area, we will briefly examine some of the cellular and molecular events that may be involved in protection of fetuses by folic acid against neural tube defects. The neural folds in cultured rat embryos failed to close in the absence of methionine (Coelho and Klein, 1990). The main function of methionine appears to be post-translations methylation of arginine, histidine, and lysine residues of microfilament proteins to form methylated derivatives which are involved in neural tube closure. Mills et al. (1996) suggest that neural tube defects in children are the result of a metabolic defect in the enzyme methionine synthase, which along with vitamin B_{12}, is involved in the methylation of homocysteine to methionine. The vitamin appears to be an independent risk factor. These considerations imply that in addition to cited effects on cell membranes,

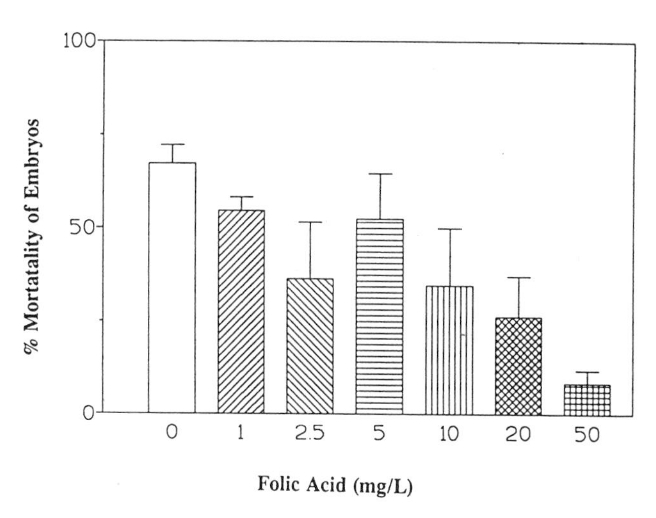

Figure 5. Protective effect of folic acid against α-chaconine-induced mortality of frog embryos. Conditions: embryos were exposed for 24 h to α-chaconine (2.5 mg/L) in the absence and presence of folic acid (Friedman et al., 1997b).

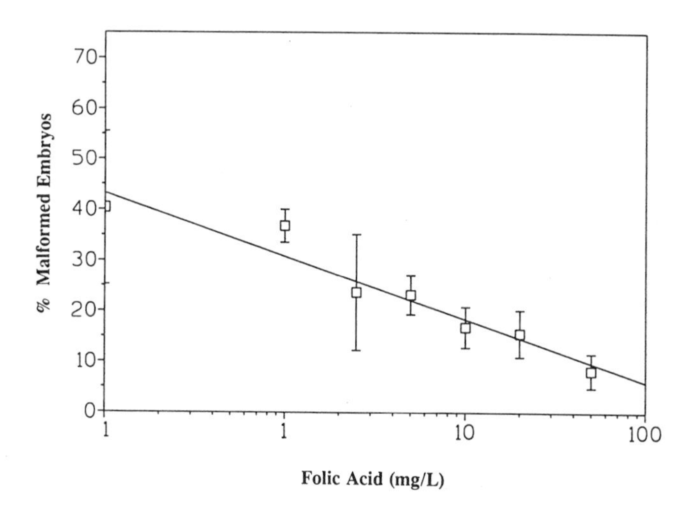

Figure 6. Protective effect of folic acid against α-chaconine-induce malformations in frog embryos. The plot shows the relationship of log folic acid concentration versus percent malformation in animal exposed for 24 h to α-chaconine (2.5 mg/L). Increasing folic acid concentration resulted in fewer malformations among the surviving embryos (Friedman et al., 1997b).

glycoalkaloids may influence sulfur amino acid metabolism (Friedman, 1994; Smolin and Benevenga, 1989) in eliciting a teratogenic response. It may therefore be worthwhile to find out whether cysteine, cystine, reduced glutathione, methionine, and related compounds can ameliorate adverse effects of glycoalkaloids.

5. REPRESSION OF GENES ENCODING ENZYME INVOLVED IN GLYCOALKALOID BIOSYNTHESIS

As part of multidiscipinary studies, we explored how glycoalkaloids are synthesized and degraded in the plant with the goal of reducing, through molecular biological means, the levels of the most toxic compounds. The final step in the biosynthesis of solanaceous glycoalkaloids is the glycosylation of the aglycone by a UDP-glucosyl transferase. In order to inhibit this enzyme, we first needed to clone the gene encoding the enzyme. This was accomplished by cloning and suppressing, through anti-sense RNA methodology, the enzyme UDP-glucosyl transferase. Initial results suggest that this strategy leads to a decrease in the activity of this potato enzyme, which is involved in the biosynthesis of glycoalkaloids (Stapleton et al., 1991, 1992; Moehs et al., 1997; Zimowski, 1997). Characterization of the enzymes and genes involved in glycoalkaloid biosynthesis may facilitate their inactivation and consequent reduction in post-harvest synthesis of glycoalkaloids (Love et al., 1996).

The above discussion of dietary and safety aspects of glycoalkaloids suggests the need to minimize the synthesis of UDPglucosyl transferase and related enzymes both in the plant and in the tuber after harvest. A possible approach to accomplish this post-harvest would be through sulfhydryl-disulfide interchange which alters the structure and function of proteins and which we previously found to be effective in inactivating plant protease inhibitors (Friedman and Gumbmann, 1991; Friedman et al., 1984). The same approach should also work for disulfide-containing toxic proteins produced by human pathogens.

A data base on glycoalkaloid formation after harvest is accumulating which contributes to our understanding of the factors that favor or minimize glycoalkaloid formation. The following is a brief overview of these factors.

6. POSTHARVEST CHANGES

6.1. Effect of Storage Temperature and Humidity

The influence of storage temperature on glycoalkaloid formation is not clear-cut, possibly because humidities varied widely in many temperature-storage studies. Immersion of potatoes in water may reduce glycoalkaloid formation (Mondy and Chandra, 1987; Friedman and Dao, 1992). Little is known about the effects of soaking or spraying with water. Since humidity could influence glycoalkaloid formation during storage, a need exists to define the combined effects of storage temperature and humidity on changes in glycoalkaloid levels of potatoes.

Storage temperature may affect potatoes both adversely and beneficially (Griffiths et al., 1997; Hwang and Lee, 1984; Lisinska and Leszczynski, 1989; Stoddard, 1992; Wunsch and Munzert, 1994). It influences sprouting, respiratory rate, disease control, sweetening, and internal and external blackspot formation. Since these events may accompany glycoalkaloid formation (e.g., bruising induces both glycoalkaloid and polyphenol formation), they are relevant to the theme of this paper. Here, we will briefly describe two events which influence the quality of potatoes: sweetening and browning discolorations.

Sweetening is caused by an accumulation of sugars in potatoes stored at low temperatures. Sugars and starch exist together in the tuber and undergo continual enzyme-catalyzed transformations as shown schematically below in equations 1 and 2:

$$\text{Sucrose} \leftrightarrow \text{Glucose} + \text{Fructose} \tag{1}$$

$$\text{Starch} \leftrightarrow \text{Glucose} \tag{2}$$

At above 10°C, the sugars and starch remain in balance, with the sugars either reforming into starch or being used up in other reactions. Below 10°C, however, reducing sugars start to accumulate in the tuber. This is undesirable because when the tubers are cooked or fried, the sugars can participate with free amino acids (which increase during storage) and proteins in nonenzymatic Maillard browning reactions. This results in the formation of darkened and off-flavor products and loss in nutritional value (Brierley et al., 1996; Friedman, 1996b).

During storage, potatoes are also susceptible to a variety of discolorations which may adversely affect quality and safety (Friedman, 1997). Internal discolorations can result from enzymatic browning, whereby the amino acid tyrosine is first hydroxylated to dihydrxyphenylalanine (DOPA), which is then oxidized to dopaquinone. Both events are catalyzed by polyphenol oxidase (PPO). Dopaquinone polymerizes to red and brown pigments in the presence of oxygen. Such browning-initiated discolorations may be increased during storage, sorting, packing, and transportation of potatoes.

Friedman and colleagues (Friedman and Bautista, 1995; Friedman et al., 1992a; Molnar-Perl and Friedman, 1990) demonstrated the potential of several different SH-containing amino acids and peptides, including cysteine, cysteine ethyl ester, cysteine methyl ester, N-acetyl-L-cysteine, and reduced glutathione to inhibit enzymatic and nonenzymatic browning in fresh and dehydrated potatoes. As mentioned earlier, these and other sulfite substitutes may also inactivate through sulfhydryl-disulfide interchange enzymes catalyzing the biosynthesis of glycoalkaloids as well as essential enzymes of bacterial pathogens infecting potatoes, and possibly also human pathogens. Such inhibition should lead to suppression of post-harvest synthesis of glycoalkaloids and to improved potatoes.

6.2. Effect of Light

Exposure of post-harvest potato tubers to light, whether incandescent, fluorescent, or natural, can dramatically enhance glycoalkaloid synthesis both during growth and after harvest (Dimenstein et al., 1997). Generally, the increases in chlorophyll and glycoalkaloid synthesis seem to depend on the wavelength of the light to which the tubers are exposed (Petermann and Morris, 1985). For example, exposure of the cultivar Sebago to a 15 watt incandescent lamp for 10 days resulted in an increase in glycoalkaloid content from 4.8 to 19 mg/100 g fresh weight (Zitnak, 1981). Exposure of peeled Russet Burbank potato slices to fluorescent light of 200-foot candles for 48 h caused an increase from 0.2 to 7.4 mg/100 g fresh weight.

Exposure of commercial White Rose potatoes for 20 days induced a time-dependent greening of potato surfaces (Dao and Friedman, 1994). In addition to increases in chlorophyll content, chlorogenic and glycoalkaloid levels (Figure 7) also increased, but no

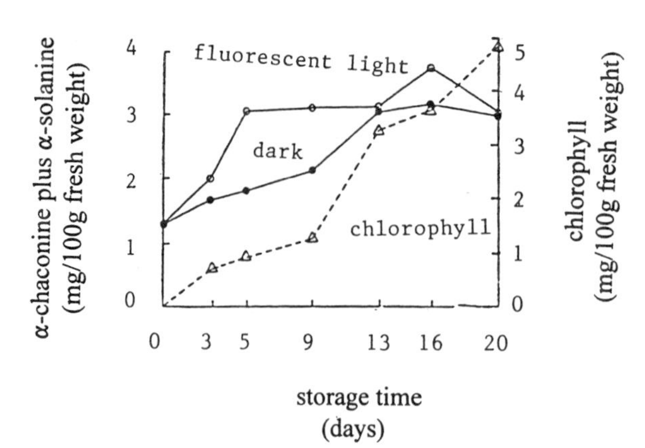

Figure 7. Chlorophyll and total glycoalkaloid content of White Rose potatoes stored under fluorescent light or in the dark (Dao and Friedman, 1994).

changes were observed in the content of inhibitors of the digestive enzymes carboxypeptidase A, chymotrypsin, and trypsin. Since potato cultivars differ significantly in their ability to produce greening-related glycoalkaloids (Dale et al., 1993), it should be possible to find and use varieties with low rates of post-harvest glycoalkaloid synthesis.

6.3. Effect of γ-Radiation

γ-Radiation effectively prevents sprouting and greening and protects potatoes during storage against damage by fungi and other phytopathogens (Mondy and Seetharaman, 1990; Swallow, 1991). This is a desirable objective since when potatoes sprout they decrease in weight, quality, and market value. Sprouts may also present a health hazard since their glycoalkaloid content in quite high (Table 1). Japan appears to be the only country where potatoes are currently being irradiated on a commercial scale (Thomas, 1984).

In reviewing the effect γ-radiation on the polyphenolic content of potatoes, Friedman (1997) noted that different investigators report different results. According to Dale et al. (1997), this is also true for various studies on the effect of γ-radiation on glycoalkaloids. To better define the possible impact of γ-radiation on potatoes, Dale and colleagues evaluated the effect of irradiation on chlorophyll and glycoalkaloid content of seven potato cultivars. They observed significant differences among genotypes in their susceptibility to radiation. Overall, irradiation significantly reduced the accumulation of glycoalkaloids. γ-Radiation also reduced the synthesis of chlorophyll, but to different degrees than observed for glycoalkaloids. The authors conclude that it is unlikely that any of the cultivars could accrue toxic levels of glycoalkaloids following irradiation and on prolonged exposure to light without any greening due to accompanying light-induced synthesis of chlorophyll. It is relevant to note that although irradiation, storage, and cooking all induced a reduction in vitamin C content of potatoes, cooking did not markedly reduce the ascorbic acid of stored irradiated potatoes compared to non-irradiated ones (Graham and Stevenson, 1997).

These observations reinforce the need to assess relative susceptibilities of different cultivars to adverse and beneficial post-harvest changes to radiation and other stress factors mentioned in this paper. Such information will serve as a guide for potato growers and processors to minimize adverse post-harvest changes in potatoes for various end uses and help in the selection of specific potato cultivars which show the greatest resistance to stress-induced compositional changes. Another need is to define possible mechanisms of the reported influence of radiation on the biosynthesis of glycoalkaloids. Possibilities include inactivation of biosynthetic enzymes and, depending on dose, radiation-induced modification of the glycoalkaloids.

6.4. Effect of Mechanical Damage

Bruising, cutting, and slicing of potato tubers induces the formation of glycoalkaloids (Mondy and Gosselin, 1988; Mondy et al., 1987). Glycoalkaloid production increases with the extent of injury and is cultivar related (Olsson, 1986). For example, Fitzpatrick et al. (1977, 1978) showed that the glycoalkaloid content of potato slices increased from 5.5 to 99.4 mg/100 g of fresh weight after storage for four days. It appears, therefore, that injury such as slicing (widely used in the home) before storage induces a burst of glycoalkaloid synthesis over time. It is therefore evident that storing whole tubers and cutting them just before cooking is much preferred over cutting and then storing them prior to cooking. As already noted, soaking sliced potatoes in water also minimizes postharvest glycoalkaloid formation. It is generally advisable to eliminate tubers that have been injured during harvest, transport, or storage, as enough time would have passed to induce formation of high levels of glycoalkaloids in these tubers.

6.5. Pest Resistance

Fungi such as *Fusarium solani and Phoma foreata* damage potatoes by causing storage rot (Olsson, 1987). Fewell and Roddick (1997) found that the antifungal property of α-chaconine was greater than that of α-solanine and that synergism between these two potato glycoalkaloids in other organisms, tissues, cells, and membrane-bound structures was also evident. Olsson (1987) studied the effects of initial glycoalkaloid levels and ability to respond to potato damage (by increasing glycoalkaloid synthesis) on the resistance of various potato cultivars to fungi. There was a direct correlation between the extent of damage and the initial glycoalkaloid content. A genotype with a high initial glycoalkaloid content resulted in a greater increase than in one with a low initial level. Cultivars most susceptible to mechanical injury showed the greatest increases in glycoalkaloid content. Surprisingly, the initial content of glycoalkaloids in different cultivars, which ranged from 2 to 15 mg/100 g fresh weight, did not affect resistance to infection. Some genotypes with high glycoalkaloid levels were less resistant than those with low levels. These observation suggest that selection of low-glycoalkaloid potato cultivars by breeders may not always adversely affect the resistance of the potato to some phytopathogens.

6.6. Effect of Food Processing

Since potatoes are usually not consumed raw but are subject to a variety of food processing condition including baking, boiling, broiling, frying, and microwaving, the question arises whether these conditions influence glycoalkaloid content. Table 2 summarizes the glycoalkaloid content of various potato products. The levels vary widely ranging from about 1 mg/kg for fresh french fries to about 700 mg/kg for commercial potato chips. The high range of potato chips reported by Sizer et al. (1980) was attributed to one sample that contained a significant amount of peel.

Generally, baking, broiling, and frying leave the glycoalkaloids largely unaffected (Bushway and Ponnampalam, 1980; Bushway et al., 1981, 1983; Muller, 1983; Schwardt, 1982; Zobel and Schilling, 1964). Most cooked samples had a glycoalkaloid content of

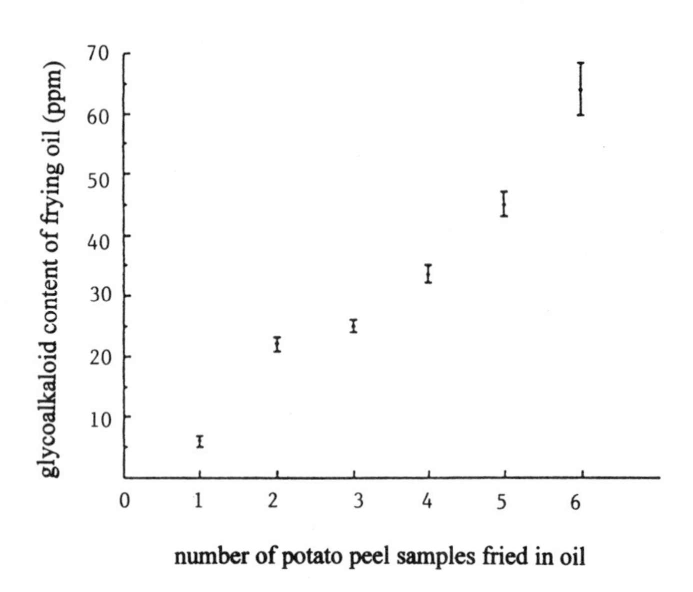

Figure 8. Glycoalkaloid content of corn oil after frying of six consecutive samples of potato peels (Adapted from Chungcharoen, 1988).

about 90–95% that of the uncooked ones. However, boiling sprouted potatoes results in diffusion of glycoalkaloids from the sprouts into the tubers (Gonmori and Shindo, 1985). Takagi et al. (1990) found that micro waving potatoes reduced their glycoalkaloid content by about 15%. The significant loss of glycoalkaloids during baking and frying reported by Ponnampalam and Mondy (1983) may have been partly due to incomplete extraction. Also noteworthy is our observation that 72% of the original amount of the tomato glycoalkaloid α-tomatine survived home processing condition used in the preparation of Southern fried green tomatoes (Friedman and Levin, 1995). It is often more difficult to extract glycoalkaloids from processed products that have lost water than from fresh samples (Duan and Zong, 1993; Friedman and McDonald, 1995b).

Takagaki et al. (1990) noted that the temperature of the oil in deep frying affected glycoalkaloid levels. They found that frying at 150°C caused little change, but frying at 210°C resulted in a 40% loss of glycoalkaloids. In related studies, Chungcharoen (1988) showed that glycoalkaloids were stable in cooking oil at 180°C. She also demonstrated a continuing diffusion of glycoalkaloids into the oil as subsequent batches of potatoes with peels were cooked in the same oil (Figure 8). This observation implies that the glycoalkaloid content of low-level glycoalkaloid potatoes cooked in oil may actually increase during frying in subsequent batches of oil, presumably due to absorption of the glycoalkaloids from the oil into the potatoes. Food safety may be enhanced by frequent changes of frying oils.

7. ANALYSIS OF GLYCOALKALOIDS

As already mentioned, many factors influence the concentration of glycoalkaloids in potatoes. These include variety, method of harvest, method of transport, light, humidity, temperature of storage, and mechanical damage. A variety of analytical methods have

Table 5. Glycoalkaloid content of fresh and processed potatoes determined by HPLC and a commercial enzyme-linked immunosorbent assay (ELISA) kit

	Glycoalakloid content (mg/kg original weight)	
Potato or potato product[a]	HPLC	ELISA
Fresh whole potatoes		
Large Russet	22.4	23.6
Yukon gold	39.0	38.4
Small purple	40.0	37.3
Small gold	105.4	112.9
Small red	101.3	128.4
Large white	125.5	132.3
Small white	203.4	208.9
Processed potato products		
Potato skins	37.2	41.0
French fries	24.1	22.7
Low-fat potato chips	16.3	11.3

[a] Purchased in a local grocery store or restaurant.

been proposed to better assess the influence of individual and combined effects of these parameters on the glycoalkaloid content of potatoes. These methods, critically evaluated elsewhere (Friedman and Levin, 1992, 1995; Friedman and McDonald, 1995a, 1997; Hellenas and Branzell, 1997), are often time consuming and relatively expensive. A simple method that can analyze a large number of samples in a reasonably short time is needed to meet the needs of plant breeders, plant molecular biologist, food processors, and scientists interested in better defining the role of glycoalkaloids in the plant, in the diet, and in medicine. A reliable immunoassay that correlates with HPLC may provide the answer. An ELISA kit for glycoalkaloids that meets these criteria should find widespread use.

To meet this need, we evaluated a prototype ELISA kit produced by EnviroLogix, Inc., Portland, Maine based on antibodies developed by Stanker et al. (1994). Our initial results show a good correlation between HPLC and the ELISA for glycoalkaloids in potato tubers and processed products (Table 5). Hopefully, this kit will provide a variety of benefits from the farm to processing, shipping, marketing, and consumption of potatoes and potato products. It should also facilitate the development of potatoes with improved compositional and processing qualities.

8. CONCLUSIONS AND RESEARCH NEEDS

Inappropriate post-harvest handling of potatoes during storage, shipping, and processing increases their glycoalkaloid content. Another major concern of food safety is whether phytochemicals such as glycoalkaloids behave differently, depending on whether they are consumed alone or part of complex interactions with each other and other dietary components. Such interactions are not well understood. A better understanding of the fate of glycoalkaloids from harvest to consumption is therefore needed to better assess the impact of glycoalkaloids on the quality, safety, and nutritional value of potatoes. A need exists to devise better conditions to minimize pre- and post-harvest production of the most toxic glycoalkaloids so as to assure that the products reaching the consumer are optimal in appearance, taste, and safety. Such information will also help guide plant breeders and plant molecular biologists in their efforts to develop improved potatoes.

In addition to recommendations made earlier to facilitate progress in order to enhance the value of the potato as a safe and nutritious food, we are challenged to respond to additional research needs outlined below:

1. Determine the *relative susceptibilities* to greening, mechanical damage, and increases in glycoalkaloid levels of newly developed and present major commercial varieties of potatoes. Recommend adoption and use of cultivars showing the greatest resistance to greening, bruising, and postharvest glycoalkaloid production.
2. Evaluate food-compatible inhibitors of enzymes that catalyze the biosynthesis of glycoalkaloids.
3. Evaluate films with built-in chromophores that absorb light for their ability to protect potatoes against greening, browning, and spoiling.
4. Develop improved sampling, extraction, and analytical methods for glycoalkaloids and metabolites.
5. Define relative biological and toxicological potencies of structurally different glycoalkaloids and metabolites. Most of the pharmacological and toxicological studies have been done with either α-chaconine or α-solanine. Very little data is available for the hydrolysis products (metabolites) of the glycoalkaloids. Almost nothing is known about possible synergism among structurally different glycoalkaloids.
6. Define and optimize beneficial anti-carcinogenic, cholesterol-lowering, and antibiotic effects of glycoalkaloids (Cham et al., 1991; Friedman et al., 1998; Thorne et al., 1985).

   Generally, the overlapping objectives of needed safety evaluations are as follows:

   a. To define relative potencies of potato, tomato, and eggplant glycoalkaloids.
   b. To define combinations that maximize or minimize biological effects.
   c. To use molecular modeling to predict potencies of mixtures of known and unknown glycoalkaloids.
   d. To assess the predictive value of *in vitro* assays for *in vivo* toxicity and prevention.
   e. To assess the ability of nutrients to reduce the toxic potential of glycoalkaloids.

   Expected benefits from safety evaluation studies include the following:

   a. Development of a potency ranking scale of structurally different glycoalkaloids.
   b. Development of a data base to guide the creation of new plant varieties with low content of the most toxic glycoalkaloids and setting limits for the glycoalkaloid content of foods.

7. Using the available information and new knowledge derived from the suggested studies, make recommendations for a standard protocol for sampling and handling of potatoes to minimize glycoalkaloid biosynthesis before and after harvest.

REFERENCES

Azim, A.; Shaikh, H. A.; Ahmad, R. Effect of feeding greened potatoes on different visceral organs and blood palsma of rabbits. *J. Sci. Food Agric.* **1982**, *33*, 1275–1279.

Blankemeyer, J. T.; Stringer, B. K.; Rayburn, J. R.; Bantle, J. A.; Friedman, M. Effect of potato glycoalkaloids α-chaconine and α-solanine on membrane potential of frog embryos. *J. Agric. Food Chem.* **1992**, *40*, 2022–2026.

Blankemeyer, J. R.; Atherton, R.; Friedman, M. Effect of potato glycoalkaloids α-chaconine and α-solanine on sodium active transport in skin. *J. Agric. Food Chem.* **1995**, *43*, 636–639.

Blankemeyer, J. T.; White, J. B.; Stringer, B. K.; Friedman, M. Effect of α-tomatine and tomatidine on membrane potential of frog embryos and active transport in frog skin. *Food Chem. Toxicol.* **1997**, *35*, 639–647.

Blankemeyer, J. T.; McWilliams, M. L.; Rayburn, J. R.; Weissenberg, M.; Friedman, M. Developmental toxicology of solamargine and solasonine glycoalkaloids in frog embryos. *Food Chem. Toxicol.* **1998**, *36*, 383–389.

Brierley, E. R.; Bonner, P. L. R.; Cobb, A. H. Factors influencing the free amino acid content of potato (*Solanum tuberosum L.*) tubers during prolonged storage. *J. Sci. Food Agric.* **1996**, *47*, 515–525.

Bushway, R. J.; Ponnampalam, R. α-Chaconine and α-solanine content of potato products and their stability during several modes of cooking. *J. Agric. Food Chem.* **1981**, *29*, 814–817.

Bushway, A. A.; Bushway, A. W.; Belyea, P. R.; Bushway, R. J. The proximate composition and glycoalkaloid content of three potato meals. *Am. Potato J.* **1981**, *58*, 498.

Bushway, R. J.; Bureau, J. L.; McGann, D. F. α-Chaconine and α-solanine content of potato peels and potato peel products. *J. Food Sci.* **1983**, *48*, 84–86.

Caldwell, K. A.; Grosjean, O. K.; Henika, P. R.; Friedman, M. Hepatic ornithine decarboxylase induction by potato glycoalkaloids in rats. *Food Chem. Toxicol.* **1991**, *29*, 531–535.

Camire, M. E.; Zhao, J.; Dougherty, M. P; Bushway, R. J.; *In vitro* binding of benz(a)pyrene by extruded potato peel. *J. Agric. Food Chem.* **1995**, *43*, 970–973.

Cham, B. E.; Daunter, B.; Evans, R. A. Topical treatment of malignant and premalignant skin lesions by very low concentrations of a standard mixture (BEC) of solasodine glycoalkaloids. *Cancer Lett.* **1991**, *59*, 55–58.

Chungcharoen, A. *Glycoalkaloid Content of Potatoes Grown under Controlled Environments and Stability of Glycoalkaloids during Processing.* Ph. D. Thesis, University of Wisconsin, Madison, WI. **1988.**

Cieslik. E. Glycoalkaloids - toxic substances in plants. *Zywnosc. Technologia. Jakosc.* **1997**, *1 (10)*, 21–29. (Polish)

Coelho, C. N. D.; Klein, N. W. Methionine and neural tube closure in rat embryos: morphological and biochemical analyses. *Teratology* **1990**, *42*, 437–451.

Coxon, T. The glycoalkaloid content of potato berries. *J. Sci. Food Agric.* **1981**, *32*, 412–414.

Dale, M. F. B.; Grfiffiths, D. W.; Bain, H.; Todd, D. Glycoalkaloid increase in *Solanum tuberosum* on exposure to light. *Ann. Appl. Biol.* **1993**, *123*, 411–418.

Dale, M. F. B.; Griffiths, D. W.; Bain, H.; Goodman, B. A. The effect of gamma irradiation on glycoalkaloid and chlorophyll synthesis in seven potato cultivars. *J. Sci. Food Agric.* **1997**, *75*, 141–147.

Dao, L.; Friedman, M. Chlorogenic acid content of fresh and processed potatoes determined by ultraviolet spectrophotometry. *J. Agric. Food Chem.* **1992**, *40*, 2152–2156.

Dao, L.; Friedman, M. Chlorophyll, chlorogenic acid, glycoalkaloid, and protease inhibitor content of fresh and green potatoes. *J. Agric. Food Chem.* **1994**, *42*, 633–639.

Dao, L.; Friedman, M. Comparison of glycoalkaloid content of fresh and freeze-dried potato leaves determined by HPLC and colorimetry. *J. Agric. Food Chem.* **1996**, *44*, 2287–2291.

Davies, A. M.; Blincow, P. J. Glycoalkaloid content of potatoes and potato products sold in the U. K. *J. Sci. Food Agric.* **1984**, *35*, 553–557.

Dimenstein, L.; Lisker, N.; Kedar, N.; Levy, D. Changes in the content of steroidal glycoalkaloids in potato tubers grown in the field and in the greenhouse under different conditions of light, temperature and daylength. *Physiol. Mol. Plant Pathol.* **1997**, *50*, 391–402.

Domek, J. M.; Cantelo, W. W.; Wagner, R. M.; Li, B. W.; Miller-Ihli, N. J. Nutritional composition of potato foliage. *J. Agric. Food Chem.* **1995**, *43*, 1512–1515.

Duan, G. M.; Zong, H. Effect of different solvent systems on extraction of potato glycoalkaloids. *Plant Physiol. Commun.* **1993**, *29*, 365–368. (Chinese)

Fewell, A. M.; Roddick, J. G. Potato glycoalkaloid impairment of fungal development. *Mycol. Res.* **1997**, *101*, 597–603.

Filadelfi, M. A.; Zitnak, A. Preparation of chaconines by enzymatic hydrolysis of potato berry alkaloids. *Phytochemistry* **1982**, *21*, 250–251.

Fitzpatrick, T. J.; Herb, S. F.; Osman, S. F.; McDermott, J. A. Potato glycoalkaloids: increases in variations of ratios in aged slices over prolonged storage. *Am. Potato J.* **1977**, *54*, 539–544.

Fitzpatrick, T. J.; MacDermott, J. A.; Osman, S. F. Evaluation of injured commercial potato samples for total glycoalkaloid content. *J. Food Sci.* **1978**, *43*, 1617–1618.

Friedman, M. Composition and safety evaluation of potato berries, potato and tomato seeds, potatoes, and potato alkaloids. *ACS Symp. Ser.* **1992**, *484*, 429–462.

Friedman, M. Improvement in the safety of foods by SH-containing amino acids and peptides. *J. Agric. Food Chem.* **1994**, *42*, 3–20.

Friedman, M. Nutritional value of proteins from different food sources. *J. Agric. Food Chem.* **1996a**, *44*, 6–20.

Friedman, M. Food browning and its prevention. *J. Agric. Food Chem.* **1996b**, *44*, 631–653.

Friedman, M. Chemistry, biochemistry, and dietary role of potato polyphenols. *J. Agric* .Food Chem. **1997**, *45*, 3–20.

Friedman, M.; Bautista, F. F. Inhibition of polyphenol oxidase by thiols in the absence and presence of potato tissue suspensions. *J. Agric. Food Chem.* **1995**, *43*, 69–76.

Friedman, M.; Dao, L. Distribution of glycoalkaloids in potato plants and commercial potato products. *J. Agric. Food Chem.* **1992**, *40*, 419–423.

Friedman, M.; Henika, P. R. Absence of genotoxicity of potato alkaloids α-chaconine, α-solanine, and solanidine in the Ames *Salmonella* and adult and foetal erythrocyte micronucleus assays. *Food Chem. Toxicol.* **1992**, *30*, 689–694.

Friedman, M.; Gumbmann, M. R. Nutritional improvement of legume proteins through disulfide interchange. In *Nutritional and Toxicological Significance of Enzyme Inhibitors in Foods*; Friedman, M., Ed.; Plenum: New York, 1989; pp 357–390.

Friedman, M.; Levin, C. E. Reversed-phase high-performance liquid chromatographic separation of potato glycoalkaloids and hydrolysis products on acidic columns. *J. Agric. Food Chem.* **1992**, *40*, 2157–2163.

Friedman, M.; Levin, C. E. α-Tomatine content in tomatoes and tomato products determined by HPLC with pulsed amperometric detection. *J. Agric. Food Chem.* **1995**, *43*, 1507–1511.

Friedman, M.; Levin, C.E. Dehydro tomatine content in tomatoes. *J. Agric. Food Chem.* **1998**, *46*, 4571–4576.

Friedman, M.; McDonald, G. M. Acid catalyzed partial hydrolysis of carbohydrate groups of the potato glycoalkaloid α-chaconine in alcoholic solutions. *J. Agric. Food Chem.* **1995a**, *43*, 1501–1506.

Friedman, M.; McDonald, G. M. Extraction efficiency of various solvents for glycoalkaloid determination in potatoes and potato products. *Am. Potato J.* **1995b**, *72*, 66A.

Friedman, M.; McDonald, G. M. Potato glycoalkaloids: chemistry, analysis, safety, and plant physiology. *Crit. Rev. Plant Sci.* **1997**, *16*, 55–132.

Friedman, M.; McDonald, G. M. Steroidal glycoalkaloids. In *Naturally Occurring Glycosides: Chemistry, Distribution and Biological Properties*. R. Ikan, Ed.; John Wiley and Sons: New York and London, **1999**; pp. 311–342.

Friedman, M.; Grosjean, O. K.; Gumbmann, M. R. Nutritional improvement of soy flour. *J. Nutr.* **1984**, *114*, 2241–2246.

Friedman, M.; Rayburn, J. R.; Bantle, J. A. Developmental toxicology of potato alkaloids in the frog embryo teratogenesis assay-*Xenopus* (FETAX). *Food Chem. Toxicol.* **1991**, *29*, 537–547.

Friedman, M.; Rayburn, J. R.; Bantle, J. A. Structural relationships and developmental toxicity of *Solanum* alkaloids in the frog embryo teratogenesis assay-*Xenopus* (FETAX). *J. Agric. Food Chem.* **1992a**, *40*, 1617–1624.

Friedman, M.; Molnar-Perl, I.; Knighton, D. Browning prevention in fresh and dehydrated potatoes by SH-containing amino acids. *Food Addit. Contam.* **1992b**, *9*, 499–503.

Friedman, M.; McDonald, G. M.; Haddon, W. F. Kinetics of acid-catalyzed hydrolysis of potato glycoalkaloids α-chaconine and α-solanine. *J. Agric. Food Chem.* **1993**, *41*, 1397–1406.

Friedman, M.; Henika, P. R.; Mackey, B. E. Feeding potato, tomato, and eggplant alkaloids affects food consumption and body and liver weights of mice. *J. Nutr.* **1996**, *126*, 989–999.

Friedman, M.; Kozukue, N.; Harden, L. A. Structure of the tomato glycoalkaloid tomatidenol-3-β-lycotetraose (dehydrotomatine). *J. Agric. Food Chem.* **1997a**, *45*, 1541–1547.

Friedman, M.; Burns, C. F.; Butchko, C. A. Blanakemeyer, J. T. Folic acid protects against potato glycoalklaoid α-chaconine-induced disruption of frog embryo cell membranes and developmental toxicity. *J. Agric. Food Chem.* **1997b**, *45*, 3991–3994.

Friedman, M.; Fitch, T. E.; Levin, C. E.; Yokoyoma, W. H. Reduction of dietary cholesterol, plasma LDL cholesterol and triglycerides in hamsters fed green and red tomatoes. Presented at the ACS Meeting, Las Vegas, NE. Abstract AGFD 67. **1997c**.

Friedman, M.; Bautista, F.F.; Stanker, L.H.; Larkin, K. Analysis of potato glycoalkaloids by a new ELISA kit. *J. Agric. Food Chem.* **1998**, *46*, 5097–5102.

Gee, J.M.; Wortley, G. M.; Johnson, I. T.; Prince, K. R.; Rutten, A. A. J. J. L.; Houben, G. F.; Penninks, A. H. Effect of saponins and glycoalkaloids on the permeability and viability of mammalian intestinal cells and the integrity of tissue preparations *in vitro*. *Toxicol. in Vitro* **1996**, *10*, 117–128.

Gonmori, K.; Shindo, S. Effect of cooking on the concentration of solanine in potato. *Res. Pract. Forens. Med.* **1985**, *28*, 91–93.

Gonmori, K.; Yoshioka, N. The risk of solanine poisoning in a folk remedy. *Proc. 31st Meeting of the International Association of Forensic Toxicologists;* Mueller, R. K., Ed., Leipzig: Germany, **1994**; pp 247–251.

Graham, W. D.; Stevenson, M. H. Effect of irradiation on vitamin C content of strawberries and potatoes in combination with storage and with further cooking in potatoes. *J. Sci. Food Agric.* **1997**, *75*, 371–377.

Griffiths, D. W.; Dale, M. F. B.; Bain, H. The effect of cultivar, maturity and storage on photo-induced changes in total glycoalkaloid and chlorophyll contents of potatoes (*Solanum tuberosum*). *Plant Sci.* **1994**, *98*, 103–109.

Griffiths, W. D.; Bain, H.; Finlay, M.; Dale, B. The effect of low-temperature storage on the glycoalkaloid content of potato (*Solanum tuberosum*) tubers. *J. Sci. Food Agric.* **1997**, *74*, 301–307.

Hellenas, K. E. *Glycoalkaloids in Potato Tubers - Aspects of Analysis, Occurrence and Toxicology.* Dissertation, Swedish University of Agricultural Sciences, Department of Food Science, Report 12, Uppsala: Sweden. **1994.**

Hellenas, K. E.; Branzell, C. K. Liquid chromatographic determination of the glycoalkaloids α-solanine and α-chaconine in potato tubes: NMKL interlaboratory study. *J. AOAC Int.* **1997**, *80*, 549–554.

Hopkins, J. The glycoalkaloids: naturally of interest (but a hot potato?). *Food Chem. Toxicol.* **1995**, *33*, 323–328.

Hwang, C. S.; Lee, S. W. Change in glycoalkaloids of potatoes during storage. *Kor. J. Food Sci. Technol.* **1984**, *16*, 388–391.

Johns, T.; Keen, S. L. Taste evaluation of potato glycoalkaloids by the Ayamara: a case study in human chemical ecology. *Human Ecol.* **1986**, *14*, 437–452.

Jones, P. G.; Fenwick, G. R. The glycoalkaloid content of some edible *Solanaceous* fruits and potato products. *J. Sci. Food Agric.* **1981**, *32*, 419–421

Jones, R. Challenging success. *Am. Veg. Grower* **1998**, *46*, *No 1*, 46–47.

Kaaber, L. Glycoalkaloids, green discoloration and taste development during storage of some potato varieties *(Solanum tuberosum)*. *Norwegian J. Agric. Sci.* **1993**, *7*, 221–229.

Kozukue, N.; Kozukue, E.; Mizuno, S. Glycoalkaloids in potato plants and tubers. *HortSci.* **1987**, *22*, 294–296.

Kritchevsky, D. Dietary fiber. *Ann. Rev. Nutr.* **1988**, *8*, 301–328.

Kubo, I.; Fukuhara, K. Steroidal glycoalkaloids in Andean potatoes. In *Saponins Used in Food and Agriculture.* Waller, P., Ed.; Plenum Press: New York, **1996**; pp 405–417.

Lazarov, K.; Werman, M. J. Hypocholesterolaemic effect of potato peel as a dietary fiber source. *Med. Sci. Res.* **1996**, *24*, 581–582.

Lisinska, G.; Leszczynski, W. *Potato Science and Technology.* Elsevier: London and New York, **1989.**

Louise, C. B.; Obrig, T. J. Specific interaction of *Escherichia coli* 0157:H7-derived Shiga-like toxin with human renal endothelial cells. *J. Infect. Dis.* **1995**, *172*, 1397–1401.

Love, S. L.; Baker, T. P.; Thompson-Johns, A.; Werner, P. K. Induced mutations for reduced tuber glycoalkaloid content in potatoes. *Plant Breeding* **1996**, *115*, 119–122.

Mills, J. L.; Scott, J. M.; Kirks, P. N.; McPartlin, J.M.; Conley, M. R.; Weir, D.; Molloy, A. M.; Lee, Y. J. Homocysteine and neural tube defects. *J. Nutr.* **1996**, *126*, 756S-760S.

Moehs, C. P.; Allen, P. V.; Friedman, M.; Belknap, W. R. Cloning and expression of solanidine UDP-glucose glucosyltransferase (SGT) from potato. *Plant J.* **1997**, *11*, 101–110.

Molanr-Perl, I.; Friedman, M. Inhibition of food browning by sulfur amino acids. 3. Apples and potatoes. *J. Agric. Food Chem.* **1990**, *38*, 1652–1656.

Mondy, N. I.; Chandra, S. Reduction of glycoalkaloid synthesis in potato slices by water soaking. *HortSci.* **1979**, *14*, 173–174.

Mondy, N. I.; Gosselin, B. Effect of peeling on total phenols, total glycoalkaloids, discoloration and flavor of cooked potatoes. *J. Food Sci.* **1988**, *53*, 756–759.

Mondy, N. I.; Seetharaman, K. Effect of irradiation on total glycoalkaloids in Kennebec and Russet Burbank potatoes. *J. Food Sci.* **1990**, *55*, 1740–1742.

Mondy, N. I.; Leja, M.; Gosselin, B. Changes in total phenolic, total glycoalkaloid, and ascorbic acid content of potatoes as a result of bruising. *J. Food Sci.* **1987**, *52*, 631–635.

Morris, S. C.; Lee, T. H. The toxicity and teratogenicity of *Solanaceae* glycoalkaloids, particularly those of the potato (*Solanum tuberosum*). *Food Technol. Austral.* **1984**, *36*, 118–124.

Muller, K. Glycoalkaloids in native and processed potatoes. *Der Kartoffelbau* **1983**, *43*, 310–312.

Nigg, H. N.; Ramos, L. E.; Graham, E. M.; Sterling, J.; Brown, S.; Cornell, J. A. Inhibition of human plasma and serum butyryl cholinesterase by α-chaconine and α-solanine. *Fund. Appl. Toxicol.* **1996**, *33*, 272–281.

Olsson, K. The influence of genotype and the effects of impact damage on the accumulation of glycoalkaloids in potato tubers. *Potato Res.* **1986**, *29*, 1–12.

Olsson, K. The influence of glycoalkaloids and impact damage on resistance of *Fusarium solani* var. *coeruleum* and *Phooma exigua* var. *foveata* in potato tubers. *J. Phytopathol.* **1987**, *118*, 347–357.

Onyeneho, S-N.; Hettiaachchy, N. S.; Antioxidant activity, fatty acid and phenolic acid composition of potato peels. *J. Sci. Food Agric.* **1993**, *62*, 345–350.

Panovska, Z.; Hajslova, J.; Kosinkiva, P.; Cepl, J. Glycoalkaloid content of potatoes sold in Czechia. *Nahrung* **1997**, *41*, 146–149.

Petermann, J. B.; Morris, S. C. The spectral response of chlorophyll and glycoalkaloid synthesis in potato tubers (*Solanum tuberosum*). *Plant Sci.* **1985**, *39*, 105–110.

Phillips, B. J.; Hughes, J. C.; Phillips, D. G.; Walters, D. G.; Anderson, D.; Tahourdin, C. S. M. A study of the toxic hazard that might be associated with the consumption of green potato tops. *Food Chem. Toxicol.* **1996**, *34*, 439–448.

Ponnampalam, R.; Mondy, N. Effect of cooking on the total glycoalkaloid content of potatoes. *J. Agric. Food Chem.* **1986**, *34*, 686–688.

Rayburn, J. R.; Bantle, J. A.; Friedman, M. Role of carbohydrate side chains of potato glycoalkaloids in developmental toxicity. *J. Agric. Food Chem.* **1994**, *42*, 1511–1515.

Rayburn, J. R.; Friedman, M.; Bantle, J. A. Synergism of potato glycoalkaloids α-chaconine and α-solanine in the developmenal toxicity of *Xenopus* embryos. *Food Chem. Toxicol.* **1995a**, *33*, 1013–1019.

Rayburn, J. R.; Bantle, J. A.; Qualls, C. W., Jr.; Friedman, M. Protective effects of glucose-6-phosphate and NADP against α-chaconine-induced developmental toxicity in *Xenopus* Embryos. *Food Chem. Toxicol.* **1995b**, *33*, 1021–1025.

Rodriguez de Sotillo, D.; Hadley, M.; Holm, E. T. Potato peel waste; stability and antioxidant activity of a freeze-dried extract. *J. Food Sci.* **1994**, *59*, 1031–1033.

Rodriguez-Saona, L. E.; Wrolstad, R. E. Influence of potato composition on chip color quality. *Am. Potato J.* **1997**, *74*, 87–106.

Schwardt, E. Changes in glycoalkaloid content in industrial treatment processes for potatoes. *Kartoffelforschung* **1982**, *4*, 48–53.

Sinden, S. L.; Deahl, K. L.; Aulenbach, B. B. Effect of glycoalkaloids and phenolics on potato flavor. *J. Food Sci.* **1976**, *41*, 520–523.

Sizer, C. E.; Maga, J. A.; Craven, C. J. Total glycoalkaloids in potatoes and potato chips. *J. Agric. Food Chem.* **1980**, *28*, 578–579.

Slanina, P. Solanine (glycoalkaloids) in potatoes: toxicological evaluation. *Food Chem. Toxicol.* **1990**, *28*, 759–761.

Smolin, L. A.; Benevenga, N. H. Methionine, homocyst(e)ine metabolic interrelationships. In *Absorption and Utilization of Amino Acids*; Friedman, M., Ed.; CRC: Boca Rato, FL, 1989; Vol. 1, pp 157–187.

Stanker, L. H.; Kampos-Holtzapple, C.; Friedman, M. Development and characterization of monoclonal antibodies that differentiate between potato and tomato glycoalkaloids. *J. Agric. Food Chem.* **1994**, *42*, 2360–2366.

Stapleton, A.; Allen, P. V.; Friedman, M.; Belknap, W. R. Purification and characterization of solanidine glucosyltransferase from the potato (*Solanum tuberosum*). *J. Agric. Food Chem.* **1991**, *39*, 1187–1203.

Stapleton, A.; Allen, P. W.; Tao, H. P.; Belknap, W. R.; Friedman, M. Partial amino acid sequence of solanidine UDP-glucose glucosyltransferase purified by anion exchange and size exclusion media. *Protein Express. Purif.* **1992**, *3*, 85–92.

Stoddard, L. M. *Glycoalkaloid Synthesis during Storage of Potatoes*. Thesis, Department of Food Science, The University of Leeds, UK, **1992.**

Swallow, A. Wholesomeness and safety of irradiated foods. In *Nutritional and Toxicological Consequences of Food Processing*; Friedman, M., Ed.; Plenum Press: New York, **1991**, pp 1–31.

Takagi, K; Toyoda, M.; Fujiyama, Y.; Saito, Y. Effect of cooking on the contents of α-chaconine and α-solanine of potatoes. *J. Food Hyg. Soc. Japan* **1990**, *31*, 67–73.

Thomas, P. Radiation preservation of foods of plant origin. Part 1. Potatoes and other tuber crops. *CRC Crit. Rev. Food Sci. Nutr.* **1984**, *19*, 327–379.

Thorne, H. V.; Clarke, G. F.; Skuce, R. The inactivation of herpes simplex virus by some *Solanaceae* glycoalkaloids. *Antiviral Res.* **1985**, *5*, 335–343.

Vazquez, A.; Gonzalez, G.; Ferreira, F.; Moyna, P.; Kenne L. Glycoalkaloids of *Solanum commersonii* Dun. ex Poir. *Euphytica* **1997**, *95*, 195–201.

Willard, M. Potato processing: past, present and future. *Am. Potato J.* **1993**, *70*, 405–418.

Wunsch, A.; Munzert, M. Effect of storage and cultivar on the distribution of glycoalkaloids in potato tuber. *Potato Res.* **1994**, *37*, 3–10.

Zhao, J.; Camire, M. E.; Bushway, R. J.; Bushway, A. A. Glycoalkaloid content and *in vitro* glycoalkaloid solubility of extruded potato peels. *J. Agric. Food Chem.* **1994**, *42,* 2570–2573.

Zimowski, J. Synthesis of γ-chaconine and γ-solanine are catalyzed in potato by two separate glycosyltransferases: UDP-glucose: solanidine glucosyltransferase and UDP-galactose: solanidine galactosyltransferase. *Acta Biochem. Polonica* **1997**, *44*, 209–214.

Zitnak, A. Photoinduction of glycoalkaloids in cured potatoes. *Am. Potato J.* **1981**, *58*, 415–421.

Zitnak, A.; Filadelfi, M. A. Estimation of taste thresholds of three potato glycoalkaloids. *J. Can. Inst. Food Sci. Technol.* **1985**, *18*, 337–339.

Zitnak, A.; Filadelfi-Keszi, M. A. Isolation of β_2-chaconine, a potato bitterness factor. *J. Food Biochem.* **1988**, *12*, 183–190.

Zobel, M.; Schilling, J. Behavior of solanine in potatoes with various preparation metods. *Z. Lebensm. Unters. Forsch.* **1964**, *124*, 327–333.

10

LYSINOALANINE IN FOOD AND IN ANTIMICROBIAL PROTEINS

Mendel Friedman

Western Regional Research Center
Agricultural Research Service, U.S. Department of Agriculture
800 Buchanan Street, Albany, California 94710

1. ABSTRACT

Heat and alkali treatment of food proteins widely used in food processing results in the formation of crosslinked amino acids such as lysinoalanine, ornithinoalanine, lanthionine, and methyl-lanthionine and concurrent racemization of L-amino acid isomers to D-analogues. The mechanism of lysinoalanine formation is a two-step process: first, hydroxide ion-catalyzed elimination of cysteine and serine residues to a dehydroalanine intermediate; second, reaction of the double bond of dehydroalanine with the ϵ-NH_2 group of lysine to form a lysinoalanine crosslink. The corresponding elimination-addition reaction of threonine produces methyl-dehydroalanine, which then reacts with the NH_2 and SH groups to form methyl-lysinoalanine and methyl-lanthionine, respectively. The crosslinked amino acids lanthionine and methyl-lanthionine are formed by analogous nucleophilic addition reactions of the SH group of cysteine to dehydroalanine and methyl-dehydroalanine, respectively. Processing conditions that favor these transformations include high pH, temperature and exposure time. Factors which minimize lysinoalanine formation include the presence of SH-containing amino acids such as cysteine, N-acetyl-cysteine, and glutathione, dephosphorylation of O-phosphoryl esters, and acylation of ϵ-NH_2 groups of lysine side chains. The presence of lysinoalanine residues along a protein chain decreases digestibility and nutritional quality in rodents but enhances nutritional quality in ruminants. Protein-bound and free lysinoalanines are reported to induce enlargement of nuclei of rat kidney cells. All of the mentioned dehydro and crosslinked amino acids also occur naturally in certain peptide and protein antibiotics. These include duramycin, cinnamycin, epidermin, subtilin and the widely used food preservative nisin. Mechanistic rationalizations are offered for the observed antimicrobial activities of these compounds in relation to their structures. The cited findings and new research to better define the chemistry and dietary and antimicrobial roles of lysinoalanine and related compounds should lead to better and safer foods.

Impact of Processing on Food Safety, edited by Jackson et al.,
Kluwer Academic / Plenum Publishers, New York, 1999.

2. INTRODUCTION

Food has been exposed to alkali and heat for preparing protein concentrates, meat analogue vegetable (soy) protein, olives, tortillas, etc.; for peeled fruits and vegetables; and for destroying microorganisms. Such treatment, however, may cause undesirable changes. These include formation of new amino acids such as lysinoalanine and lanthionine. Foods containing these crosslinked amino acids are widely consumed (Sternberg and Kim, 1977). These observations cause some concern about the nutritional quality and safety of alkali-treated foods. The chemistry leading to the formation of crosslinked amino acids during alkali treatment of proteins needs to be studied and explained. The nutritional and toxicological significance of these changes needs to be defined. Appropriate strategies to minimize or maximize these reactions need to be developed. Although the crosslinked and dehydro amino acids are unnatural amino acids formed on exposure of proteins to certain processing conditions, they also appear naturally in certain antibiotic peptides and proteins. This overview emphasizes mechanistic aspects related to (a) the factors that influence lysinoalanine formation in food proteins; (b) possible approaches to minimize lysinoalanine formation; (c) the chemistry and microbiology of crosslinked and dehydro amino acids in natural antibiotics; and (d) research needs designed to develop new antimicrobial compounds against human pathogens.

3. FACTORS GOVERNING LYSINOALANINE FORMATION

3.1. Mechanism of Lysinoalanine Formation

Figure 1 depicts a postulated mechanism of lysinoalanine formation (Asquith and Otterburn, 1977; Friedman and Noma, 1986; Patchornik and Sokolovsky, 1964). The mechanism involves a hydroxide ion-catalyzed transformation of the ϵ -NH_2 group of lysine to a lysinoalanine side chain via elimination and crosslink formation. The rate-determining second-order elimination reaction thus depends directly on the concentration of both hydroxide ions and susceptible lysine side chains. This elimination reaction generates a dehydroalanine residue whose conjugated carbon-carbon double bond then reacts with the ϵ-NH_2 of lysine to a form a lysinoalanine crosslink. This nucleophilic addition reaction is governed not only by the number of available amino groups but also by the location of the amino groups and reactive dehydroalanine groups in the protein chain.

After neighboring sites have reacted, additional lysinoalanine (or other) crosslinks form less readily. Each protein has a limited fraction of sites for forming lysinoalanine residues (Hasegawa et al., 1981). The number of such sites is dictated by the protein's size, amino acid composition, conformation, chain mobility, steric factors, and extent of ionization of reactive amino groups. In principle, two types of lysinoalanine protein crosslinks are possible: intramolecular and intermolecular. The introduction of intramolecular crosslinks leaves the molecular weight of the treated protein largely unchanged, whereas the molecular weight increases proportionately with the number of intermolecular crosslinks. Nutritional and biological properties of lysinoalanine-containing proteins are probably strongly influenced by the relative numbers of the two types of crosslinks.

Since the nucleophilic addition reaction may take place on either side of the carbon-carbon double bond of dehydroalanine, the resulting product is a mixture of L- and D-isomers (LL- and LD-lysinoalanines). Moreover, since some of the original L-lysine residues can undergo a hydroxide ion-catalyzed racemization to D-lysine before lysinoalanine for-

DISULFIDE

DEHYDROALANINE

PERSULFIDE

THIOL (ANION)

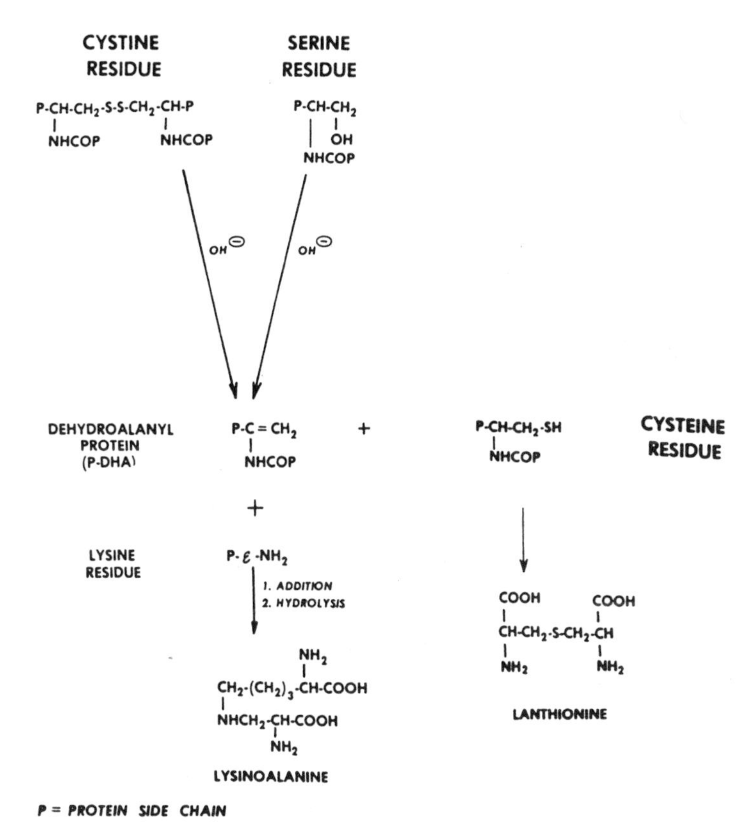

Figure 1. Top. Base-catalyzed formation of one dehydroalanine residue and one persulfide ion from a protein disulfide bond. The persulfide ion can further decompose to a cysteine anion and elemental sulfur. Bottom. Hydroxide-ion-catalyzed β-elimination reactions of cystine and serine residues to dehydroalanine, which can then react with an ϵ-NH_2 group of lysine to produce lysinoalanine and/or with an SH group of cysteine to form lanthionine.

Table 1. Effect of pH on lysinoalanine (LAL) content (mole %) of soybean protein. Conditions: 1% protein; 75° C; 3 hr

	pH								
	8	9	9.5	10	10.5	10.9	12	12.5	13.9
LAL	0	0.28	0.4	0.61	0.68	0.95	1.14	1.86	1.47

mation (Friedman and Gumbmann, 1989; Friedman and Liardon, 1985), the D-lysine can, in principle, generate two additional isomers (DD- and DL-lysinoalanines). Four lysinoalanine isomers are therefore theoretically possible: DD, DL, LD, and LL (Liardon et al., 1991; Tas and Kleipool, 1979). These have different chemical and biological properties (De Weck-Gaudard et al., 1988; Feron et al., 1977; Friedman and Pearce, 1989).

Interaction between the double bond of threonine-derived methyl dehydroalanine with the ϵ-NH_2 of lysine can, in principle, produce eight methyl-lysinoalanine isomers. The stereochemistry of these and other crosslinked amino acids is described in detail elsewhere (Friedman, 1977).

3.2. Effect of pH

Table 1 illustrates the influence of pH on lysinoalanine content of soybean proteins. The results show that lysinoalanine began to appear at pH 9 and increased continually with pH up to pH 12.5, and then decreased at pH 13.9. At the very high pH, lysinoalanine is evidently both formed and degraded. The following amino acids were also degraded or modified during the alkaline treatment of soy proteins: arginine, cystine, lysine, serine, and threonine. It should be noted that at high temperatures (100° C), lysinoalanine formation in casein begins to appear at pH 5 (Sternberg and Kim, 1977).

3.3. Effect of Reaction Time

Table 2 shows that when a 1% solution of soy protein was heated in 0.1 N NaOH (pH 12.5) at 75° C, lysinoalanine formation progressively increased for about 3 hours. Beyond that time lysinoalanine formation leveled off, then started to decrease. These results and those mentioned above for the pH-dependence of lysinoalanine formation indicate that for each protein, conditions may exist where lysinoalanine is formed as fast as it is destroyed. The nature of the lysinoalanine degradation products is not known.

3.4. Effect of Reaction Temperature

Table 3 shows that exposure of a 1% solution of soy protein at pH 12.5 for 3 hours at temperatures ranging from 25° C to 85° C caused a progressive disappearance of the fol-

Table 2. Effect of time (min) of treatment on lysinoalanine (LAL) content (mole %) of soybean protein. Conditions : 1% protein; 75° C; pH 12.5

	Time							
	10	20	40	60	120	180	300	480
LAL	0.46	0.63	1.01	1.10	1.75	2.39	2.98	2.05

Table 3. Effect of temperature (°C) on lysinoalanine (LAL), lysine, arginine, serine, and threonine content of soybean protein. Conditions: 1% protein; pH 12.5

		Temperature						
	Dialyzed control	25	35	45	55	65	75	85
LAL (mole %)	0	0.29	0.41	0.79	0.85	1.40	1.86	2.24
LAL (weight %)	0	0.69	0.81	1.04	1.64	2.64	3.66	4.13
Lysine (mole %)	5.48	5.32	5.08	4.97	4.64	4.13	3.68	3.24
Lysine (weight %)	5.54	4.91	4.88	4.63	4.29	3.72	3.46	2.86
Arginine (mole %)	5.77	5.86	5.81	5.67	5.54	5.11	4.33	3.15
Arginine (weight %)	6.96	6.49	6.52	6.29	6.11	5.48	4.86	3.30
Serine (mole %)	6.57	6.33	6.24	6.08	6.13	5.14	4.97	2.73
Serine (weight %)	4.78	4.47	4.48	4.07	4.08	3.32	2.69	1.73
Threonine (mole %)	4.12	4.49	4.32	4.29	4.16	3.87	2.92	2.56
Threonine (weight %)	3.40	3.39	3.35	3.25	3.00	2.83	2.24	1.84

lowing labile amino acids: arginine, lysine, serine, and threonine. Disappearance of arginine and lysine started at about 35° C and of serine and threonine at about 45° C. The treatment also induced the progressive loss of cystine residues (not shown) and the appearance of lysinoalanine residues. Lysinoalanine residues started to appear at 25° C (0.69 weight %) and continuously increased up to 4.13 weight % at 85° C.

The δ-amino group of ornithine, a degradation product of arginine, can react with dehydroalanine to form ornithinoalanine, which is sometimes seen in chromatograms of amino acid hydrolysates (Asquith and Otterburn, 1977). Analogous interaction of the NH_2 group of phenylethylamine, a biogenic amine present in some foods, produces phenylethylaminoalanine (Friedman and Noma, 1986).

4. INHIBITING LYSINOALANINE FORMATION

4.1. SH-Containing Amino Acids and Peptides

The double bond of dehydroalanine, which is part of an activated conjugated double-bond system, reacted 34 to 5000 times more rapidly with the SH group of cysteine in the pH range 7 to 12 than with the ε-NH_2 group of α-N-acetyl-L-lysine (Snow et al., 1976; Finley et al., 1977). In related studies, Friedman et al. (1977) showed that dehydroalanine derivatives converted lysine side chains in casein, bovine albumin, lysozyme, wool, and polylysine to lysinoalanine residues at pH 9 to 10. These studies demonstrated that lysinoalanine residues can also be introduced into a protein by chemical modification under relatively mild conditions without strong alkaline treatment. We also showed that treatment of protein SH groups with dehydroalanine transformed all of the cysteine residues to lanthionine side chains. These model studies suggested that by adding thiols such as cysteine or reduced glutathione it may be possible to competitively trap the dehydroalanine intermediate in alkali-treated proteins and thus prevent the formation of lysinoalanine residues. This expectation was realized as demonstrated in Tables 4 and 5. Structurally different SH-containing compounds partly inhibited lysinoalanine formation during alkali-treatment of proteins. The added cysteine and derivatives evidently combined at a faster rate with the double bond of dehydro- proteins (to form lanthionine crosslinks) than did the amino groups of lysine residues (to form lysinoalanine crosslinks) (Friedman, 1994).

Table 4. Effect of thiols (1 mM) on the lysinoalanine content (mole %) of alkali-treated soybean proteins. Conditions: 1% protein; pH 12.5; 65° C; 3 hr

SH-compound	Lysinoalanine
None	1. 09
L-cysteine	0.36
N-acetyl-L-cysteine	0.38
Reduced glutathione	0.38
DL-penicillamine	0.60

Our studies (Masri and Friedman, 1982) also revealed the presence of significant amounts of dehydroalanine residues in alkali-treated casein (Table 6). To demonstrate this result, we developed a procedure for detecting dehydroalanine residues in alkali-treated proteins based on the formation of S-β-(2-pyridylethyl) cysteine (2-PEC) from protein dehydroalanine side chains and added 2-mercaptoethylpyridine. The 2-PEC along with all other amino acids can be assayed after acid protein hydrolysis by ion exchange chromatography (Friedman et al., 1979, 1980).

4.2. Sodium Sulfite

Table 6 shows the lysinoalanine, lanthionine, and lysine content of four proteins exposed to pH 11.6 in the absence and presence of sodium sulfite (Friedman, 1977). The data show that the amount of lysinoalanine formed under similar conditions varied greatly among the four proteins tested and that the presence of sodium sulfite resulted in significant decreases in the lysinoalanine content. The reduction for casein was 55%, for wool 68%, for lysozyme 73%, and for bovine trypsin inhibitor 84%. Comparison of these results with those listed in Tables 4 and 5 indicates that sulfite ions may be more effective in inhibiting lysinoalanine formation than are sulfhydryl compounds such as cysteine. Significant amounts of lanthionine were found only on amino acid chromatograms of alkali-treated wool. Sodium sulfite completely prevented lanthionine formation.

Sulfite ions probably prevent lysinoalanine formation by the following mechanisms: suppressing dehydroalanine formation and/or trapping dehydroalanine. First, by cleaving protein disulfide bonds, the added sulfite ions can diminish a potential source of dehydroalanine, since cystine residues would be expected to undergo β-elimination reactions more readily than negative charged cysteine ($P\text{-}S^-$) or sulfo-cysteine ($P\text{-}S\text{-}SO^-$) protein side

Table 5. Lysinoalanine content (g/16 g N) of casein and soy protein isolates prepared in the absence and presence of L-cysteine[a]

Protein source	Protein isolate	Lysinoalanine
Commercial soy isolate		0.027
Soy flour	soy isolate	0.087
Soy flour plus cysteine	soy isolate	0.001
Commercial sodium caseinate		0.21
Skim milk	sodium caseinate	0.160
Skim milk plus cysteine	sodium caseinate	0.006

[a]Adapted from Finley et al., (1977).

Table 6. Dehydroalanine content of alkali-treated casein and acetylated casein[a]. Conditions: 1% proteins; pH 12.5; 70°C; 3 hr

Protein	Dehydroalanine (g/16 g N)
Casein, untreated	0
Acetylated casein	0
Casein, alkali-treated	0.33
Acetylated casein, alkali-treated	1.39

[a] Adapted from Masri and Friedman (1982).

chains produced by sulfite ion-catalyzed cleavage of protein disulfide bonds (Friedman, 1994; Friedman and Gumbmann, 1986). Second, since sulfite ions also inhibit lysinoalanine formation in casein which has no cystine residues, sulfite ions also probably trap dehydroalanine residues by nucleophilic addition to their double bonds, as mentioned earlier for SH groups of thiols. The presence of thiols and sulfites during alkali-treatment of soy proteins affects their rheological properties and spinnability (Katsuta and Hayakawa, 1984).

4.3. Dephosphorylation of Proteins

In addition to disulfide bonds of cystine residues and hydroxyl groups of serine and threonine residues, O-glycosyl and O-phosphoryl groups of glycoproteins (e.g., antifreeze protein) and phosphorylated proteins (e.g., phosphitin) also undergo hydroxide ion-induced β-elimination reactions to form dehydroalanine residues (Whitaker and Feeney, 1977). Meyer et al. (1981) found that the amount of lysinoalanine produced from enzymatically dephosphorylated casein was significantly less than from native casein with intact phosphate esters. This finding can be rationalized by postulating a more rapid elimination of the phosphoryl groups from native casein to form dehydroalanine than of the hydroxyl groups of serine residues from dephosphorylated casein. It is also worth noting that phosphate salts facilitate lysinoalanine formation in wool (Touloupis and Vassiliadis, 1977).

Table 7. Effect of sodium sulfite on lysinoalanine, lanthionine, and lysine content (μmoles/g) of proteins treated at pH 11.6. Conditions: 60° C; 3 hr[a]

Protein	Lysinoalanine	Lanthionine	Lysine
Casein, untreated	0	0	482.7
Casein, pH 11.6	145.2	0	294.0
Casein, pH 11.6, Na_2SO_3	65.7	0	373.0
Lysozyme, untreated	0	0	397.3
Lysozyme, pH 11.6	135.2	0	222.2
Lysozyme, pH 11.6, Na_2SO_3	35.6	0	317.2
Bovine trypsin inhibitor, untreated	0	0	319.3
Bovine trypsin inhibitor, pH 11.6	235.1	0	129.2
Bovine trypsin inhibitor, pH 11.6, Na_2SO_3	36.8	0	239.0
Wool, untreated	0	0	222.5
Wool, pH 11.6	58.7	119.5	139.0
Wool, pH 11.6, Na_2SO_3	19.1	0	176.9

[a] Adapted from Friedman (1977).

4.4. Modification of Protein Amino Groups

Since formation of lysinoalanine from lysine requires the participation of an ϵ-NH_2 group of a lysine side chain, modification of amino groups by, for example, acetylation or peptide bond formation should reduce lysinoalanine formation if the protected amino groups survived the alkali treatment. This turned out to be the case since our studies revealed that acetylation (with acetic anhydride) of soybean and wheat proteins minimized or prevented lysinoalanine formation (Friedman, 1978; Friedman et al., 1984). The nutritional quality (protein efficiency ratios (PER) and nitrogen digestibilities) of native and acetylated soy proteins was the same. These findings imply that prior acetylation of a protein's amino groups should reduce or prevent or minimize lysinoalanine formation. Modification of the ϵ-amino group of lysine through peptide bond formation can also minimize nonenzymatic browning during food processing (Friedman, 1996a; Friedman and Finot, 1990).

5. NUTRITION AND SAFETY

5.1. Nutritional Quality

The nutritional quality of any protein depends on amino acid composition, digestibility, and utilization of the released amino acids (Friedman, 1996b). Alkali-treated proteins have less digestibility and bioavailability as compared to untreated proteins (Van Beek et al., 1974). For example, Friedman et al. (1981) demonstrated an inverse relationship between lysinoalanine content of casein and extent of *in vitro* proteolysis by trypsin.

The biological utilization of lysinoalanine as a source of lysine was determined in a growth assay in weanling male mice in which all lysine in a synthetic amino acid diet was replaced by a molar equivalent of lysinoalanine (Friedman et al., 1982a). The replacement produced an amount of weight gain equivalent to that expected from a diet containing 0.05% L-lysine. On a molecular equivalent basis, lysinoalanine was 3.8% as potent as lysine in supporting weight gain in mice. Robbins et al. (1980) reported that lysinoalanine is completely unavailable as a source of lysine to the rat although it is 37% available to the chick.

Generally, the extent of nutritional damage of alkali-treatment associated with loss of lysine may depend on the original lysine content of a protein. Thus, a partial decrease in lysine content due to lysinoalanine formation in a high-lysine protein such as soy protein or casein may have a less adverse effect than in a low-lysine protein such as wheat gluten, where lysine is a nutritionally limiting amino acid.

In contrast, the lower digestibility of lysinoalanine-containing proteins reduces the rate of degradation of the modified proteins in the rumen of cattle by bacterial enzymes (Nishino and Uchida, 1995). Such reduction is beneficial for ruminant nutrition since it improves nitrogen retention and the nutritional quality of the proteins consumed by cattle and sheep (Friedman et al., 1982b).

5.2. Antigenicity

Since soybean proteins are often processed under alkaline conditions, we evaluated the influence of pH in the range 8 to 12.5 on the antigenic activity of the Kunitz soybean trypsin inhibitor (KTI) using an immunoassay (ELISA) (Brandon et al., 1988, 1989; Friedman et al., 1989). The set of titration curves in Figure 2 suggests that antigenic, functional,

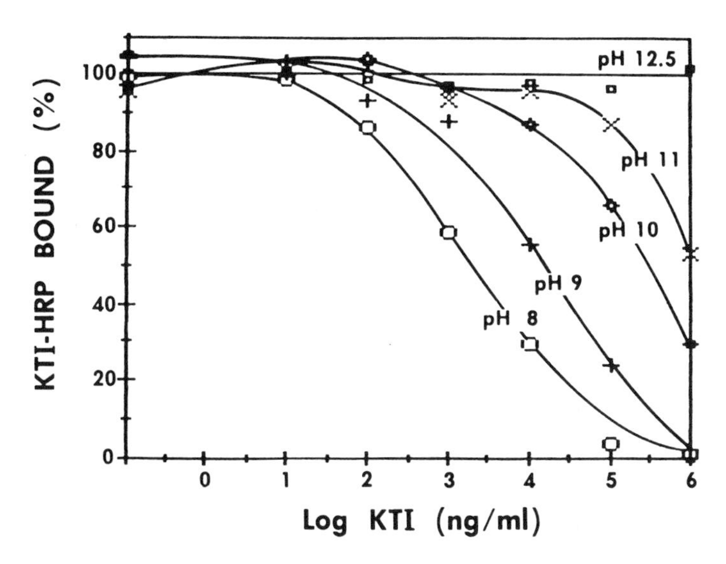

Figure 2. ELISA of the Kunitz soybean trypsin inhibitor (KTI) exposed at 65°C to solutions of increasing pH (Brandon et al., 1988, 1989; Friedman et al., 1989).

and structural changes in KTI progressively increased with pH. These observations and related studies with heat-treated proteins imply that an ELISA test can be used to follow inactivation of KTI and the soybean Bowman-Birk Inhibitor (BBI) during food processing and possibly also the allergenicity and immunotoxicity of food proteins. Although we did not measure the lysinoalanine content of the KTI samples, the trend in lysinoalanine content as a function of pH probably parallels that for the soy protein isolate shown in Table 1.

5.3. Nephrocytomegaly

Feeding alkali-treated proteins to rats induces changes in kidney cells. These changes are characterized by enlargement of the nucleus and cytoplasm and disturbances in DNA synthesis and mitosis. These lesions, which have been attributed to lysinoalanine (Gould and MacGregor, 1977; Karayiannis et al., 1979; Woodard et al., 1975), are designated as nephrocytomegaly (karyomegaly). The affected cells are epithelial cells of the straight portion (*pars recta*) of the proximal renal tubules. Renal cytomegaly is also induced by feeding rats synthetic lysinoalanine.

These observations were confirmed by Kolonkaya (1986) who fed rats a commercial soy protein diet containing a small amount of lysinoalanine. The renal tubular epithelial kidney cells of all animals increased in both size and in DNA content. Necrosis of the cells was characterized by cytoplasmic edema and vacuolization, loss of microvilli, and increased lysosomal and cytoplasmic inclusions.

Lysinoalanine has been found to be a sensitive indicator of heat damage of commercial milk-based infant formulas (Pompei et al., 1987). It is also reported to be a useful marker for distinguishing natural from imitation cheeses (Pellegrino et al., 1996; Pearce et al., 1988). Although infant milk formulas contain up to 300 ppm of lysinoalanine (Antilla, 1987), Langhendries et al. (1992) found that short-term feeding of lysinoalanine- and Maillard product-containing formulas to healthy preterm babies did not appear to induce tubular kidney damage, as determined by urinary excretion of four kidney-derived enzymes. However, the formula diets did induce a general increase in urinary microprotein levels. The authors conclude that the 10-day feeding study may be too short to cause significant changes in renal function. Whether the described histological changes in kidney tissues lesions are species-specific to rats is not known.

5.4. Metal Ion Chelation

Because the structure of lysinoalanine contains two amino, one imino, and two carboxyl groups which can serve as potential metal ion chelating sites (Friedman, 1974), I suggested that some of the biological properties of the molecule may be due to metal ion chelation (Friedman, 1977). This prediction was later confirmed by several investigators (Hayashi, 1982; Friedman et al., 1986; Furniss et al., 1985, 1989; Rehner and Walter, 1991; Sarwar et al., this volume). To further demonstrate this possibility, we have examined lysinoalanine (a mixture of the LD and LL isomers as well as the individual isomers) for its affinity towards a series of metal ions, of which copper (II) was chelated the most strongly. On this basis, we have suggested a possible mechanism for kidney damage in the rat involving lysinoalanine interaction with copper within the epithelial cells of the proximal tubules.

As described in detail elsewhere (Pearce and Friedman, 1988; Friedman and Pearce, 1989), it is possible to predict the *in vivo* equilibria between histidine, the major low-molecular weight copper carrier in plasma, and competing chelating agents such as lysinoalanine. A mathematical analysis was used to calculate predicted lysinoalanine plasma levels needed to displace histidine as the major copper carrier *in vivo*. The calculated values were: 27 μM for LD-LAL, 100 μM for LL-LAL, and 49 μM for the mixture of the two.

These considerations suggest that LD-lysinoalanine would be a better competitor for copper (II) *in vivo* than the LL-isomer, i.e., it will take about one fourth as much LD-LAL as LL-LAL to displace the same amount of histidine from copper-histidine. This difference could explain the greater observed toxicity of LD-LAL (Feron et al., 1977). The apparent direct relationship between the observed affinities of the two LAL isomers for copper (II) ions *in vitro* and their relative toxicities in the rat kidney is consistent with our suggestions that LAL exerts some of its biological effects through chelation to copper and other metal ions in body fluids and tissues.

6. ANTIMICROBIAL COMPOUNDS

Lysinoalanine, lanthionine, methyl-lanthionine, dehydroalanine, and methyl-dehydroalanine are not formed only chemically during food processing, but also naturally as a result of enzyme-catalyzed post-translational modifications during the biosynthesis of certain antimicrobial compounds (Gross, 1977). These include cinnamycin, duramycin, nisin, and subtilin. Because some of these antibiotics are widely used in food preservation, this aspect is also relevant to an assessment of the role of crosslinked and dehydro amino acids in the diet, especially in relation to food safety. This section (a) briefly reviews the chemistry of the antimicrobial compounds; (b) discusses possible mechanisms of the antimicrobial effects in relation to the structures of the antibiotics; (c) describes proposed mechanisms for antimicrobial activities of related processing-induced Maillard (browning) products derived from amino acid-carbohydrate reactions; and (d) proposes new research to assess the possible value of lysinoalanine-containing peptides and proteins as antimicrobial agents for human pathogen reduction.

6.1. Natural Peptide Antibiotics

The following is a brief review of the literature on lantibiotics, small protein antibiotics which are produced by and primarily act on gram-positive bacteria (Jung, 1991; Liu and Hansen, 1993, 1993; Kaletta et al., 1991; Morris et al., 1984; Sahl et al., 1995; Zimmermann et al., 1993).

a. The structures of these compounds contain intra-molecular rings formed by lanthionine, methyl-lanthionine, and lysinoalanine, as well as the dehydrated amino acids 2,3-didehydroalanine (dehydroalanine) and 2,3-didehydrobutyrine (methyl-dehydroalanine (Figure 3).
b. Dehydroalanine and methyl-dehydroalanine are formed by enzyme-catalyzed site-specific dehydration of serine and threonine residues, respectively; lanthionine is formed by addition of the SH group of a neighboring cysteine residue to the double bond of dehydroalanine; the corresponding addition to methyl-dehydroalanine produces methyl-lanthionine; lysinoalanine is generated from the nucleophilic addition of an ϵ-NH_2 group of a neighboring lysine to dehydroalanine.
c. The crosslinked bridges may stabilize the spatial structures of the antibiotics and the dehydroamino acids may act as alkylating agents of essential functional groups of the bacterial cells.
d. The mechanism of antimicrobial action appears to involve (1) interference with energy transduction (depolarization) of membranes, which results in formation of membrane channels through which low-molecular weight compounds of bacterial cells may pass; (2) aggregation of the lipid components of vesicles such as lysophosphatidylethanolamine, enhancing permeability and causing hemolysis of the vesicles; and (4) alkylation of SH groups of membrane proteins and enzymes by the dehydroalanines. NMR studies (Hosoda et al., 1996; Wakamatsu et al., 1990) suggest that the imino (NH) group of lysinoalanine probably binds to the phosphate group of the lipid during complex formation.

6.2. Antibiotic Maillard Browning Products

Some amino acid-carbohydrate and amino acid-quinone nonenzymatic and enzymatic browning reaction products formed during food processing are also reported to have antimicrobial properties (Friedman, 1996a, 1997). These have been extensively evaluated by Einarsson (1987) and Einarsson et al. (1983, 1988). The following is a brief summary of some of their findings.

Examination of the effectiveness of the test compounds against 20 strains of pathogenic and spoilage organisms present in foods showed that (a) gram-positive *Bacillus subtilis* and *Staphylococcus* strains were strongly inhibited; (b) the susceptibility to inhibition of different *Escherichia coli* strains varied markedly; and (d) gram-negative enterobacteria *Salmonella* strains were not inhibited to any great extent.

Potential targets for the action of the antimicrobial compounds include cellular membranes, bacterial enzymes, and genetic material. The evidence supports the involvement of all three targets. First, the Maillard products act as iron chelating agents that influence the solubility and availability of this important trace element. Second, because iron in bacterial cells is a cofactor in enzymes involved in metabolism of oxygen, the presence of the inhibitors also inhibits oxygen uptake. Third, the inhibitors may alter energy metabolism by preventing uptake of glucose and serine. Fourth, the ability of the inhibitors to precipitate proteins suggests another pathway for the inhibition of bacterial growth.

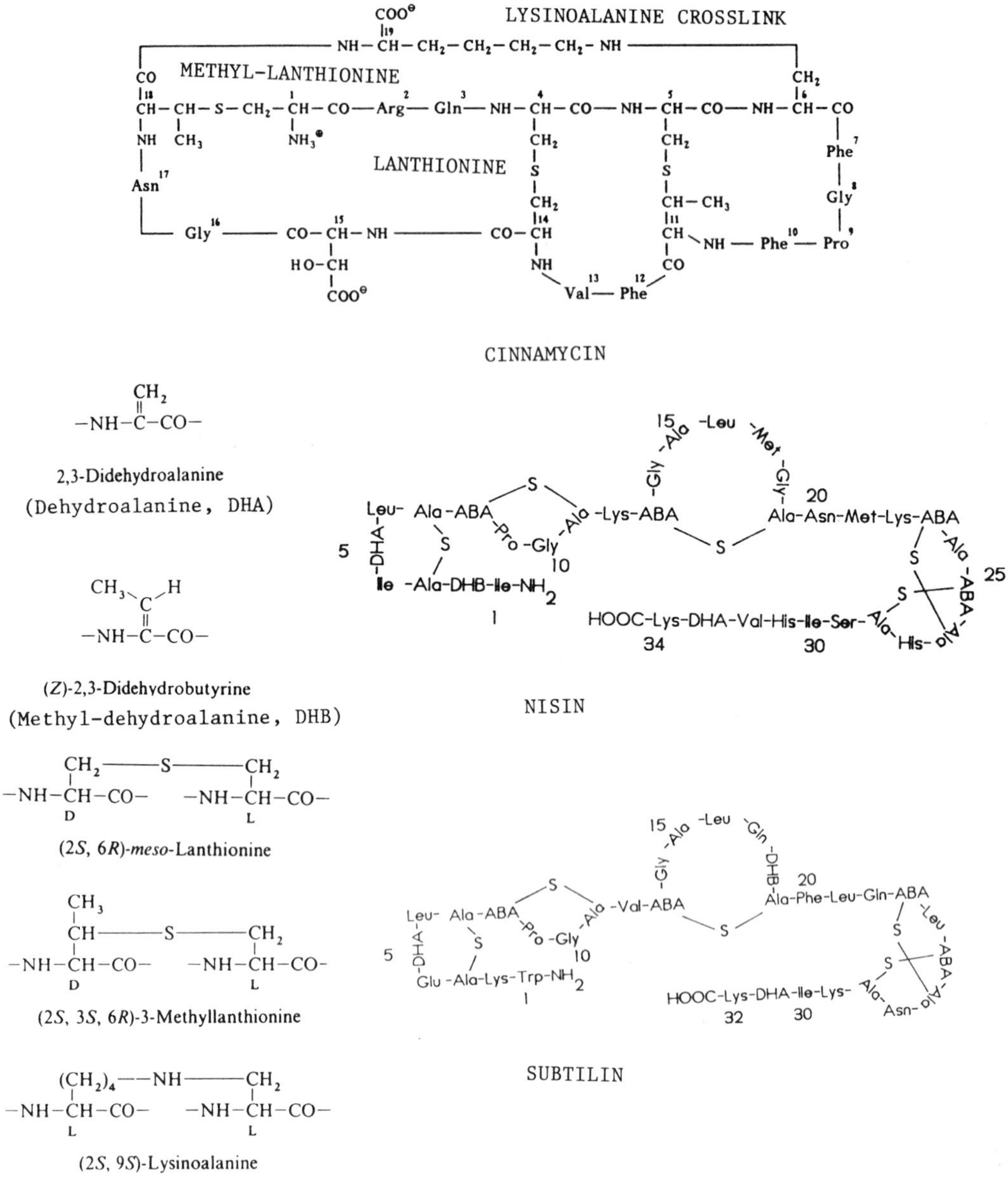

LYSINOALANINE CROSSLINK

METHYL-LANTHIONINE

LANTHIONINE

CINNAMYCIN

2,3-Didehydroalanine
(Dehydroalanine, DHA)

(*Z*)-2,3-Didehydrobutyrine
(Methyl-dehydroalanine, DHB)

(2*S*, 6*R*)-*meso*-Lanthionine

(2*S*, 3*S*, 6*R*)-3-Methyllanthionine

(2*S*, 9*S*)-Lysinoalanine

NISIN

SUBTILIN

Figure 3. Structures of peptide antibiotics containing the unusual amino acids dehydroalanine, methyl-dehydroalanine, lanthionine, methyl-lanthionine, and lysinoalanine (Gross, 1977; Jung, 1991; Kaletta et al., 1993; Liu and Hansen, 1993).

To what extent each of these inhibition mechanisms operate individually, additively, and/or synergistically in different microorganisms is not known.

6.3. Research Needs

Since, as mentioned earlier, lysinoalanine has a strong affinity for essential metal ions such as cobalt, copper, iron, and zinc, it is quite possible that metal-ion chelation by lysinoalanine-containing antibiotics such as cinnamycin and duramycin and by the browning products contributes to the antimicrobial activity. Another possibility is that in addition to SH groups, other functional groups of bacterial cell membranes such NH_2 and NH groups associated with proteins and with DNA may also be alkylated by the dehydroalanines of the antibiotics. These considerations also suggest that free lysinoalanine and lysinoalanine-containing peptides and food proteins may also possess antimicrobial properties. These possibilities merit study.

7. CONCLUSIONS

Commercial and home processing of foods employ heat, radiation, sunlight, ultraviolet light, acids, alkali, oxidizing and reducing agents, and combinations of these. The purpose of such treatments is to make food edible, to alter texture and flavor, to destroy toxins, and to kill microorganisms. One by-product of such treatments may be the occasional formation of undesirable new amino acid- and protein-derived food ingredients such as lysinoalanine. An important objective of research in food science is to more fully understand the underlying chemistry and the resulting nutritional and toxicological consequences of such changes in order to optimize processing parameters which minimize adverse effects and maximize beneficial ones. Understanding food processing conditions that govern lysinoalanine formation makes it possible to minimize or maximize the lysinoalanine content of foods and feeds depending on dietary needs. It may also facilitate the development of new lysinoalanine-, lanthionine-, and dehydroamino acid- containing antimicrobial peptides effective against human pathogens for the benefit of food safety and health.

REFERENCES

Antilla, P. The formation and determination of lysinoalanine in foods containing milk proteins. *Meijerritierteellinen-Aikakauskirja* **1987**, *45*, 1-12. [Finnish]

Asquith, R. S.; Otterburn, M. S. Cystine-alkali reactions in relation to protein crosslinking. *Adv. Exp. Med. Biol.* **1977**, *86B*, 93-121.

Brandon, D. L.; Bates, A. H.; Friedman, M. Enzyme-linked immunosorbent assay of soybean Kunitz trypsin inhibitor using monoclonal antibodies. *J. Food Sci.* **1988**, *53*, 97-101.

Brandon, D. L.; Bates, A. H.; Friedman, M. Monoclonal antibody-based immunoassay of Bowman-Birk protease inhibitor of soybeans. *J. Agric. Food Chem.* **1989**, *37*, 1192-1196.

De Weck-Gaudard, D.; Liardon, R.; Finot, P. A. Stereomeric composition of urinary lysinoalanine after ingestion of free or protein-bound lysinoalanine in rats. *J. Agric. Food Chem.* **1988**, *36*, 717-721.

Einarsson, H. The effect of pH and temperature on the antibacterial effect of Maillard reaction products. *Lebensm. Wiss. Technol.* **1987**, *20*, 56-58.

Einarsson, H.; Goran Snygg, B. G.; Eriksson, C. Inhibition of bacterial growth by Maillard reaction products. *J. Agric. Food Chem.* **1983**, *31*, 1043-1047.

Einarsson, H.; Eklund, T.; Nes, I. F. Inhibitory mechanisms of Maillard reaction products against bacteria. *Microbios* **1988**, *53*, 27-36.

Feron, V. J.; van Beek, L.; Slump, P.; Beems, R. B. Toxicological aspects of alkali-treatment of food proteins. In *Biological Aspects of New Protein Foods*; Alder Nissen, J., Ed.; Pergamon: Oxford, England, **1977**.

Finley, J. W.; Snow, J. T.; Johnston, P. H.; Friedman, M. Inhibition of lysinoalanine formation in food proteins. *J. Food Sci.* **1978**, *43*, 619-621.

Friedman, M., Ed. *Protein-Metal Interactions*. Plenum Press, New York, **1974**.

Friedman, M. Crosslinked amino acids -- stereochemistry and nomenclature. In *Protein Crosslinking : Nutritional and Medical* Consequences; Friedman, M. Ed., Plenum Press, New Yor. Adv. *Exp. Med. Biol.* **1977**, *86B*, 1-27.

Friedman, M. Inhibition of lysinoalanine synthesis by protein acylation. In *Nutritional Improvement of Food and Feed Proteins*; Friedman, M., Ed.; Plenum Press: New York. *Adv. Exp. Med. Biol.* **1978**, *105*, 613-648.

Friedman, M. Improvement in the safety of foods by SH-containing amino acids and peptides. *J. Agric. Food Chem.* **1994**, *42*, 3-20.

Friedman, M. Food browning and its prevention. *J. Agric. Food Chem.* **1996a**, *44*, 631-653.

Friedman, M. Nutritional value of proteins from different food sources. *J. Agric. Food Chem.* **1996b**, *44*, 6-29.

Friedman, M. Chemistry, biochemistry, and dietary role of potato polyphenols. *J. Agric.Food Chem.* **1997**, *45*, 1523-1540.

Friedman, M.; Finot, P. A. Nutritional improvement of bread with lysine and γ-glutamyl-lysine. *J. Agric. Food Chem.* **1990**, *38*, 2011-2020.

Friedman, M.; Gumbmann, M. R. Nutritional improvement of soy flour through inactivation of trypsin inhibitors by sodium sulfite. *J. Food Sci.* **1986**, *51*, 1239-1241.

Friedman, M.; Gumbmann, M. R. Dietary significance of D-amino acids. In *Absorption and Utilization of Amino Acids*. Friedman, M., Ed.; CRC Press; Boca Raton, FL, **1989**, Vol. 2, pp. 173-190.

Friedman, M., ; Liardon, R. Racemization kinetics of amino acid residues in alkali-treated food proteins. *J. Agric. Food Chem.* **1985**, *33*, 666-672.

Friedman, M.; Noma, A. T. Formation and analysis of phenylethylaminoalanine in food proteins. *J. Agric. Food Chem.* **1986**, 497-502.

Friedman, M.; Pearce, K. N. Copper (II) and cobalt (II) affinities of LL- and LD-lysinoalanine diastereoisomers: implications for food safety and nutrition. *J. Agric. Food Chem.* **1989**, *37*, 123-127.

Friedman, M.; Finley, J. W.; Yeh, Lai-Sue. Reactions of proteins with dehydroalanine. *Adv. Exp. Med. Biol.* **1977**, *86B*, 213-224.

Friedman, M.; Noma, A. T.; Wagner, J. R. Ion-exchange chromatography of sulfur amino acids on a single-column amino acid analyzer. *Analyt. Biochem.* **1979**, *98*, 293-304.

Friedman, M.; Zahnley, J. C.; Wagner, J. R. Estimation of the disulfide content of trypsin inhibitors as S-β-(pyridylethyl)-L-cysteine. *Analyt. Biochem.* **1980**, *106*, 27-34.

Friedman, M.; Zahnley, J. C.; Masters, P. M. Relationship between *in vitro* digestibility of casein and its content of lysinoalanine and D-amino acids. *J. Food Sci.* **1981**, *46*, 127-131.

Friedman, M.; Gumbmann, M. R.; Savoie, L. The nutritional value of lysinoalanine as a source of lysine. *Nutr. Rep. Int.* **1982a**, *26*, 937-943.

Friedman, M.; Diamond, M. J.; Broderick, G. L. Dimethylolurea as a tyrosine reagent and protein protectant against ruminal degradation. *J. Agric. Food Chem.* **1982b**, *30*, 72-77.

Friedman, M.; Levin, C. E.; Noma, A. T. Factors governing lysinoalanine formation in soybean proteins. *J. Food Sci.* **1984**, *49*, 1282-1288.

Friedman, M.; Grosjean, O. K.; Zahnley, J. C. Inactivation of metalloenzymes by food constituents. *Food Chem. Toxicol.* **1986**, *24*, 497-502.

Friedman, M.; Gumbmann, M. R.; Brandon, D. L.; Bates, A. H. Inactivation and analysis of soybean inhibitors of digestive enzymes. In *Food Proteins*; Kinsella, J. E.; Soucie, W. G., Eds.; The American Oil Chemists' Society, Champaign: Illinois, 1989; pp 296-328.

Furniss, D. E.; Hurrell, R. F.; De Weck, D.; Finot, P. A. The effect of lysinoalanine and N-ϵ-fructose lysine on kidney, liver and urine trace elements in the rat. In *Trace Elements in Man and Animals*; Mills, C. F.; Bremmer, I.; Chesters, J. K., Eds.; Commonwealth Agricultural Bureau: Slough, U. K. **1985**.

Furniss, D. E.; Vuichoud, J.; Finot, P. A.; Hurrell, R. F. The effect of Maillard reaction products on zinc metabolism in the rat. *Br. J. Nutr.* **1989**, *62*, 739-749.

Gross, E. α , β-Unsaturated amino acids in peptides and proteins. In *Protein Crosslinking: Biochemical and Molecular* Aspects; Friedman, M., Ed.; Plenum Press: New York. *Adv. Exp. Med. Biol.* **1977**, *86A*, 131-153.

Gould, D. H.; MacGregor, J.. T Biological effects of alkali-treated protein and lysinoalanine: an overview. *Adv. Exp. Med. Biol.* **1977**, *86B*, 29-48.

Hasegawa, K.; Okamoto, N.; Ozawa, H.; Kitajima, S; Takado, Y. Limits and sites of lysinoalanine formation in lysozyme, α-lactalbumin and α_{s1}- and β-caseins by alkali treatment. *Agric. Biol. Chem.* **1981**, *45*, 1645-1651.

Hayashi, R. Lysinoalanine as a metal ion chelator. An implication for toxicity. *J. Biol. Chem.* **1982**, *45*, 1430-1431.

Hosoda, K.; Ohya, M.; Kohno, T.; Maeda, T.; Endo, S.; Wakamatsu, K. Structure determination of an immunopotentiator peptide, cinnamycin, complexed with lysophosphatidylethanolamine by ^{1}H-NMR. *J. Biochem.* **1996**, 226-230.

Jung, G. Lantibiotics - ribosomally synthesized biologically active polypeptides containing sulfide bridges and α, β-didehydroamino acids. *Angew. Chem. Engl. Ed.* **1991**, *30*, 1051-1068.

Kaletta, C.; Entian, K. D.; Jung, G. Prepeptide sequence of cinnamycin: the first structural gene of a duramycin-type lantibiotic. *Eur. J. Biochem.* **1991**, *199*, 411-415.

Karayiannis, N. I.; MacGregor, J. T.; Bjeldanes, L. F. Biological effects of alkali-treated soy protein and lactalbumin in the rat and mouse. *Food Cosmet. Toxicol.* **1979**, *17*, 585-590.

Katsuta, K.; Hayakawa, I. Effects of reducing agents on rheological properties, inhibition of lysinoalanine formation, and spinnability of soy protein fibers. *Agric. Biol. Chem.* **1984**, *48*, 2927-2933.

Kolonkaya, D. Renal toxicity of soybean protein containing lysinoalanine. *DOGA TU Bio D.* **1986**, 394-402. [Turkish]

Langhendries, J. P.; Hurrell, R. F.; Furniss, D. E.; Hirschenhuber, C.; Finot, P. A.; Bernard, A.; Battisti, O.; Bertrand, J. M.; Senterre, J. Maillard reaction products and lysinoalanine: urinary excretion and the effects on kidney function of preterm infants fed heat-processed milk formula. *J. Pediatric Gastroentorol. Nutr.* **1992**, *14*, 62-70.

Liardon, R.; Friedman, M; Philippossian, G. Racemization kinetics of free and protein bound lysinoalanine (LAL) in strong acid media. Isomeric composition of protein bound LAL. *J. Agric. Food Chem.* **1991**, *39*, 531-537.

Liu, W.; Hansen, J. N. The antimicrobial effects of a structural variant of subtilin against outgrowing *Bacillus cereus* T spores and vegetative cells occurs by different mechanisms. *Appl. Env. Microbiol.* **1993**, *59*, 648-651.

Masri, M. S.; Friedman, M. Transformation of dehydroalanine to S-β-(2-pyridylethyl)-L-cysteine side chains. *Biochem. Biophys. Res. Commun.* **1982**, *104*, 321-325.

Meyer, M.; Klostermeyer, H.; Kleyn, D. H. Reduced formation of lysinoalanine in enzymatically dephosphorylated casein. *Z. Lebensm.-Untersuch. Forsch.* **1981,** *172*, 446-448.

Morris, S.; Walsh, R. C.; Hansen, J. N. Identification and characterization of some bacterial membrane sulfhydryl groups which are targets of bacteriostatic and antibiotic action. *J. Biol. Chem.* **1984**, *259*, 13590-13594.

Nishino, N.; Uchida, S. Formation of lysinoalanine following alkaline processing of soya bean meal in relation to the degradability of protein in the rumen. *J. Sci. Food Agric.* **1995**, *68*, 59-64.

Patchornik, A.; Sokolovsky, M. Chemical interaction between lysine and dehydroalanine in modified bovine pancreatic ribonuclease. *J. Am. chem. Soc.* **1964**, *86*, 1860-1861.

Pearce, K. N.; Friedman, M. The binding of copper and other metal ions by lysinoalanine and related compounds. *J. Agric. Food Chem.* **1988**, *36*, 707-717.

Pearce, K. N.; Karahalios, D.; Friedman, M. Ninhydrin assay for proteolysis in ripening cheese. *J. Food Sci.* **1988**, *52*, 432-435.

Pellegrino, L.; Resmini, P.; DeNoni, I.; Masotti, F. Sensitive determination of lysinoalanine for distinguishing natural from imitation mozzarella cheese. *J. Dairy Sci.* **1996,** *79*, 725-734.

Pompei, C.; Rossi, M.; Mare, F. Protein quality in commercial milk-based infant formulas. *J. Food Quality* **1987**, *10*, 375-391.

Rehner, G.; Walter, T. H. Effect of Maillard products and lysinoalanine on the bioavailability of iron, copper and zinc. *Z. Ernahrungswiss.* **1991**, *30*, 50-55.

Robbins, K. R.; Baker, D. H.; Finley, J. W. Studies on the utilization of lysinoalanine and lanthionine. *J. Nutr.* **1980**, *110*, 907-914.

Sahl, H. G.; Jack, R. W.; Bierbaum, G. Biosynthesis and biological activities of lantibiotics with unique post-translational modifications. *Eur. J. Biochem.* **1995**, *230*, 827-853.

Snow, J. T.; Finley, J. W.; Friedman, M. Relative reactivities of sulfhydryl groups with N-acetyl dehydroalanine and N-acetyl dehydroalanine methyl ester. *Int. J. Peptide Protein Res.* **1976**, *7*, 461-466.

Sternberg, M.; Kim, C. Y. Lysinoalanine formation in protein food ingredients. *Adv. Exp. Med. Biol.* **1977**, *86B*, 73-84.

Tas, A. C.; Kleipool, R. J. C. The stereoisomers of lysinoalanine. *Lebensm. Wiss. Technol.* **1979**, *9*, 360-363.

Touloupis, C.; Vassiliadis, A. Lysinoalanine formation in wool after treatments with some phosphate salts. *Adv. Exp. Med. Biol.* **1977**, *86B*, 187-195.

Van Beek, L.; Feron, V. J.; de Groot, A. P. Nutritional effects of alkali-treated soy protein in rats. *J. Nutr.* **1974**, *104*, 1630-1634.

Wakamatsu, K.; Choung, S. Y.; Kobayashi, T.; Inoue, K.; Higashijima, T.; Miyazawa, T. Complex formation of peptide antibiotic RoO9-098 with lysophosphatidylethanolamine. ^{1}H NMR analysis in dimethyl sulfoxide solution. *Biochemistry* **1990**, *29*, 113-118.

Whitaker, J. R.; Feeney, R. E. Behavior of O-glycosyl and O-phosphoryl proteins in alkaline solution. *Adv. Exp. Med. Biol.* **1977**, *86B*, 155-175.

Woodard, J. C.; Short, D. D.; Alvarez, M. R.; Reyniers, J. Biologic effects of lysinoalanine. In *Protein Nutritional Quality of Foods and Feeds*; Friedman, M., Ed.; Marcel Dekker: New York, 1975; pp 595-616.

Zimmermann, N.; Freund, S.; Fredenhagen, A.; Jung, G. Solution structure of lantibiotics duramycin B and C. *Eur. J. Biochem.* **1993**, *216*, 419-428.

11

INFLUENCE OF FEEDING ALKALINE/HEAT PROCESSED PROTEINS ON GROWTH AND PROTEIN AND MINERAL STATUS OF RATS

G. Sarwar,[1] M. R. L'Abbé,[1] K. Trick,[1] H. G. Botting,[1] and C. Y. Ma[2*]

[1]Nutrition Research Division, Health Protection Branch, Health Canada
Banting Research Building (AL:2203C)
Tunney's Pasture, Ottawa, Ontario Canada K1A OL2
[2]Centre for Food and Animal Research, Agriculture and Agri-Food Canada
Ottawa, Ontario Canada K1A 0C6

1. ABSTRACT

Effects of feeding alkaline (0.1 N NaOH) and heat treated (75° C for 3 h) proteins (lactalbumin and soybean protein isolate, SPI) on growth, and protein and mineral status of rats have been determined. The untreated and alkaline/heat treated lactalbumin contained 0.10 and 4.42 g lysinoalanine (LAL)/100 g protein, respectively. Similarly, the untreated and treated SPI contained 0.03 and 1.94 g LAL/100 g protein, respectively. The formation of LAL in the treated proteins was accompanied with a loss of cystine (73–77%), threonine (35–45%), serine (18–30%) and lysine (19–20%). The alkaline/heat treatments caused significant ($P < 0.05$) reductions in protein digestibility of lactalbumin (99 vs. 73%) and SPI (96 vs. 68%). The processing treatments also caused a drastic negative effect on protein quality, as measured by rat growth methods such as relative protein efficiency ratio (RPER) and relative net protein ratio (RNPR). The RPER and RNPR values of untreated lactalbumin and SPI were 89–91 and 56–64%, respectively. But the RPER and RNPR values of the treated lactalbumin and SPI were 0%. The mineral status of rats was also compromised by feeding alkaline/heat treated proteins. Liver iron levels in male rats (165–180 μg/g dry weight) and female rats (306–321 μg/g dry weight) fed the treated proteins were about half the levels in male rats (229–257 μg/g dry weight) and female rats (578–697 μg/g dry weight) fed the untreated proteins. The kidney iron contents of rats fed the treated proteins were also lower than that of rats fed the untreated pro-

* Present address: Department of Botany, University of Hong Kong, Pokfulam Road, Hong Kong, China.

Impact of Processing on Food Safety, edited by Jackson et al.,
Kluwer Academic / Plenum Publishers, New York, 1999.

teins. Liver copper levels of male and female rats fed the treated proteins were up to three fold higher than those found in rats fed the untreated proteins. The data suggested that LAL, an unnatural amino acid derivative formed during processing of foods, may produce adverse effects on growth, protein digestibility, protein quality and mineral bioavailability and utilization. The antinutritional effects of LAL may be more pronounced in sole-source foods such as infant formulas and formulated liquid diets which have been reported to contain significant amounts (up to 2400 ppm of LAL in the protein) of LAL.

2. INTRODUCTION

During processing of foods, protein products are treated with heat and alkali for many purposes, such as to sterilize/pasteurize, to improve flavour or texture, to destroy toxic or antinutritional factors, to promote desirable physical properties, and to solubilize proteins during the preparation of protein isolates and meat analogs and substitutes (Friedman et al., 1984). Formation of crosslinked peptide chains in protein such as lysinoalanine (LAL), ornithine and lanthionine, formation of Maillard reaction products, and racemization of L-amino acids have been reported to occur when proteins are subjected to heat and alkaline conditions (Friedman et al., 1981; 1984; Robbins et al., 1980). The formation of LAL was also reported in a variety of proteins when heated under nonalkaline conditions (Codex Alimentarius Commission, 1982). LAL (an unnatural amino acid derivative) is formed during alkaline treatment of proteins, mainly by the addition of an ϵ-amino group of a lysine residue to the double bond of a dehydroalanine residue that has been generated by the β-elimination reaction of cystine, phosphoserine or glycoserine residues (Friedman et al., 1984). The quantity of LAL formed is dependent upon many factors such as temperature, concentration of alkali, time of exposure to alkali, type of protein, and type of cations in the solution (Codex Alimentarius Commission, 1982; Struthers et al., 1979).

LAL is present in significant amounts in infant formulas and formulated liquid diets. The liquid concentrate forms of milk-based infant formulas and commercially available formulated liquid diets were found to contain up to 1200 and 2400 ppm of LAL in the formula/diet protein, respectively (G. Sarwar, unpublished data).

The health concerns associated with LAL are two fold. First, LAL formation in processed foods results in a loss of essential amino acids (such as lysine and cysteine) and reduced protein digestibility and quality. Secondly, LAL can cause kidney damage (Codex Alimentarius Commission, 1982; ILSI, 1976; 1989; Sternberg et al., 1975; Struthers et al., 1979). Nerphrocytomegaly (i.e. enlarged kidney cells) and nephrokaryomegaly (enlarged nuclei) are unique lesions induced in rats by LAL. The level of dietary LAL needed to induce nephrocytomegaly depends on whether LAL is fed as the free amino acid or bound in a protein. Enlarged nuclei have been reported in rats by feeding as little as 1200–1400 ppm protein-bound LAL (Gould and MacGregor, 1977; Karayiannis et al., 1979). In comparison, feeding of free LAL was found to produce nephrocytomegaly at much lower levels (100–250 ppm) (DeGroot et al., 1976; Woodard, 1975). L-lysyl-D-alanyl-LAL, the most potent isomer of the four optical isomers of LAL, induced nephrocytomegaly when fed at levels as low as 30 ppm, whereas D-lysyl-D-alanyl-lysinoalanine did not produce lesions at less than 1000 ppm (Slump, 1978).

The cause of the kidney damage induced by LAL is not known. Based on *in vitro* studies, it has been suggested that LAL acts as a chelator of essential trace minerals, and may exert its toxic effect by binding metal in renal tubule cells (Hayashi, 1982). Extracts from human kidney cells were reported to be less effective in metabolizing LAL than cor-

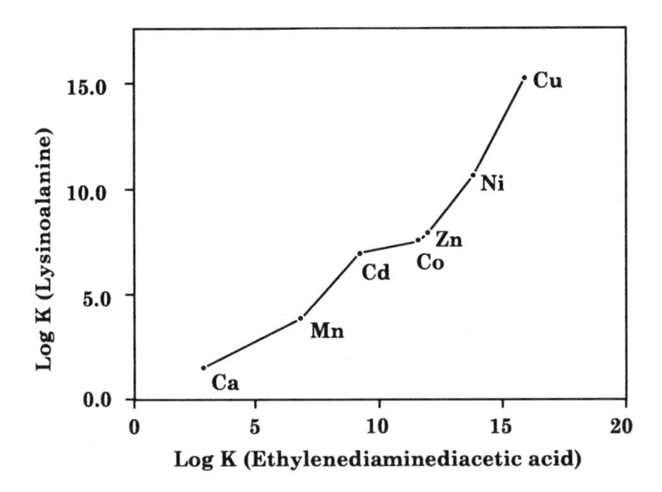

Figure 1. Comparison of the stability constants for LAL and EDDA complexes of divalent metal ions. (from Pearce and Friedman 1988, with permission).

responding extracts from several animal species including rats, mice, hamsters, dogs and gerbils (Kawamura and Hayashi, 1987), suggesting that human kidney cells may be more susceptible to kidney damage by LAL than those from rats or other animal species tested. The metal-binding properties of LL- and LD-lysinoalanine and ethylenediaminediacetic acid (EDDA, a commercial chelating agent) have been compared using spectrophotometric titrations (Figure 1) (Pearce and Friedman, 1988).

The binding of minerals with LAL almost parallelled binding with EDDA. High-specificity binding of Cu^{2+} and other divalent cations by racemic LAL was observed, mainly as 1:1 complexes. The mechanism of toxicity of LAL has been reviewed (ILSI, 1989). It was concluded that the susceptibility of humans to the nephrotoxic effect of LAL is unknown. Although LAL is present in many foods consumed by humans, its concentration is thought to be sufficiently low and that the risk is low. However, further analytical data are required for assessment of the actual quantity of LAL ingested. Moreover, the influence of chronic consumption of alkaline-treated foods high in LAL on the balance of copper and other minerals should be examined, especially in sole-source foods such as infant formulas and enteral foods..

The effects of feeding two alkaline/heat treated proteins, lactalbumin and soybean protein isolate (SPI) on the mineral status of male and female rats have been studied in our laboratory (L'Abbé et al., 1998). To our knowledge, this was the first *in vivo* report about the effect of LAL on mineral status. The effects of alkaline/heat treatment of proteins on protein digestibility and quality were also examined (Sarwar, 1997). The data are reviewed in this manuscript.

3. AMINO ACID COMPOSITION OF ALKALINE/HEAT TREATED PROTEINS

Two protein sources (lactalbumin and SPI) were subjected to alkaline-treatment with 0.1N NaOH at room temperature for 1 h, followed by heat treatment at 75°C for 3 h, neutralization with 10 N HCl to pH 7.5, ultrafiltration to remove salts and spray drying of the ultrafiltered retentate (L'Abbé., 1998). The treated and untreated protein sources were hy-

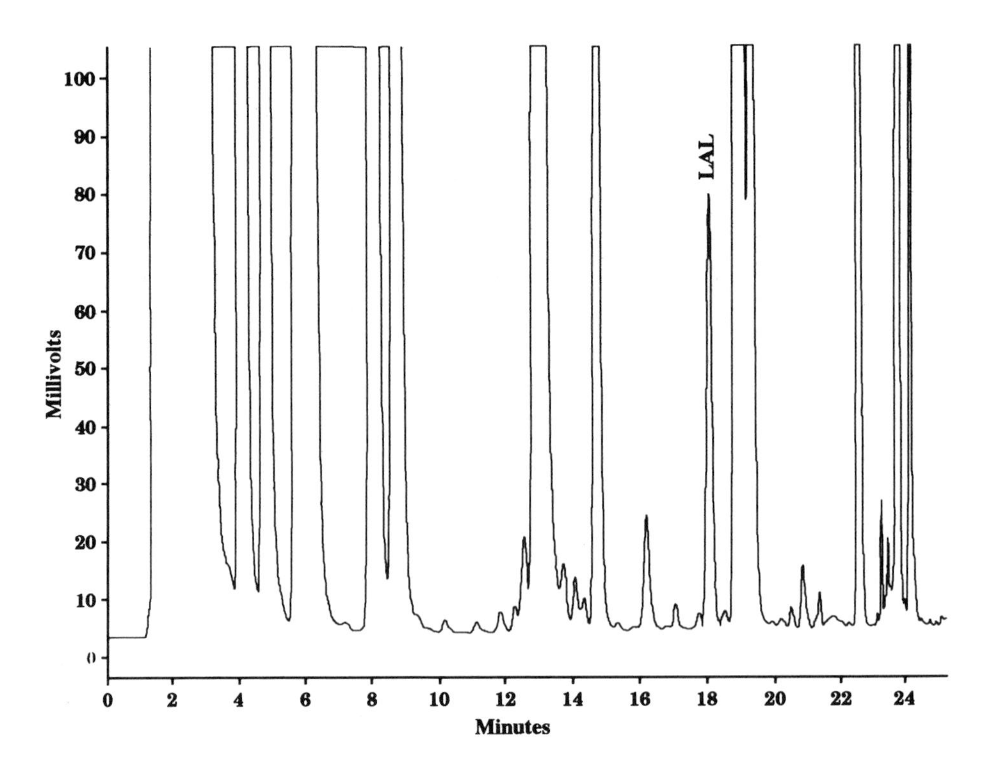

Figure 2. Chromatogram of the LAL standard as the dansyl chloride derivative.

drolysed with 6 N HCl at 110° C for 22 h for the determination of all amino acids except sulfur amino acids and tryptophan (AOAC, 1990). Hydrolysis with 4.2N NaOH was used for quantitative determination of tryptophan, while hydrolysates for determination of sulfur amino acids, methionine as methionine sulfone and cyste(i)ne as cysteic acid, were prepared by performic acid oxidation of protein followed by hydrolysis with 6N HCl (AOAC, 1990). All amino acids in protein hydrolysates were determined by liquid chromatography of precolumn phenylisothiocyanate derivatives (Sarwar et al., 1988). Tryptophan in alkaline hydrolysates was determined by a liquid chromatography method requiring no derivatization (Sarwar et al., 1988). A portion of the 6 N HCl hydrolysates was derivatized with dansyl chloride for the determination of LAL by liquid chromatography (Wood-Rethwill and Warthesen, 1980), using a Waters HPLC system with Jasco flourescence detector and Waters 717 autosampler. A chromatogram showing separation of LAL standard, as dansyl chloride derivative is shown in Figure 2. Similarly, a chromatogram showing separation of LAL (as dansyl chloride derivative) from a hydrolysate of the alkaline/heat-treated lactalbumin, is shown in Figure 3. Satisfactory separation of LAL from the control and the treated protein was completed in about 18 minutes.

Amino acid compositions of untreated and alkaline/heat treated protein sources are shown in Table 1. The treated proteins contained considerably higher levels of LAL compared to the untreated proteins. The amount of LAL in the treated lactalbumin was more than two-fold higher than in the treated SPI. As expected, the formation of LAL in the treated proteins was associated with a loss of lysine (19–20%), cystine (73–77%), and serine (18–30%). There was also a loss of threonine (35–45%) in the treated proteins (Table 1). Most other amino acids were not greatly affected by the alkaline treatment of the two

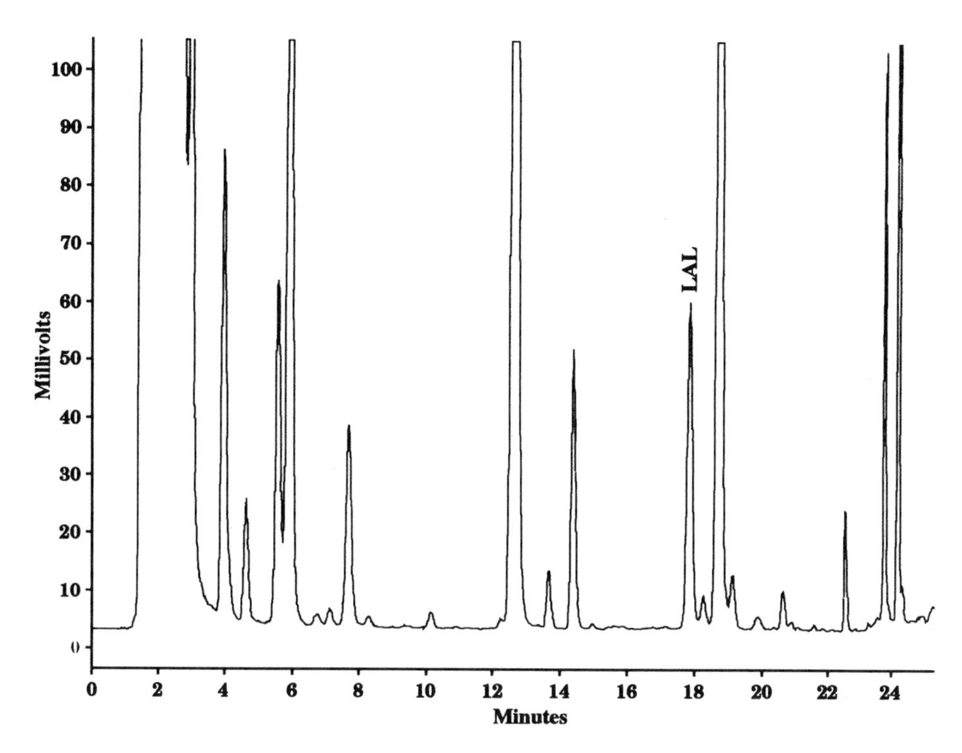

Figure 3. Chromatogram of a hydrolysate from alkaline/heat treated lactalbumin after reaction with dansyl chloride.

proteins. Since the amino acid methodology used did not distinguish between D- and L-forms of amino acids, the influence of the processing treatments on the formation of D-amino acids could not be determined.

4. PROTEIN DIGESTIBILITY AND QUALITY OF ALKALINE/HEAT TREATED PROTEINS

A rat balance and growth study was conducted to determine protein digestibility and quality of processed protein products (Sarwar, 1997). Protein quality was assessed by rat growth methods such as relative protein efficiency ratio (RPER) and relative net protein ratio (RNPR) and by the protein digestibility-corrected amino acid score (PDCAAS) method based on rat growth and human growth patterns of amino acid requirements. The PDCAAS method has recently replaced the PER method for evaluating protein quality of foods except infant formulas in the United States.

The protein digestibility and protein quality data for untreated and alkaline/heat treated lactalbumin and SPI are shown in Table 2. Casein (both unsupplemented and supplemented with methionine), untreated lactalbumin and untreated SPI had high true protein digestibility values (96–100%). The alkaline/heat treatment had significant ($P < 0.05$) negative effects on the protein digestibility of lactalbumin (99 vs. 73%) and SPI (96 vs. 68%). The alkaline treatment also had a drastic negative effect on the RPER and RNPR values of lactalbumin (89 vs. 0%; 91 vs. 0%) and SPI (56 vs. 0%; 64 vs. 0%).

Table 1. Amino acid compositions of untreated and alkaline/heat treated lactalbumin and soybean protein isolate (SPI) (from L'Abbé et al., 1998, with permission)

Amino acid, g/100 g protein	Lactalbumin, untreated	Lactalbumin, treated	SPI, untreated	SPI, treated
LAL	0.10	4.42	0.03	1.94
Arginine	3.43	3.12	7.84	7.56
Histidine	2.20	1.90	2.51	2.77
Isoleucine	6.02	6.25	5.08	5.38
Leucine	13.68	14.29	8.15	8.97
Lysine	10.50	8.35	6.08	4.94
Methionine	2.71	2.60	1.47	1.50
Cyst(e)ine	2.81	0.76	1.16	0.27
Phenylalanine	4.26	4.64	5.42	5.98
Tyrosine	4.45	4.69	3.85	4.25
Threonine	5.73	3.13	3.98	2.57
Tryptophan	2.12	2.12	1.35	1.30
Valine	6.29	6.62	5.12	5.78
Alanine	5.81	6.17	4.17	4.63
Aspartic acid	11.20	12.41	11.05	11.96
Glutamic acid	17.60	12.42	18.84	20.60
Glycine	2.24	2.52	3.93	4.45
Proline	5.69	5.77	5.21	5.71
Serine	4.93	3.46	5.12	4.16

Table 2. Protein digestibility (%), protein digestibility-corrected amino acid score (PDCAAS, %), relative protein efficiency ratio (RPER, %) and relative net protein ratio (RNPR, %) of untreated and alkaline/heat treated proteins[a]

Product	True protein digestibility	PDCAAS (rat)	PDCAAS (human)	RPER	RNPR
Casein+Met	100	100	100	100	100
Casein	99	85	100	80	84
Lactalbumin, untreated	99	100	100	89	91
Lactalbumin, treated	73	55	67	0	0
SPI, untreated	96	62	100	56	64
SPI, treated	68	44	49	0	0

[a] Abstracted from Sarwar (1997). True protein digestibility values were calculated using the following equation: True protein digestibility = PI- [FP-MFP]/PI X 100, where PI= protein intake, FP=fecal protein and MFP=metabolic fecal protein. The amount of protein in the feces of rats fed the protein-free diet was used as the estimate for MFP. The PDCAAS was calculated as follows:PDCAAS (%)= True protein digestibility X amino acid score (or the lowest amino acid ratio). Amino acid ratios (mg of an essential amino acid in 1.0 g of test protein/mg of the same amino acid in 1.0 g of reference protein X 100) for 9 essential amino acids (histidine, isoleucine, leucine, lysine, methionine+cystine, phenylalanine+tyrosine, tryptophan and valine) were calculated using a rat growth pattern of amino acid requirements (for calculating PDCAAS based on rat's requirements) and a human pattern of amino acid requirements as the reference pattern (for calculating PDCAAS based on human's requirements).RPER and RNPR values (2-wk) were calculated using the following equations:RPER= [PER of test diet/PER of control diet] X 100,RNPR=[NPR of test diet/NPR of control diet] X 100,where PER (protein efficiency ratio)= weight gain of test rat/protein consumed by test rat, and NPR (net protein ratio)= (weight gain of test rat+weight loss of non-protein rat)/ (protein consumed by test rat).

Due to the higher amino acid requirements for rat growth compared to those for humans (especially sulfur amino acids), the PDCAAS based on rat's requirements of protein products were lower compared to those based on human amino acid requirements (Table 2). The differences between the PDCAAS (based on rat's requirements) and RNPR or RPER of casein, untreated lactalbumin and untreated SPI were small (about 10%). But the PDCAAS (based on rat's requirements) for alkaline/heat treated lactalbumin and alkaline/heat treated SPI were considerably higher compared to the RPER or RNPR values of these products. This comparison indicated that the PDCAAS method clearly overestimated protein quality of the treated lactalbumin (PDCAAS of 55–67 vs. RPER or RNPR of 0) and the treated SPI (PDCAAS of 44–49 vs. RPER or RNPR of 0). The PDCAAS score method also overestimated the quality of other protein sources which contained antinutritional factors such as mustard flour (PDCAAS of 84–92 vs. RPER or RNPR of 0), raw black beans (PDCAAS of 45–72 vs. RPER or RNPR of 0), and overheated skim milk powder (PDCAAS of 29–31 vs. RPER/RNPR of 0–5) (Sarwar, 1997).

The inferior protein digestibility and protein quality of the alkaline/heat treated lactalbumin and SPI compared to the untreated products (Table 2) could be due to the formation of D-amino acids and crosslinked peptide chains (such as LAL and lanthionine) which result in lower protein digestibility and amino acid bioavailability (Friedman et al., 1980; 1984; Robbins et al., 1980; Sarwar, 1997). To be utilized, orally administered D-amino acids must be absorbed from the gut and then converted to the corresponding L-amino acids, which involves the D-amino acid oxidase-catalyzed conversion of D-amino acids to α-keto compounds and transaminative synthesis of the L-amino acid from its keto analog (Baker, 1986; Friedman and Gumbmann, 1984). The amino acid oxidase system, which varies in amount and specificity of oxidases in different animal species, may become saturated when high amounts of D-amino acids are consumed, resulting in reduced utilization of D-amino acids.

The utilization of orally administered D-amino acids has been reviewed (Friedman et al., 1991). D-isomers of Met, Phe and Tyr are utilized efficiently by chicks and rats while D-Met is inefficiently utilized by humans. It is generally agreed that humans have less capacity to convert D-Met to L-Met than do other mammals. D-Trp is utilized by pigs but inefficiently by humans, mice and chicks. The D-isomers of Leu, Ile and Val are utilized efficiently by chicks but poorly by rats. D-His is not utilized by rats but slightly by chicks. The D-isomers of Lys, Thr, Arg and Cys are not utilized by either rats or chicks.

The *in vitro* digestibility of a series of model epimeric tripeptides occurring in β-casein (Ala-Met-Ala, Ala-D-Met-Ala, Val-Met-Phe, and Val-D-Met-Phe) and soybean glycinine (Thr-Met-Arg, Thr-D-Met-Arg, and Thr-Met-Lys) by intestinal mucosal peptidases showed that none of the D-amino acids was released (Paquet et al., 1985; 1987; Sarwar et al., 1985). In fact, neither the amino-terminal nor the carboxy-terminal L-amino acid residue was released when D-Met, D-Asp, D-Glu, or D-Phe was the internal residue. This suggested that racemization not only affected utilization of racemized amino acids but also L-amino acids located adjacent to racemized amino acids in a protein structure. Although peptides containing L-amino acids were totally hydrolysed after 24 h, there were marked differences in the initial rates of hydrolysis. The initial rates of hydrolysis of peptides with bulky side chains (Val-Met-Phe and Val-Asp-Val) were considerably lower than the rates of the corresponding tripeptides with light side chains (Ala-Met-Ala and Ala-Asp-Ala). Similarly, the bioavailability of Met in tripeptides with the bulky amino acids (Val-Met-Phe, Thr-Met-Arg, and Thr-Met-Lys) was lower than in the unhindered tripeptide (Ala-Met-Ala) (Table 3).

D-Met on internal sites of these tripeptides was considerably less bioavailable than Met, and completely unavailable in bulky peptides (Val-D-Met-Phe and Thr-D-Met-Arg). The methionine bioavailability data (based on rat growth) ranked the Met-containing

Table 3. Net protein ratio (NPR) and bioavailability values of some Met-containing tripeptides, based on rat growth [a]

Diet	NPR	Met bioavailability, %
Basal (Met deficient)	1.17	—
Basal + Met (reference)	3.82	100
Basal + D-Met	3.81	100
Basal + tripeptides		
Ala-Met-Ala	3.05	71
Ala-D-Met-Ala	2.37	45
Val-Met-Phe	2.71	58
Val-D-Met-Phe	1.09	0
Thr-Met-Arg	2.64	55
Thr-D-Met-Arg	1.15	0
Thr-Met-Lys	1.13	0

[a] Abstracted from Sarwar et al. (1985). Met bioavailability = (NPR of test diet- NPR of basal diet)/ (NPR of reference diet- NPR of basal diet) X 100; NPR = (weight gain of test rat + weight loss of nonprotein rat)/ (protein consumed by test rat).

tripeptides in the following order: Ala-Met-Ala > Val-Met-Phe = Thr-Met-Arg > Ala-D-Met-Ala > Thr-D-Met-Arg = Thr-Met-Lys = Val-D-Met-Phe (Table 3).

5. EFFECTS OF FEEDING ALKALINE/HEAT TREATED PROTEINS ON GROWTH, SOME BLOOD PARAMETERS AND MINERAL STATUS

L'Abbé et al. (1998) studied the mineral status of rats fed untreated and alkaline/heat treated lactalbumin and SPI. Each diet was fed to 8 individually caged female and 8 male weanling Sprague-Dawley rats for a period of six weeks. The control was a casein-based AIN-93G diet (Reeves et al., 1993). Alkaline/heat treated or untreated lactalbumin or SPI was added at 15% to the control diet. All diets met or exceeded the nutrient requirements for rat growth. Data on growth, blood serum urea nitrogen (BUN), serum glucose, serum hemoglobin, liver iron, kidney iron, and liver copper were obtained.

5.1. Effects on Growth

The antinutritional factors formed during alkaline/heat treatment caused a significant ($P < 0.05$) reduction in weight gains of rats (especially male rats) fed the treated lactalbumin or SPI diets compared to of those fed the untreated diets. The weight gain of male rats fed the untreated and treated diets were 41–42 and 32 g/100 g food consumed, respectively.

5.2. Effects on BUN

The data on BUN are shown in Figure 4. The levels of BUN in male or female rats fed the alkaline/heat treated diets (lactalbumin and SPI) were significantly ($P < 0.05$) higher compared to those fed the untreated diets. High levels of BUN in rats fed the treated diets suggest kidney damage and inferior protein quality.

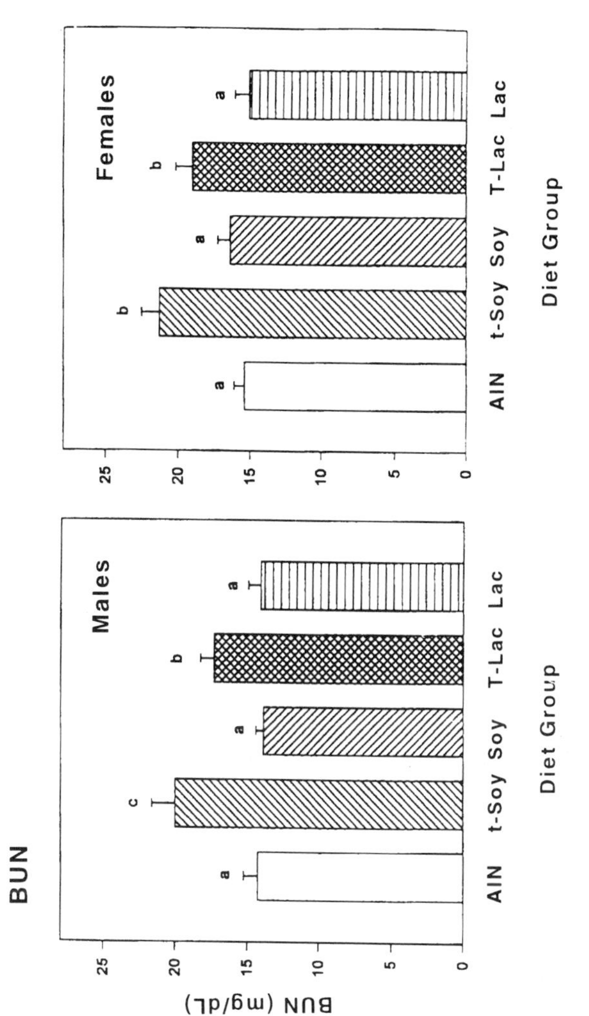

Figure 4. Levels of blood urea nitrogen (BUN) in male and female rats fed control (AIN), untreated SPI (Soy), alkaline/heat treated SPI (t-Soy), untreated lactalbumin (Lac) and alkaline/heat treated lactalbumin (t-Lac) diets (from L'Abbé et al., 1998, with permission).

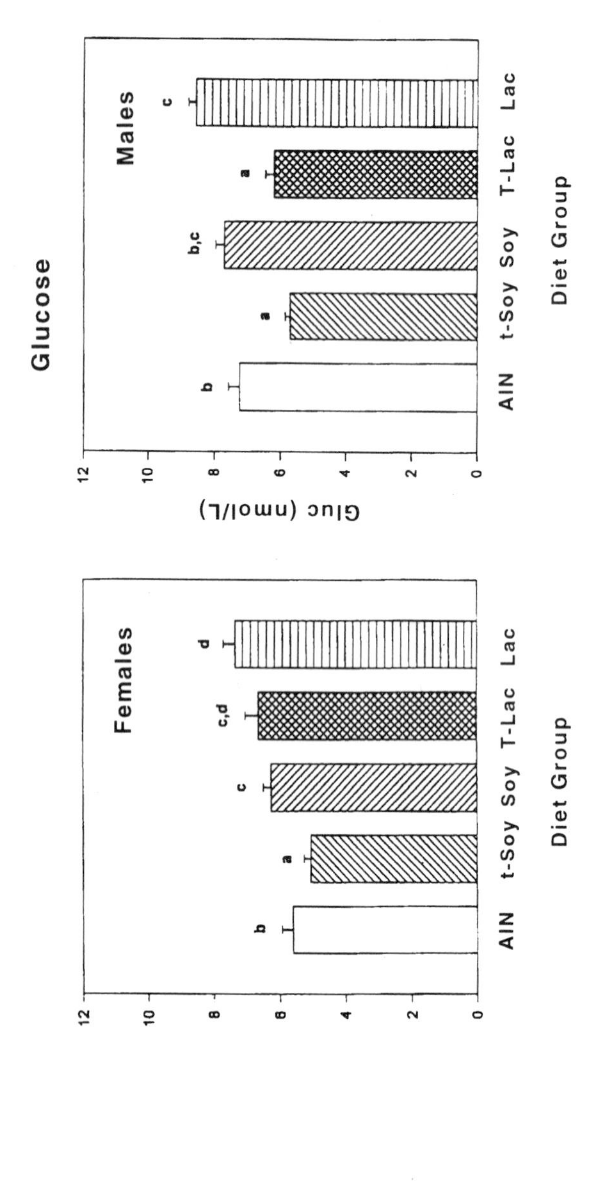

Figure 5. Levels of serum glucose in male and female rats fed control (AIN), untreated SPI (Soy), alkaline/heat treated SPI (t-Soy), untreated lactalbumin (Lac) and alkaline/heat treated lactalbumin (t-Lac) diets (from L'Abbé et al., 1998, with permission).

5.3. Effects on Serum Glucose

The data on serum glucose are shown in Figure 5. The alkaline/heat treatment had a significant ($P < 0.05$) negative effect on the levels of serum glucose, especially in the case of males, where the levels were lower for the alkaline/heat treated lactalbumin and SPI diets compared to the untreated diets. In the case of females, significant differences were only found between the treated and the untreated SPI diets.

5.4. Effects on Serum Hemoglobin

The data on serum hemoglobin are shown in Figure 6. The levels in male rats fed the alkaline/heat treated lactalbumin diet were significantly ($P < 0.05$) lower compared to the levels in those fed the untreated lactalbumin diet. In females, such differences were, however, not significant. The levels in male rats fed the alkaline/heat treated SPI diet tended to be lower compared to the levels in those fed the untreated SPI diet, but the difference was not significant ($P > 0.05$).

5.5. Effects on Liver Iron

The data on liver iron are shown in Figure 7. In both sexes, the levels were significantly ($P < 0.05$) lower in animals fed the alkaline/heat treated diets compared to the feeding of the untreated diets. Low liver iron and marginally low hemoglobin (Figure 6) in rats fed the treated diets would suggest that LAL formed during the alkaline/heat treatment is interfering with either the absorption or metabolism of iron. Since liver iron (first site after absorption) is low, LAL is probably interfering with absorption of iron. Slightly lower serum hemoglobin in rats fed the alkaline-treated diets compared to untreated diets supports this observation; keeping in mind that hemoglobin is the last symptom of iron depletion and is only seen after liver stores have been depleted.

5.6. Effects on Kidney Iron

The data on kidney iron are shown in Figure 8. Although not as dramatic as noted in the case of liver iron, the levels of iron in kidneys of rats fed the alkaline/heat treated diets were significantly ($P < 0.05$) lower compared to the levels in rats fed the untreated diets.

5.7. Effects on Liver Copper

The data on liver copper are shown in Figure 9. The most dramatic differences were observed in the case of liver copper. In males, the levels of liver copper in rats fed the alkaline/heat treated diets were two-to-three fold higher compared to the levels in rats fed the untreated diets. Similar results were noted in the case of females. The very high liver copper levels in rats fed the treated diets would agree with the *in vitro* observations of Pearce and Friedman (1988) that LAL (formed during alkaline treatment of proteins) had the highest affinity for copper among the minerals tested. Therefore, any copper entering the liver may be being sequestered by LAL. If so, LAL may be holding on to the copper so tightly that it may not be available for incorporation into copper-containing enzymes such as superoxide dismutase (SOD), cytochrome c oxidase (CCO), and ceruloplasmin (CP). This situation may be analogous to that for metallothionein (L'Abbé and Fischer, 1984). High dietary zinc induces metallothionein which has a much higher affinity for copper

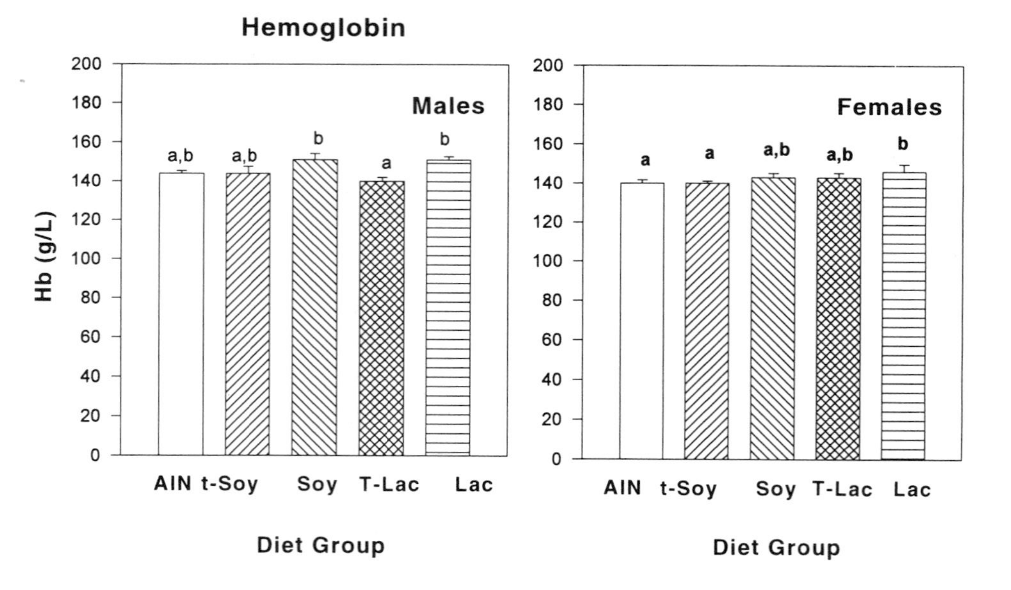

Figure 6. Levels of serum hemoglobin (Hb) in male and female rats fed control (AIN), untreated SPI (Soy), alkaline/heat treated SPI (t-Soy), untreated lactalbumin (Lac) and alkaline/heat treated lactalbumin (t-Lac) diets (from L'Abbé et al., 1998, with permission).

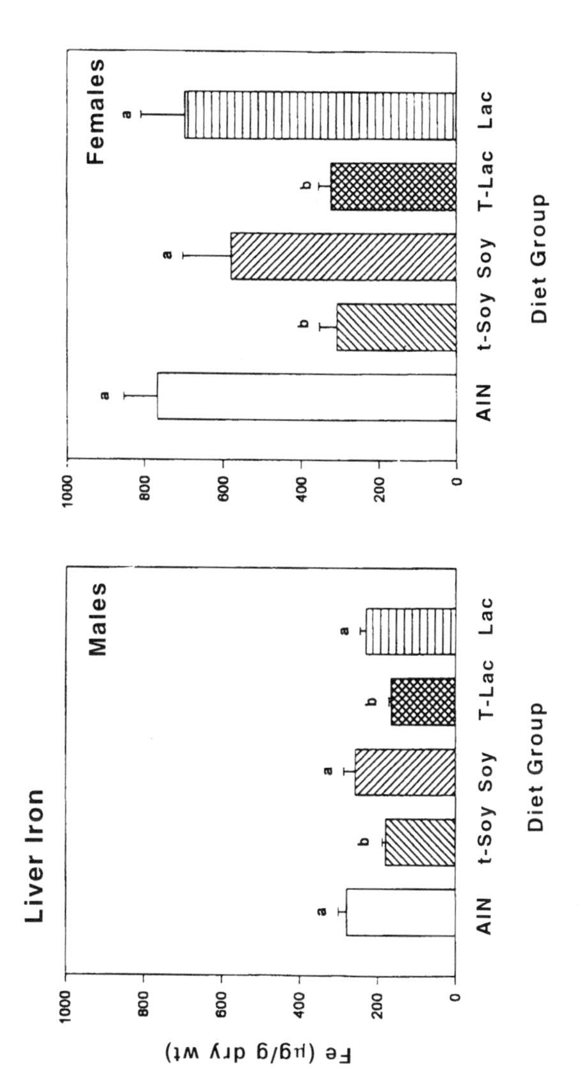

Figure 7. Levels of liver iron in male and female rats fed control (AIN), untreated SPI (Soy), alkaline/heat treated SPI (t-Soy), untreated lactalbumin (Lac) and alkaline/heat treated lactalbumin (t-Lac) diets (from L'Abbé et al., 1998, with permission).

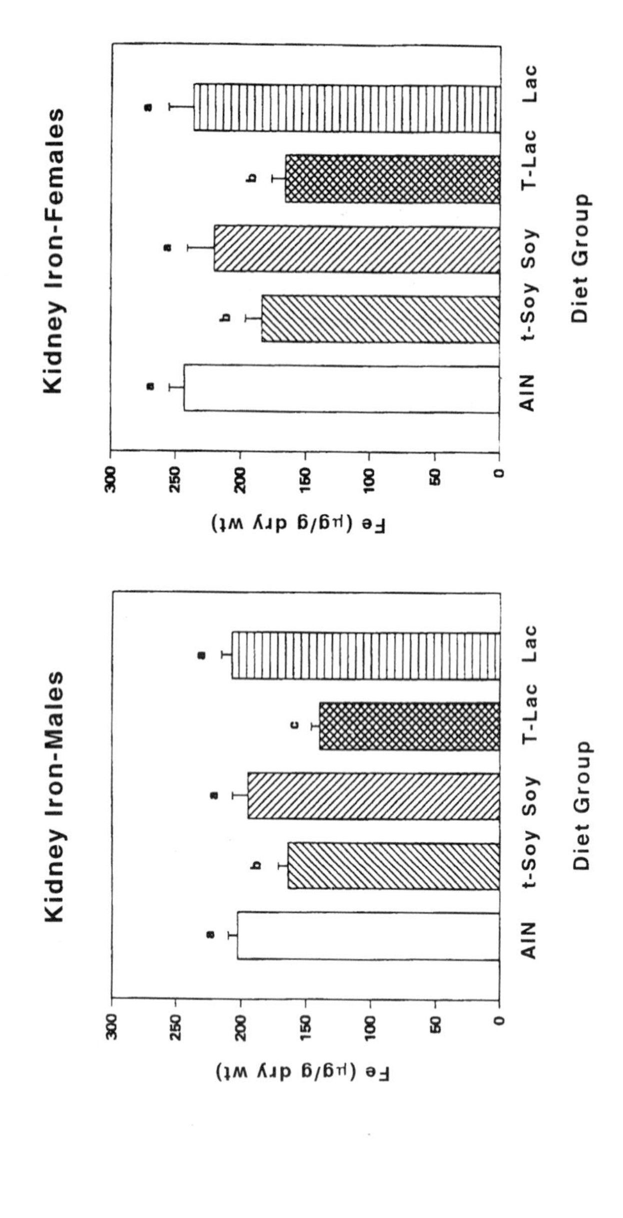

Figure 8. Levels of kidney iron in male and female rats fed control (AIN), untreated SPI (Soy), alkaline/heat treated SPI (t-Soy), untreated lactalbumin (Lac) and alkaline/heat treated lactalbumin (t-Lac) diets (from L'Abbé et al., 1998, with permission).

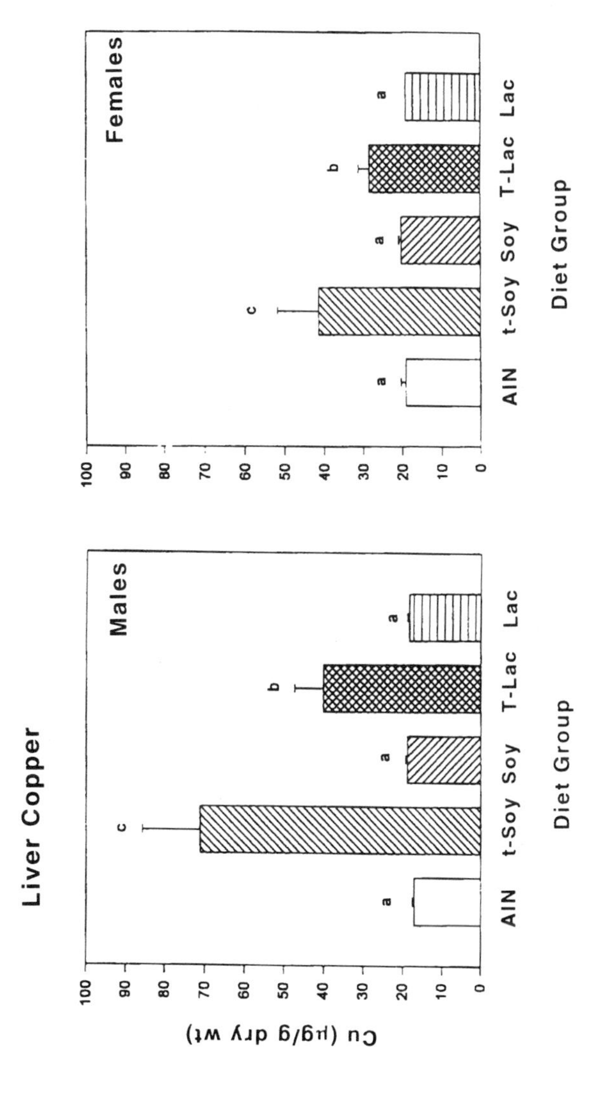

Figure 9. Levels of liver copper in male and female rats fed control (AIN), untreated SPI (Soy), alkaline/heat treated SPI (t-Soy), untreated lactalbumin (Lac) and alkaline/heat treated lactalbumin (t-Lac) diets (from L'Abbé et al., 1998, with permission).

than zinc, thereby sequestering copper. The copper bound to metallothionein is then not available for incorporation into copper-containing enzymes. In another experiment with high dietary zinc, we saw high liver copper but low activity of copper containing enzymes (L'Abbé and Fischer, 1984). This has potential health ramifications. It can have detrimental effects on handling of free radicals (SOD), iron metabolism (Ceruloplasmin), energy metabolism and neurotransmitters.

It has been suggested that the damage observed in the proximal renal tubules in rats fed LAL, DAPA (DL-2,3-diaminopropanoic acid, a well known bidentate metal ion chelator) or D-serine (formed during processing of foods) may arise from interaction of these compounds with copper (II) within the epithelial cells (Pearce and Friedman, 1988). LAL may exert its effect partly by inactivating the metalloenzyme catalase and therefore potentiate peroxide formation and the liberation of copper (II). If this is true, then copper status, water intake, and urine volume would influence the incidence and severity of lesions. In turn, LAL would affect copper nutritional status by altering copper retention and redistribution (Pearce and Friedman, 1988).

6. SUMMARY AND CONCLUSIONS

The formation of LAL during alkaline/heat treatment of proteins resulted in a significant loss of essential amino acids (cystine, lysine and threonine), and reduced protein digestibility and quality. The reduction in protein digestibility was more pronounced in old rats (20 months of age) compared to young rats (6-weeks of age), suggesting higher susceptibility of the elderly to the antinutritional effects of dietary LAL. Dietary LAL formed during alkaline/heat treatment of proteins has also been reported to have an adverse effect on mineral status. The liver iron content of rats fed the LAL-containing treated proteins was about half that of the rats fed the untreated proteins. Kidney iron levels were also significantly reduced. In contrast, liver copper levels were up to 3 times higher in the rats fed the treated proteins. The large reductions in liver and kidney iron levels are of particular concern, as iron is the mineral in which status is often already reduced in infants and the elderly, the groups most likely to consume diets composed of exclusively formula-type foods. Additional research and analytical data are needed for examining the influence of chronic consumption of alkali-treated food products on the balance of iron, copper and other minerals, and in estimating an acceptable daily intake of LAL.

REFERENCES

Association of Official Analytical Chemists. Official methods of Analysis, 15th Ed., AOAC, Arlington, VA., **1990.**

Baker, D.H. Utilization of isomers and analogs of amino acids and other sulfur-containing compounds. *Prog. Food Nut. Sci.* **1986**, 10, 133.

Codex Alimentarius Commission. Working group's report, on Lysinoalanine Toxicity, to the second session of Codex Committee on vegetable Proteins (CCVP), FAO, Rome, Italy & WHO, Geneva, Switzerland. **1982**.

DeGroot, A.P.; Slump, P.; Feron, W.J.; Van Beek, L. Feeding of alkali-treated proteins: feeding studies with free and protein-bound lysinoalanine in rats and other animals. *J. Nutr.* **1976**, 106, 1527–15

Friedman, M. Formation, nutritional value and safety of D-amino acids. In *Nutritional and Toxicological Consequences of Food Processing*, Friedman, M. Ed.; Plenum Press: New York, N.Y. **1991**, pp 447–481

Friedman, M.; Gumbmann, M.R. The utilization and safety of isomeric sulfur-containing amino acids in mice. *J. Nutr.* **1984**, 144, 2301.

Friedman, M.; Gumbmann, M.R.; Masters, P.M. Protein-alkali reactions: chemistry, toxicology, and nutritional consequences. In *Nutritional and Toxicological Aspects of Food Safety*; Friedman, M., Ed.; Plenum Press: New York, N.Y. **1984**; pp 367–412.

Friedman, M.; Zahnley, J.C.; Masters, P.M. Relationship between in vitro digestibility of casein and its content of lysinoalanine and D-amino acids. *J. Food Sci.* **1981**, 46, 127–131.

Gould, D.H.; MacGregor, J.T. Biological effects of alkali-treated protein and lysinoalanine: an overview. In *Protein Crosslinking: Nutritional and Medical Consequences*; Friedman, M., Ed; Plenum Press: New York, N.Y. **1977**; pp 29–48.

Hayashi, R. Lysinoalanine as a metal chelator. *J. Biol. Chem.* **1982**, 257, 13896–13898.

International Life Sciences Institute. Processed protein foods and lysinoalanine. *Nutr. Rev.* **1976**, 34(4), 120–122.

International Life Sciences Institute. Mechanism of toxicity of lysinoalanine. *Nutr. Rev.* **1989**, 47(11), 362–364.

Karayiannis, N.; MacGregor, J.T.; Bjeldanes, L.F. Biological effects of alkali-treated soy protein and lactalbumin in the rat and mouse. *Food Cosmet. Toxicol.* **1979**, 17, 591–604.

Kawamura, Y.; Hayashi, R. Lysinoalanine-degrading enzymes of various animal kidneys. *Agric. Biol. Chem.* **1987**, 51, 2289–2290.

L'Abbé, M.R.; Fischer, P.F.W. The effects of dietary zinc on the activity of copper-requiring metalloenzymes in the rat. *J. Nutr.* **1984**, 114, 823–828.

L'Abbé, M.R.; Sarwar, G.; Trick, K.; Botting, H.G.; Ma, C.Y. Dietary lysinoalanine formed during processing of proteins exerts adverse effects on mineral status of rats. *Lancet* **1998** (submitted for publication).

Paquet, A.; Thresher, W.C.; Swaisgood, H.E. Further studies on in vitro digestibility of some epimeric tripeptides. *Nutr. Res.* **1987**, 7, 581.

Paquet, A.; Thresher, W.C.; Swaisgood, H.E.; Catignani, G.L. Synthesis and digestibility determinations of some epimeric tripeptides occurring in dietary proteins. *Nutr. Res.* **1985**, 5, 893–904.

Pearce, K.N.; Friedman, M. The binding of copper (II) and other metals by lysinoalanine and related compounds and its significance for food safety. *J. Agric. Food Chem.* **1988**, 36, 707–717.

Reeves, P.G.; Nielsen, F.H.; Fehey, G.C., Jr. AIN-93 purified diets for laboratory rodents: final report of the American Institute of Nutrition ad hoc writing committee on the reformulation of the AIN-76A rodent diet. *J. Nutr.* **1993**, 123, 1939–1951.

Robbins, K.R.; Baker, D.H.; Finley, J.W. Studies on the utilization of lysinoalanine and lanthionine. *J. Nutr.* **1980**, 110, 907–915.

Sarwar, G. The protein digestibility-corrected amino acid score method overestimates quality of proteins containing antinutritional factors and of poorly digestible proteins supplemented with limiting amino acids in rats. *J. Nutr.* **1997**, 127, 758–764.

Sarwar, G.; Botting, H.G.; Peace, R.W. Complete amino acid analysis in hydrolysates of foods and feeds by liquid chromatography of precolumn phenylisothiocyanate derivatives. *J. Assoc.Off. Anal. Chem.* **1988**, 71, 1172–1175.

Sarwar, G.; Paquet, A.; Peace, R.W. Bioavailability of methionine in some tripeptides occurring in dietary proteins as determined by rat growth. *Nutr. Res.* **1985**, 5, 905–912.

Slump, P. Lysinoalanine in alkali treated proteins and factors influencing its biological activity. Annales de la Nutr. et de l'Alimentation. **1978**, 32, 271–279.

Sternberg, M.; Kim, C.Y.; Schwende, F.J. Lysinoalanine: presence in foods and food ingredients. *Science* **1975**, 190, 992–994.

Struthers, B.J.; Dahlgren, R.R.; Hopkins, D.T.; Raymond, M.L. Lysinoalanine: biological effects and significance. In *Soy Protein and Human Nutrition*; Wilcke, H.L.; Hopkins, D.T.; Waggle, D.H., Ed; Academic Press, New York, N.Y. **1979**; pp 235–260.

Woodard, J.C. Renal toxicity of N ε-DL (2-amino-2-carboxyethyl)-L-lysine, lysinoalanine. *Vet. Path.* **1975**, 12, 65–66.

Wood-Rethwill, J.C.; Warthesen, J.J. Lysinoalanine determination in proteins using high-pressure liquid chromatography. *J. Food Sci.* **1980**, 45, 1637–1640.

12

FOOD HEATING AND THE FORMATION OF HETEROCYCLIC AROMATIC AMINE AND POLYCYCLIC AROMATIC HYDROCARBON MUTAGENS/CARCINOGENS

Mark G. Knize, Cynthia P. Salmon, Pilar Pais, and James S. Felton

Biology and Biotechnology Research Program
Lawrence Livermore National Laboratory, University of California
P. O. Box 808, Livermore, California 94551-9900

ABBREVIATIONS

B[*a*]A= benzo[*a*]anthracene, B[*a*]P=benzo[*a*]pyrene, B[*b*]F=benzo[*b*]fluoranthene, B[*k*]F=benzo[*k*]fluoranthene, DBA=dibenzo[*a,h*]anthracene, DiMeIQx=2-amino-3,4,8-trimethylimidazo[4,5-*f*]quinoxaline, Indenopyrene=indeno[1,2,3-*c,d*]pyrene, MeIQx=2-amino-3,8-dimethylimidazo[4,5-*f*]quinoxaline, PhIP=2-amino-1-methyl-6-phenylimidazo [4,5-*b*]pyridine.

1. ABSTRACT

Heterocyclic aromatic amines (HAA) and polycyclic aromatic hydrocarbons (PAH) are mutagens and animal carcinogens sometimes formed when foods are heated or processed. Determining their role in cancer etiology depends on comparing human exposures and determining any significant dose-related effect. Chemical analysis of foods shows that flame-grilling can form both PAH and HAA, and that frying forms predominantly HAA. With detection limits of about 0.1 ng/g, amounts found in commercially processed or restaurant foods range from 0.1 to 14 ng/g for HAA, and levels of PAH up to 1 ng/g in a liquid smoke flavoring. Laboratory fried samples have greater amounts of PAH, up to 38 ng/g in hamburgers, and high levels of HAA, over 300 ng/g, are measured in grilled chicken breast. Understanding the processing conditions that form PAH and HAA can lead to methods to greatly reduce their occurrence in processed foods.

Impact of Processing on Food Safety, edited by Jackson et al.,
Kluwer Academic / Plenum Publishers, New York, 1999.

2. INTRODUCTION

Diet has been associated with varying cancer rates in human populations for many years, yet the causes of the observed variation in cancer patterns have not been adequately explained (Wynder and Gori, 1977). Along with the effect of diet on human cancer incidence is the strong evidence that mutations are the initiating events in the cancer process (Vogelstein and Kinzler, 1992). Some of the genotoxic carcinogens that form during heating of foods have been identified, and are found most notably in muscle meats. They fall into two chemical classes: heterocyclic aromatic amines (HAA) and polycyclic aromatic hydrocarbons (PAH).

The observed higher cancer rates at organ sites such as breast and colon in those populations consuming a "Western diet" high in meat have been attributed to high fat or low fiber in the diet. HAA and PAH are also associated with this diet and the meat it contains, and unlike fat or fiber, HAA and PAH have clear genotoxic reactivity leading to the initiating events in the cancer process. There is ample evidence that many of these compounds are complete carcinogens in rodents.

Heterocyclic aromatic amines are among the most potent mutagenic substances ever tested in the Ames/*Salmonella* mutagenicity test (Wakabayashi *et al.*, 1992). Both HAA and PAH cause tumors in rodents at multiple sites (Ohgaki *et al.*, 1991; Chu and Chen, 1985; Gold *et al.*, 1993) many of which are common tumor sites in people on a Western diet. An HAA, PhIP (2-amino-1-methyl-6-phenylimidazo[4,5-*b*]pyridine), and a PAH, B[a]P (benzo[*a*]pyrene), of comparable potency caused mammary gland tumors in a recent feeding study in female rats (El-Bayoumny *et al.*, 1995). The HAA, PhIP has recently been shown to cause carcinomas in the prostate of the male rat (Shirai *et al.*, 1997).

The possibility of cancer prevention has been recently reviewed by Doll (1996). He stated that carcinogen formation during food preparation by cooking might increase the risk of cancer, but human evidence has not yet been established. Our work is supporting efforts to estimate the human dietary dose from these rodent carcinogens.

First, we estimate human exposure to food carcinogens by quantifying the amounts present in foods. Determining the importance of the HAA and PAH food carcinogens in human health requires accurate dietary intake data to determine the amounts and types of carcinogens to which humans are exposed. This exposure information must then be combined with the rodent carcinogenic potency assessment for calculating estimates of human cancer risk. Besides the usefulness for determining the human dose of these heterocyclic amines in the diet, the quantitative chemical analysis can also be used to help devise cooking methods and preparation strategies to reduce the formation of these compounds in foods.

3. FORMATION

The cooking process is responsible for the formation of HAA and PAH from natural constituents in foods, with cooking time and temperature being important determinants in both the qualitative and the quantitative formation of these compounds (Knize *et al.*, 1985; Gross and Grüter, 1992; Skog *et al.*, 1995). Higher temperatures and longer cooking times favor the formation of HAA. A number of studies have shown the precursors for the formation of the HAA to be amino acids, such as phenylalanine, threonine, and alanine; creatine or creatinine; and sugars (Skog, 1993). HAA are frequently formed in muscle meats during frying, broiling, and grilling. Stewing, boiling, and baking usually do not

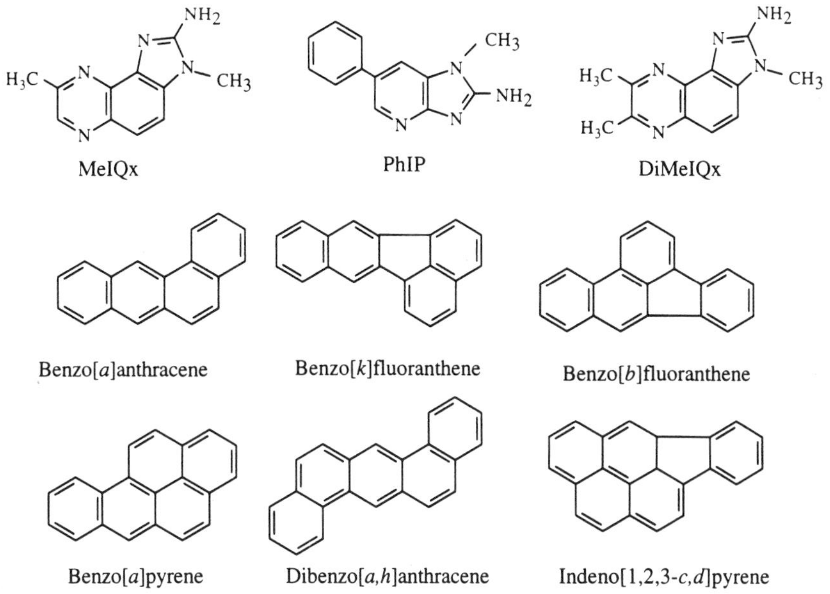

MeIQx PhIP DiMeIQx

Benzo[*a*]anthracene Benzo[*k*]fluoranthene Benzo[*b*]fluoranthene

Benzo[*a*]pyrene Dibenzo[*a,h*]anthracene Indeno[1,2,3-*c,d*]pyrene

Figure 1. Structures of HAA and carcinogenic PAH in foods.

form HAA. Although foods appear to be the major source of human exposure to heterocyclic amines, their presence in food smoke,(Vainiotalo *et al.*, 1993; Thiebaud *et al.*, 1994), cigarette smoke,(Manabe *et al.*, 1991; Wakabayashi *et al.*, 1995) and outdoor air (Manabe *et al.*, 1993) has been reported.

PAH are products of combustion and pyrolysis of organic compounds by condensation of smaller units at high temperatures to form stable polynuclear aromatic compounds (Badger and Kimber, 1960; Lijinsky, 1961). PAH levels in foods are strongly dependent on the method of cooking, including the distance of food from the heat source, design of cooking device and fat content of the foodstuff (Larsson *et al.*, 1983; Lijinsky, 1991) In food, PAH can conceivably be formed by chemical changes in protein, carbohydrate or lipids as a result of the cooking method (Howard and Fazio, 1980). Smoke deposited on the surface of charcoal-grilled meats appears to be the major source of PAH carcinogens in food (Lijinsky, 1991). In the air, PAH are present in smoke from burning fuels, tobacco smoke, and smoke generated during the cooking or the smoke-preservation of foods. There are also occupational exposures to PAH in several industries.

The HAA and PAH carcinogens formed during cooking have stable multi-ring aromatic structures. The heterocyclic amines have an exocyclic amino group and several nitrogen heteroatoms. Structures of those compounds commonly detected in foods are shown in Figure 1. Additional heterocyclic aromatic amines have been found in foods and the whole set of HAA compounds has been the subject of several recent reviews (Robbana-Baranat *et al.*, 1996; Stavric, 1994). Over 25 PAH have been identified in curing smoke and approximately 40 others have been identified but not characterized. We have focused on analysis for six carcinogenic PAH.

The variables influencing the formation of PAH and HAA create a wide range of concentrations in food, requiring the analysis of a large number of food samples cooked under various conditions to determine the sources of carcinogens in the human diet.

4. ANALYSIS

4.1. Bacterial Mutagenic Activity Testing

The heterocyclic amines were found as natural products. Their biological activity was detected in crude food extracts before their chemical structure was determined (Nagao *et al.*, 1977). Thus, unknown mutagens can be detected with bacterial mutagenicity tests. Specific strains of bacteria and metabolic activation effects can be used to differentiate chemical classes to some degree.

Many foods and related samples have been analyzed by mutagenic activity testing. The potency of heterocyclic amines enables a mutagenic response to be determined on sub-nanogram amounts for most of the HAA compounds. A study of the formation of mutagenic activity from pan-frying meat from 16 animal species showed that all meat types used formed mutagenic activity upon cooking (Vikse and Joner, 1993). This suggests slight variations in muscle carbohydrate, fat, free amino acid and creatin(in)e levels do not greatly effect carcinogen formation.

Some extracts of foods containing unknown mutagens were characterized by mutagenicity testing of HPLC fractions. This was done for meats, (Knize *et al.*, 1987), coffee substitutes (Johansson *et al.*, 1995), and grain foods (Knize *et al.*, 1995). While this method is very useful for characterizing and comparing the unknown mutagens, the more difficult task of mutagen identification followed by chemical synthesis is essential for biological experiments. Combined with dietary dose information, measurements of biological potency enable the risk of the consumption of mutagenic aromatic amines to be estimated.

Using mutagenic potency in bacteria as an indicator of risk for humans is not warranted. But for aromatic amine chemicals there is a good correspondence between those that are mutagens in bacteria and those that are carcinogens in animals (Hatch *et al.* 1992). When food extracts exhibit mutagenic activity, and when the bacterial strain and metabolic activation characteristics suggest that those extracts contain aromatic amines, then understanding genotoxic effects and mass amounts present are important because almost all of these mutagens will have carcinogenic significance.

4.2. Chemical Analysis

There are several factors that make the analysis of carcinogens from foods a difficult problem. HAA and PAH are present in foods at low nanogram per gram levels. The low levels require that chromatographic efficiency, and both detector sensitivity and selectivity be optimized. Several of the compounds are formed under the same reaction conditions, so the number of compounds to be quantified requires that the extraction, chromatographic separation, and detection be general enough to detect several of the carcinogens in each chromatographic separation. The complexity and diversity of food samples needing to be analyzed requires a rugged method not affected by the sample matrix.

Gross (1990) developed a method to purify heterocyclic amines from foods and related products with the goal of high sample throughput and high analytical sensitivity. The key to this method is the coupling of a liquid/liquid extraction step to a cation exchange resin column (propylsulfonic acid silica) procedure, thereby concentrating the sample. Using the cation exchange properties of the column allows selective washing and elution to further purify the sample.

A single solid-phase extraction scheme was used to isolate both classes of genotoxic compounds from charcoal-grilled meat: heterocyclic amines and polycyclic aromatic hydrocarbons (Rivera *et al.*, 1996). We are adapting this scheme to analyze foods for PAH in addition to our long-standing work with HAA.

All of the food carcinogens have characteristic UV spectra and high extinction coefficients. Furthermore, most of the compounds fluoresce, making HPLC with UV absorbance and fluorescence detection a practical system. The aromatic structures of these heterocyclic amines give little fragmentation and therefore show large base peaks, making mass spectrometry a good detection method or confirmation method (Overvik *et al.*, 1989; Gross *et al.*, 1993)

Peak confirmation is crucial when working with such low levels of compounds since co-elution with other co-extracted compounds can occur. The most convenient and accessible instrument to identify heterocyclic amines on-line during an HPLC separation is the UV photodiode-array detector. Most instruments allow the recording of UV spectra even at a 0.1 nanogram level. A photodiode-array detection system efficiently prevents most false peak identifications and is essential to prevent the interpretation of false positive results. In our experience, even with modern photodiode-array detection with spectral library matching by computer, human interpretation is needed for confirmation in many cases. Other peak confirmation methods like off-line mass spectrometry or mutagenicity testing have been used successfully in our laboratory and others.

Fluorescence detection is typically used in-line as a complement to photodiode-array detection. Not all heterocyclic amines fluoresce, but PhIP, a commonly measured constituent in food shows about a nine-fold greater peak signal with fluorescence detection than photodiode-array detection, and the fluorescence signal typically shows fewer interfering peaks. The carcinogenic PAH all fluoresce. In our laboratory we still require confirmation of fluorescence peaks, so the sensitivity of the photodiode-array detector and the sample preparation procedure limit the overall sensitivity of the detection scheme. When the PAH levels are lower than 1 ng/g, the confirmation of the fluorescence peaks cannot be performed by photodiode-array detection due to its lower sensitivity. Therefore we believe the current method is limited to confirming PAH at concentrations above 1 ng/g.

5. RESULTS

5.1. Mutagenic Activity

5.1.1. Food Samples. The commercially cooked meat samples were purchased from grocery stores and restaurants in the San Francisco Bay Area. The cooking technique used for some commercially cooked samples remains unknown. Restaurant cooked meats were prepared well-done by request or unspecified, whereas grocery store products were reheated as specified on the package. All samples included every part of the meat normally eaten and were homogenized to create a homogeneous sample. Extraction for mutagenic activity testing and HPLC analysis for the HAA determination was done as previously described (Knize *et al.*, 1995) and developed by Gross and Grüter (1992).

5.1.2. Salmonella Mutagenicity Assay. The mutagenic activity of the sample extracts was determined using the standard plate incorporation assay described by Ames *et al.*, (1975) with *S. typhimurium* strain TA98 (a kind gift of Dr. B. Ames) with 2 mg of Aroclor-induced rat liver S9 protein per plate for metabolic activation as previously described (Knize *et al.*, 1995). Mutagenic activity was taken from the slope of the linear portion of

Table 1. Mutagenic activity of poultry gravies

Product type	Description	TA98 revertants colonies per gram
Chicken gravy	Liquid (jar)	NP
Turkey gravy	Liquid (jar)	NP
Chicken gravy	Liquid (can)	NP
Turkey gravy	Liquid (can)	NP
Turkey gravy	Powder (no water)	NP
Chicken gravy	Powder (no water)	NP
Chicken gravy	Powder (no water)	5
Chicken gravy	Powder-reconstituted	NP
Turkey gravy	Powder-reconstituted	NP
Chicken broth	Powder (no water)	NP
Chicken bouillon	Cubes	NP
Chicken soup mix A	Powder (no water)	NP
Chicken soup mix B	Powder (no water)	NP

NP= Not positive, no positive slope in dose-response.

dose-response curves to calculate the number of revertant colonies per gram of original sample extracted.

Mutagenic potency is a good screening method for samples to detect the potently mutagenic HAA. Table 1 shows TA98 revertant colonies per gram of poultry gravies purchased from grocery stores. The results show most samples are not positive, and that compared to many chicken samples (Sinha *et al.*, 1995), poultry gravies are not an important source of HAA-like mutagenic activity.

Table 2 shows mutagenic potency results from commercially-cooked chicken. All samples but two have less than 20 revertant colonies per gram. This is contrasted with the chicken fajita and Cajun chicken purchased in restaurants which were much more mutagenic than the others.

Related to the mutagenic HAA in cooked meats is the finding of mutagenic activity in non-meat foods. The biological response and chemical extraction results suggest that the activity is caused by heterocyclic amines. Mutagenic activity has been reported in a few baked grain foods, (Knize *et al.*, 1993) roasted grain-based beverages (Johansson *et*

Table 2. Mutagenic activity of commercially-cooked chicken

Product type	Description	Revertants/g
Chicken wing teriyaki	Baked meat w/ sauce	NP
Chicken wing Buffalo	Baked meat w/ sauce	NP
Chicken on a stick	Broiled meat w/ sauce	13
Chicken on a stick	Broiled meat w/ sauce	NP
Barbecued chicken	Baked (?) w/ sauce	NP
Cajun blackened chicken	Restaurant cooked (unknown)	130
Chicken Fajita A	Restaurant cooked (unknown)	420
Chicken Fajita B	Grocery -frozen- microwave	2
Mesquite chicken	Grocery -frozen- microwave	6
Roast chicken breast	Grocery deli roasted	7.4
Roast chicken thigh	Grocery deli roasted	9.1
Roast chicken thigh	Grocery deli roasted	8.8
Roast chicken breast	Restaurant wood fire roasted	15
Roast chicken thigh	Restaurant wood fire roasted	17

NP = Not positive, no positive slope in dose-response.

Table 3. HAA in grocery store meat products, ng/g

Food product	IQ	MeIQ	MeIQx	DiMeIQx	PhIP
Beef jerky	nd	nd	nd	nd	nd
Pork rinds A	nd	nd	0.42	0.1	nd
Pork rinds B	nd	nd	nd	nd	nd
Chili/beef	nd	nd	nd	nd	nd
Brown gravy	nd	nd	nd	nd	nd
Polish sausage	nd	nd	nd	nd	nd
Meatballs	nd	nd	nd	nd	nd

nd=Not detected.

al., 1995), and cooking oils (Shields *et al.*, 1995). Consumption of these foods also results in human exposure to bacterial mutagens that should be investigated for their chemical relationship to the heterocyclic amines found in meat.

5.2. Heterocyclic Aromatic Amines

Table 3 shows the amount of HAA in selected foods purchased in grocery stores. Only MeIQx and DiMeIQx were found, and in just one sample. This compares with Tikkanen *et al.* (1993) who analyzed commercially processed foods in Finland. Her results showed that the majority of flame broiled fish, chicken, and pork samples had detectable heterocyclic amines, (0.03 to 5.5 ng/g), but ground meat patties did not contain detectable amounts.

Table 4 shows HAA in restaurant-cooked beef, pork, and chicken samples. MeIQx was found in all samples, but at less than one ng/g. PhIP was also found at levels up to 13 ng/g. This contrasts with hamburgers, chicken, and fish cooked at fast-food restaurants, which had undetectable or low levels totaling less than 1 ng/g of HAA (Knize *et al.*, 1995). This can be explained by the thinner meat patties and short cooking times used in fast-food restaurants, which do not allow the HAA to form. In direct comparisons we have also found that ground meat made into patties produces less of the heterocyclic amines than meat steaks cooked identically.

5.3. Polycyclic Aromatic Hydrocarbons

For the PAH analysis, food samples were extracted based on the method published by Rivera *et al.* (1996) with some modifications. Briefly, the samples were ground and homogenized in NaOH, and extracted in a diatomaceous earth column using dichlo-

Table 4. HAA content of restaurant samples, ng/g

Type of sample	MeIQx	DiMeIQx	PhIP
Blackened pork	0.53	nd	3.0
Chicken fajita A	0.54	nd	6.4
Hamburger	0.89	nd	11
Blackened beef	0.48	nd	1.0
Top sirloin steak	0.87	nd	13

nd= not detected (<0.1 ng/g).

Table 5. Carcinogenic PAH in commercially cooked foods, ng/g

Sample	B[*a*]A	B[*b*]F	B[*k*]F	B[*a*]P	DBA	Indenopyrene
Cereal 1	nd	nd	nd	nd	nd	nd
Cereal 2	nd	nd	nd	nd	nd	nd
Coffee substitute	nd	nd	0.1	0.3	0.4	nd
Hot dog, smoke-flavored	0.2	nd	nd	0.3	nd	nd
Bacon, uncooked, smoke-flavored	nd	nd	0.6	nd	nd	nd
Liquid smoke flavoring	0.5	0.3	0.05	0.2	0.04	nd

nd=Not detected. Recoveries from 28 to 98%.

romethane. Further purification of the extract was performed by solid-phase extraction using a 1 g silica cartridge. The purified extracts were analyzed by HPLC with photodiode-array detection and fluorescence detection.

Because of the fatty nature of the smoked sausage and the bacon, a digestion was performed prior to the diatomaceous earth extraction. In these samples, further purification using a C_{18} cartridge was carried out. In the case of the hamburgers processed at high temperatures, the initial digestion of the sample was not necessary, but the final C_{18} purification step was not enough to obtain a clean extract that allowed the confirmation of the PAH by HPLC with photodiode-array detection. Consequently, the extract eluted from the silica cartridge was extracted with dimethylsulfoxide before the C_{18} step as described by García Falcón *et al.* (1996).

A search of the literature suggests PAH would be most likely to be found in cereal products (Dennis *et al.*, 1983; Lawrence *et al.*, 1984; Vaessen et al., 1984) and smoked foods (Howard and Fazio, 1980; García Falcón *et al.*, 1996; Lawrence and Weber, 1984; Yabiky *et al.*, 1993). Table 5 shows our results of the analysis of some products as purchased. Three food samples showed at least one carcinogenic PAH, both smoke-flavored meats and a toasted coffee substitute product. For the highest sample, total PAH was 0.8 ng/g. These results are in agreement with the data found in the literature (García Falcón *et al.*, 1996; Lawrence and Weber, 1984; Chen *et al.,* 1996; Dennis *et al.*, 1984) for the analysis of these PAH in smoked meats (levels between 0.04 and 2.8 ng/g). All PAH except indenopyrene have been detected in some breakfast cereal products (Dennis *et al.*, 1984, Lawrence and Weber, 1984, Vaessen *et al.*, 1984) at concentrations of 0.03–6.8 ng/g, but were not detected in the cereals we analyzed. A liquid smoke flavoring contained detectable PAH.

Figure 2 shows results of the HPLC analysis of hamburgers (30% fat) cooked over propane on a commercial grill. The upper chromatogram at 254 nm shows numerous peaks, while the fluorescence chromatogram (lower) shows fewer peaks that are suitable for quantification of PAH. Numbered peaks represent PAH and their UV absorbance spectra (shown in boxes) with a library spectrum. Retention time matching and spectral library matching along with peak quantitation by fluorescence detection allows some certainty in PAH identification, but further sample clean-up is needed, especially for compounds 1 (B[*a*]A) and 2 (B[*b*]F) in Figure 2.

Hamburgers cooked over propane, charcoal, or in a frying pan contained PAH and HAA (Table 6), with the propane-cooked sample having 52 ng/g of total PAH. In this experiment the average grill surface temperature for the propane (394°C) was much higher than the temperature for the charcoal grill (179°C) so a comparison of the heat source only cannot be made with these data. The PAH concentrations increased with the cooking

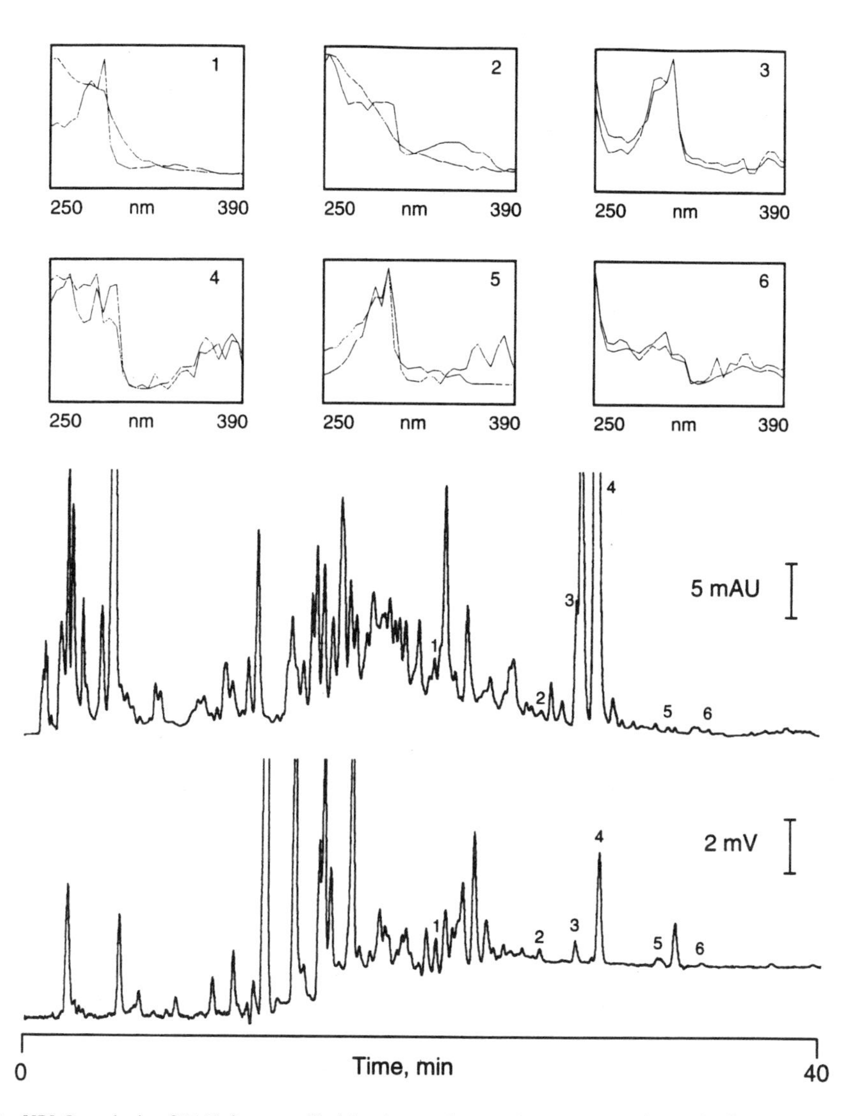

Figure 2. HPLC analysis of PAH from a grilled hamburger. Lower chromatogram shows the fluorescence signal, upper chromatogram shows the UV absorbance at 254 nm. Upper plots show sample and reference UV absorbance spectra. Compounds (excitation wavelength/emission wavelength): 1=B[*a*]A (280/389), 2=B[*b*]F (260/420), 3=B[*k*]F (260/420), 4=B[a]P (260/420), 5=DBA (296/396), 6=indenopyrene (293/498). HPLC conditions: A gradient from 50% acetonitrile in water to 100% in 30 min, flow 1 ml/min, column: Vydac TP2015415 (Hesperia, CA). HPLC system: Waters Millennium with a model 996 PDA detector and Hewlett-Packard 1046 fluorescence detector.

Table 6. Carcinogenic PAH/HAA in hamburgers, ng/g

Sample	B[*a*]A	B[*b*]F	B[*k*]F	B[*a*]P	DBA	Indenopyrene	MeIQx	PhIP
Propane grilled	5.2	18	2.0	6.2	0.5	5.1	2.2	15
Charcoal grilled	3.1	4.1	nd	0.6	nd	nd	nd	nd
Pan fried	nd	nd	nd	nd	nd	nd	3.8	16

nd = Not detected.

temperature. These results are in accordance with the data found in the literature (Larsson *et al.*, 1983; Howard and Fazio, 1980; Lawrence and Weber, 1984; Lawrence, 1986).

Comparison of the formation of PAH and HAA shows that open flames are required to make PAH, but high temperature by a variety of heat sources can form HAA (Table 6). The mass amounts of PAH and HAA are within the same order of magnitude for high temperature propane-grilling with 30% fat hamburger. Further work is needed to analyze other food types for both classes of carcinogen.

6. REDUCING THE FORMATION OF FOOD MUTAGENS/CARCINOGENS

6.1. Modifying Cooking Practices

Many studies have shown the effect of cooking time and temperature on the formation of mutagenic activity (Commoner *et al.*, 1978; Sugimura *et al.*, 1977) and specific HAA in various meats (Gross and Gruter, 1992; Skog *et al.*, 1995; Knize *et al.*, 1994). Food doneness is difficult to quantify. In our experience, measuring temperatures with thermocouples is too dependent on probe placement. Surface appearance, too, is not a good doneness indicator because color can be affected by other variables such as pH differences in meat.

Weight loss is a reasonable indicator in comparing similar methods. Weight loss of over 20% appears to be necessary at least for the higher PhIP concentrations measured in some studies (Skog *et al.*, 1995; Knize *et al.*, 1993; Salmon *et al.*, 1997).

Reducing the cooking temperature seems to be the most practical way to reduce HAA content, but avoiding the conditions where the temperatures are below those needed to kill harmful bacteria is essential. The formation of PAH can be reduced by not exposing the food directly to the heat source and resulting smoke when grilling foods (Larsson *et al.*, 1983).

6.2. Using Microwave Pretreatment

A method to reduce the amount of mutagenic/carcinogenic HAA formed during frying of ground beef was developed in our laboratory (Felton *et al.*, 1994). Beef patties received microwave treatment for various times before frying. Microwave pretreating for 2 minutes, then pouring off the resulting liquid and frying at either 200°C or 250°C for 6 minutes per side reduced HAA precursors (creatine, creatinine, amino acids, glucose), water, and fat up to 30% in the patties. The sum of the HAA shown to be present decreased 3-fold for 200°C frying or 9-fold for 250°C cooking, compared to control, non-microwave pretreated beef patties fried under identical conditions.

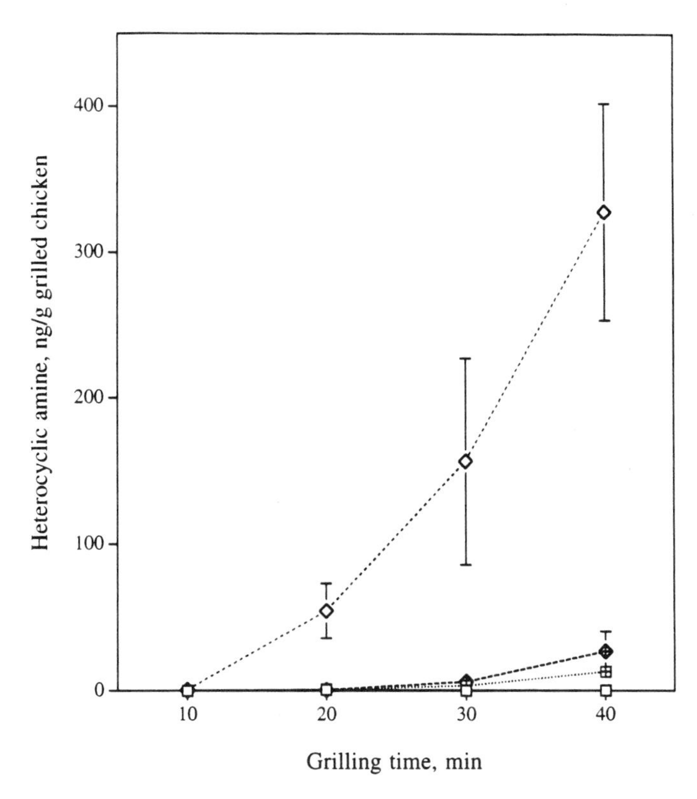

Figure 3. Formation of PhIP (diamond symbol) and MeIQx (square symbol) in marinated (filled symbol) or control (open symbol) chicken breast meat samples grilled for 10, 20, 30, or 40 minutes. Marinating was for 4 hours in a mixture of brown sugar, olive oil, cider vinegar, garlic, lemon juice, mustard and salt. Error bars represent the standard error of the mean of three experiments.

6.3. Marinating before Grilling

We recently found that the application of a marinade to chicken breast meat before grilling can greatly decrease PhIP, although MeIQx is increased at the longest cooking time (Salmon *et al.*, 1997). Figure 3 shows results from the analysis of chicken breast meat samples grilled on a propane grill for 10, 20, 30, or 40 minutes, without skin and bones. Some samples were marinated in a published recipe containing brown sugar, olive oil, lemon juice, cider vinegar, mustard, garlic, and salt. PhIP was reduced 92 to 99% after marinating and grilling for 20, 30, or 40 min. Interestingly, MeIQx showed an increasing trend with cooking time in these experiments and others, but the increase was statistically significant only at the 40 min cooking time. No reports have been found showing the effect of marinating meat prior to charbroiling or grilling on the formation of PAH.

6.4. Using Additives in Ground Meat

Schemes for reducing mutagenic activity or the specific HAA by adding substances to ground meat have been reported. Creatinase treatment was used to reduce the available creatine (Vikse and Joner, 1993) and food additives such as antioxidants (Wang *et al.*, 1982) or glucose or lactose (Skog *et al.*, 1992) were shown to lower mutagenic activity. The work with added sugars resulted in decreased mutagenic activity, contradicting our results with marinades, which suggest increased MeIQx with the sucrose we used in our marinade.

HAA are formed in trace amounts, so specifically inhibiting a reaction path without greatly affecting the quality of the cooked meat seems unlikely.

6.5. Patented Methods for Reducing Carcinogen Formation

At least one cooking grill designed to reduce the formation of carcinogens, both HAA and PAH, has been patented (Basel, 1995). Another has patents pending (Grill Away, Wichita KS). A Japanese patent (Makamura and Tsuji, 1986) suggests a method for the reduction of carcinogens in broiled meats. It involves soaking meat in a 10% solution containing any one of 7 different sugars.

7. RISK ASSESSMENT AND FUTURE STUDIES

The analysis of foods for HAA and PAH is important because there is widespread human exposure to these compounds, there is suggestive epidemiology for cause and effect, and these chemicals are potent mutagens and animal carcinogens. Exposures vary among individuals, since dietary preferences and variation in food preparation can greatly influence individual exposures. This area of research provides a unique opportunity in cancer etiology, the chance to evaluate carcinogens in human populations. The variability in the formation of these compounds also provides the opportunity for intervention, to reduce exposure if it is warranted from risk evaluation.

Which class of carcinogenic compounds and which specific compounds within those classes are the most important in human health are difficult questions to answer. All of the HAA and PAH tested are rodent carcinogens, so it could be argued that the total mass of carcinogen is the most important risk factor.

The compounds do differ in tumor-site specificity in rats, with most heterocyclic amines causing tumors in the liver and other sites. The metabolism of each class of chemical and the enzymes involved in their metabolism are known to vary, suggesting a distribution in risk, varying from individual to individual.

For PAH carcinogens, occupational studies have been used to establish risk of human exposure, with only suggestions of excessive risk at some sites (Nandon *et al.*, 1995) The health risk to the human population consuming HAA has been recently discussed (Layton *et al.*, 1995), and supports the linkage between HAA consumption and cancer risk.

ACKNOWLEDGMENTS

Pilar Pais is a postdoctoral fellow of the Ministerio de Educación y Cultura of the Spanish Goverment. This work was performed under the auspices of the U.S. Department of Energy by Lawrence Livermore National Laboratory under contract no. W-7405-Eng-48, and supported by the NCI grant CA55861 and the Breast Cancer Fund of the State of California through the Breast Cancer Research Program of the University of California, Grant Number 2RB-0126.

REFERENCES

Ames, B. N.; McCann, J.; Yamasaki E. Methods for detecting carcinogens and mutagens with the Salmonella/mammalian microsome mutagenicity test. *Mutat.Res.* **1975**, 31, 347–364.

Badger, G. M.; Kimber, R. W. L. The formation of aromatic hydrocarbons at high temperatures, Part VI. The pyrolysis of tetralin. *J. Chem. Soc.* **1960**, 51,266–270.

Basel, R. M. U.S. patent **1995**, 5,439,691.

Chen, B. H.; Wang, C. Y.; Chiu, C. P. Evaluation of analysis of polycyclic aromatic hydrocarbons in meat products by liquid chromatography. *J. Agric. Food Chem.* **1996**, 44, 2244–2251.

Chu, M. M. L.; Chen, C. W. The evaluation and estimation of potential carcinogenic risks of polynuclear aromatic hydrocarbons (PAH). *United States Environmental Protection Agency Research and Development* **1985**, 1–29.

Commoner, B.; Vithayathil, A. J.; Dolara, P.; Nair, S.; Madyastha, P.; Cuca, G. C. Formation of mutagens in beef and beef extract during cooking. *Science* **1978**, 201, 913–916.

Dennis, M. J.; Massey, R. C.; McWeeny, D. J.; Knowles, M. E.; Watson, D. Analysis of polycyclic aromatic hydrocarbons in UK total diets. *Food Chem. Toxic.* **1983**, 21, 569–574.

Dennis, M. J.; Massey, R. C.; McWeeny, D. J.; Larsson, B.; Eriksson, A.; Sahlberg, G. Comparison of a capillary gas chromatographic and a high-performance liquid chromatographic method of analysis for polycyclic aromatic hydrocarbons in food. *J. Chromatogr.* **1984**, 285, 127–133.

Doll, R. Nature and nurture: possibilities for cancer control. *Carcinogenesis* **1996**, 17, 177–184.

El-Bayoumy, K.; Chae, Y-H.; Upadhyaya, P.; Rivenson, A.; Kurtzke, C.; Reddy, B.; Hecht, S. S. Comparative tumorigenicity of benzo[*a*]pyrene, 1-nitropyrene, and 2-amino-1-methyl-6-phenylimidazo[4,5-*b*]pyridine administered by gavage to female CD rats. *Carcinogenesis* **1995,** 16, 431–434.

Felton, J. S.; Fultz, E.; Dolbeare, F. A.; Knize, M. G. Reduction of heterocyclic amine mutagens/carcinogens in fried beef patties by microwave pretreatment. *Food Chem. Toxic.* **1994**, 32, 897–903.

García Falcón, M. S.; González Amigo, S.; Lage Yusty, M. A.; López de Alda-Villaizán, M. J.; Simal Lozano, J. Enrichment of benzo[*a*]pyrene in smoked food products and determination by high-performance liquid chromatography-fluorescence detection. *J. Chromatogr. A* **1996**,753, 207–215.

Gold, L. S.; Manley, N. B.; Slone, T. H.; Garfinked, B. G.; Rohlbach, L.; Ames, B. N. The fifth plot of the carcinogenic potency database: results in animal bioassays published in the general literature through 1988 and by the National Toxicology Program through 1989. *Environ. Health Perpec.* **1993**, 100, 65–135.

Gross, G. A. Simple methods for quantifying mutagenic heterocyclic amines in food products. *Carcinogenesis* **1990**,11, 1597–1603.

Gross, G. A.; Grüter, A. Quantitation of mutagenic/carcinogenic heterocyclic aromatic amines in food products. *J. Chromatogr.* **1992**, 592, 271–278.

Gross, G. A.; Turesky, R. J.; Fay, L. B.; Stillwell, W. G.; Skipper, P. L.; Tannenbaum, S. R. Heterocyclic amine formation in grilled bacon, beef, and fish, and in grill scrapings. *Carcinogenesis* **1993**,14, 2313–2318.

Hatch, F. T.; Knize, M. G.; Moore, D. H.; Felton, J. S. Quantitative correlation of mutagenic and carcinogenic potencies for heterocyclic amine from cooked foods and additional aromatic amines. *Mutat. Res.* **1992**, 271, 269–287.

Howard, J. W.; Fazio, T. Review of polycyclic aromatic hydrocarbons in foods: analytical methodology and reported findings of polycyclic aromatic hydrocarbons in foods. *J. Assoc. Off. Anal. Chem.* **1980**, 63, 1077–1104.

Johansson, M. A. E.; Knize, M. G.; Jägerstad, M.; Felton, J. S. Characterization of mutagenic activity in instant hot beverage powders. *Environ. Molec. Mutag.* **1995**, 25, 154–161.

Knize M. G.; Andresen, B. D.; Healy, S. K.; Shen, N. H.; Lewis, P. R.; Bjeldanes, L. F.; Hatch, F. T.; Felton, J. S. Effect of temperature, patty thickness and fat content on the production of mutagens in fried ground beef. *Food Chem. Toxic.* **1985**, 23, 1035–1040

Knize M. G.; Dolbeare F. A.; Carroll K. L.; Moore II, D. H.; Felton J. S. Effect of cooking time and temperature on the heterocyclic amine content of fried-beef patties. *Food Chem. Toxic.* **1994**, 32, 595–603.

Knize, M. G.; Cunningham, P. L.; Jones, A. L.; Griffin, E. A.; Felton, J. S. Mutagenic activity and heterocyclic amine content in cooked grain food products. *Food Chem. Toxic.* **1993**, 32, 15–21.

Knize, M. G.; Shen, N. H.; Healy, S. K.; Hatch, F. T.; Felton, J. S. The use of bacterial mutation tests to monitor chemical isolation of the mutagens in cooked beef. *Devel, Ind. Microbiol.* **1987**, 28, 171–180.

Knize, M. G.; Sinha, R.; Rothman, N.; Brown, E. D.; Salmon, C. P.; Levander, O. A.; Cunningham P. L.; Felton J. S. Fast-food meat products have relatively low heterocyclic amine content. *Food Chem. Toxic.* **1995**, 33, 545–551.

Larsson, B. K.; Shalberg, G. P.; Eriksson, A. T.; Busk, L. Å. Polycyclic aromatic hydrocarbons in grilled food. *J. Agric. Food Chem.* **1983**, 31, 867–873.

Lawrence, J. F. Determination of nanogram/kilogram of polycyclic aromatic hydrocarbons in foods by HPLC with fluorescence detection. *Intern. J. Environ. Anal. Chem.* **1986**, 24, 113–131.

Lawrence, J. F.; Weber, D. F. Determination of polycyclic aromatic hydrocarbons in Canadian samples of processed vegetable and dairy products by liquid chromatography with fluorescence detection. *J. Agric. Food Chem.* **1984**, 32, 794–797.

Lawrence, J. F.; Weber, D. F. Determination of polycyclic aromatic hydrocarbons in some Canadian commercial fish, shellfish, and meat products by liquid chromatography with confirmation by capillary gas chromatography-mass spectrometry. *J. Agric. Food Chem.* **1984**, 32, 789–793.

Layton, D. W.; Bogen, K. T.; Knize, M. G.; Hatch, F. T.; Johnson, V. M.; Felton, J. S. Cancer risk of heterocyclic amines in cooked foods: An analysis and implications for research. *Carcinogenesis.* **1995**,16, 39–52.

Lijinsky, W. The formation and occurrence of food-associated polycyclic aromatic hydrocarbons associated with food. *Mutat. Res.* **1991**, 259, 251–261.

Lijinsky, W.; Raha, C. R. The pyrolysis of 2-methyl-naphthalene. *J. Org. Chem.* **1961**, 26, 3566–3567.

Makamura, T.; Ysuji, K. Japanese patent **1986**, 61–25345.

Manabe, S.; Kurihara, N.; Wada, O.; Izumikawa, S.; Asakuna, K.; Morita, M. Detection of a carcinogen, 2-amino-1-methyl-6-phenylimidazo[4,5-*b*]pyridine, in airborne particles and diesel-exhaust particles. *Environ. Pollut.* **1993**, 80, 281–286.

Manabe, S.; Tohyama, K.; Wada, O.; Aramaki, T. Detection of a carcinogen, 2-amino-1-methyl-6-phenylimidazo[4,5-*b*]pyridine (PhIP), in cigarette smoke condensate. *Carcinogenesis* **1991**, 12, 1945–1947.

Nadon, L.; Siemiatycki, J.; Dewar, R.; Krewski, D.; Gerin, M. Cancer risk due to occupational exposure to polycyclic aromatic hydrocarbons. *Am. J. Ind. Med.* **1995**, 28, 303–324.

Nagao, M.; Honda, M.; Seino, Y.; Yahagi, T.; Sugimura, T. Mutagenicities of smoke condensates and the charred surface of fish and meat. *Cancer Lett.* **1977**, 2, 221–226.

Ohgaki, H.; Takayama, S.; Sugumura, T. Carcinogenicities of heterocyclic amines in cooked food. *Mutat. Res.* **1991**, 259, 399–410.

Övervik, E.; Kleman, M.; Berg, I.; Gustafsson J-Å. Influence of creatine, amino acids and water on the formation of the mutagenic heterocyclic amines found in cooked meat. *Carcinogenesis* **1989**, 10, 2293–2301.

Rivera, L.; Curto, M. J. C.; Pais, P.; Galceran, M. T.; Puignou, L. Solid-phase extraction for the selective isolation of polycyclic aromatic hydrocarbons, azaarenes, and heterocyclic amines in charcoal-grilled meat. *J. Chromatogr. A* **1996**, 719, 85–94.

Robbana-Barnat, S.; Rabache, M.; Rialland E.; Fradin, J. Heterocyclic amines: Occurrence and prevention in cooked food. *Environ. Health Persp.* **1996**,104, 280–288.

Salmon, C. P.; Knize, M. G.; Felton, J. S. Effects of marinating on heterocyclic amine carcinogen production in grilled chicken (*Food Chem. Toxic.* **1997**, 35, 433–441).

Sheilds, P. G.; Xu, G. X.; Blot, W. J.; Fraumeni Jr., J. F.; Trivers, G. E.; Pellizzari, E. D.; Qu, Y. H.; Gao, Y. T.; Harris, C. C. Mutagens from heated Chinese and U.S. cooking oils. *J. Natl. Cancer Inst.* **1995**, 87, 836–841.

Shirai, T.; Sano, M.; Tamano, S.; Takahashi, S.; Hirose, M.; Futakuchi, M.; Hasegawa, R.; Imaida, K; Matsumoto, K-I.; Wakabayashi, K.; Sugimura, T.; Ito, N. The prostate: A target for the carcinogenicity of 2-amino-1-methyl-6-phenylimidazo[4,5-*b*]pyridine derived from cooked foods. *Cancer Res.* **1997**, 57, 195–198.

Sinha, R.; Rothman, N.; Brown, E.; Levander, O.; Salmon, C. P.; Knize, M. G.; Felton, J. S. High concentrations of the carcinogen 2-amino-1-methyl-6-imidazo[4,5-*b*]pyridine (PhIP) occur in chicken but are dependent on the cooking method. *Cancer Res.* **1995**, 55, 4516–4519.

Skog, K. Cooking procedures and food mutagens: A literature review. *Food Chem. Toxic.* **1993**, 31, 655–675.

Skog, K.; Jägerstad, M.; Laser Reuterswärd, A. Inhibitory effect of carbohydrates on the formation of mutagens in fried beef patties. *Food Chem. Toxic.* **1992**, 30, 681–688.

Skog, K.; Steineck, G.; Augustsson, K.; Jägerstad, M. Effect of cooking temperature on the formation of heterocyclic amines in fried meat products and pan residues. *Carcinogenesis* **1995**, 16, 861–867.

Stavric, B. Biological significance of trace levels of mutagenic heterocyclic aromatic amines (HAAs) in the human diet: a critical review. *Food Chem. Toxic.* **1994**, 32, 977–994.

Sugimura, T.; Nagao, M.; Kawachi, T.; Honda, M.; Yahagi, T.; Seino, Y.; Sato, S.; Matsukura, N.; Matsushima, T.; Shirai, A.; Sawamura, M.; Matsumoto, H. Mutagen-carcinogens in foods with special reference to highly mutagenic pyrolytic products in broiled foods. In *Origins of Human Cancer*; Hiatt, H.H.; Watson, J.D.; Winsten, J.A., Eds.; Cold Spring Harbor, New York, **1977**, 1561–1577.

Thiebaud, H. P.; Knize, M. G.; Kuzmicky, P. A.; Felton, J. S.; Hsieh, D. P. Mutagenicity and chemical analysis of fumes from cooking meat. *J. Agric. Food Chem.* **1994**, 42, 1502–1510.

Tikkanen, L. M.; Sauri, T. M.; Latva-Kala, K. J. Screening of heat-processed Finnish foods for the mutagens 2-amino-3,4,8-dimethylimidazo[4,5-*f*]quinoxaline, 2-amino-3,8-dimethylimidazo[4,5-*f*]quinoxaline, and 2-amino-1-methyl-6-phenylimidazo[4,5-*b*]pyridine. *Food Chem. Toxic.* **1993**, 31, 717–721.

Vaessen, H. A. M. G.; Schuller, P. L.; Jekel, A. A.; Wilbers, A. M. M. A. Polycyclic aromatic hydrocarbons in selected foods; analysis and occurrence. *Toxicol. Environ. Chem.* **1984**, 7, 297–324.

Vainiotalo, S.; Matveinen, K.; Reunamen, A. GC/MS Determination of the mutagenic heterocyclic amines MeIQx and DiMeIQx in cooking fumes. *Fresenius J. Anal. Chem.* **1993**, 345, 462–466.

Vikse, R.; Joner, P. E. Mutagenicity, creatine, and nutrient contents of pan fried meat from various animal species. *Acta Vet. Scand.* **1993**, 34, 1–7.

Vogelstein, B.; Kinzler, W. W. Carcinogens leave fingerprints. *Nature* **1992**, 355, 209–210.

Wakabayashi, K.; Kim, I-S.; Kurosaka, R.; Yamaizumi, Z.; Ushiyams, H.; Takahashi, M.; Koyota, A.; Tada, A.; Nukaya. H.; Goto, S.; Sugimura, T.; Nagao, M. In *Heterocyclic amines in cooked foods: possible human carcinogens*; Adamson, R.H.: Gustafsson, J-A.: Ito, N.: Nagao, M.; Sugimura, T.; Wakabayashi, K.; Yamazoe, Y., Eds.; Princeton Scientific Publishing, Princeton, NJ, USA, **1995**, p. 39.

Wakabayashi, K.; Nagao, M.; Esumi, H.; Sugimura T. Food-derived mutagens and carcinogens. *Cancer Res.* **1992**, 52 (suppl.), 2092s-2098s.

Wang, Y. Y.; Vuolo, L. L.; Springarn, N. E.; Weisburger, J. H. Formation of mutagens in cooked foods, V. The mutagen reducing effect of soy protein concentrates and antioxidants during frying of beef. *Cancer Lett.* **1982**, 16, 179–186.

Wynder, E. L.; Gori, G. B. Contribution of the environment to cancer incidence: an epidemiologic exercise. *J. Nat. Cancer Inst.* **1977**, 58, 825–832.

Yabiky, H. Y.; Martins, M. S.; Takahashi, M. Y. Levels of benzo[*a*]pyrene and other polycyclic aromatic hydrocarbons in liquid smoke flavour and some smoked foods. *Food Addit. Contamin.* **1993**, 10, 399–405.

13

EFFECTS OF PROCESSING ON HEAVY METAL CONTENT OF FOODS

Jeffrey N. Morgan

U.S. Environmental Protection Agency
National Exposure Research Laboratory
Microbiological and Chemical Exposure Assessment Research Division
Chemical Exposure Research Branch
26 W. Martin Luther King Dr., Cincinnati, Ohio 45268

1. ABSTRACT

Metals occur in all foodstuffs. Of particular concern is the presence of toxic metals, which include lead, cadmium, arsenic and mercury. The toxic metal content of foods is influenced by many factors ranging from environmental conditions during growth to post-harvest handling, processing, preparation and cooking techniques. For example, metal content increases in some commodities grown in contaminated soils or atmospheres while post-harvest handling steps such as washing generally remove metal contaminants. Cooking may reduce metal content although some foods can absorb metals if the cooking water is contaminated. Metals used in food processing equipment or food packaging material may contribute to food contamination. Contamination may also occur during kitchen preparation and storage. This paper will review the effects of processing of foods on toxic metal content. A broad interpretation of processing, to include aspects of food production from growth through cooking, will be taken in discussing the toxic metal content of foods. Specific examples of changes in metal content due to processing will be discussed.

2. INTRODUCTION

Metal contamination of foods, of both plant and animal origin, may occur at various stages of production. These stages include growth, post-harvest handling, in-plant processing, preparation for consumption either in the home or elsewhere, cooking and the act of consumption itself.

Impact of Processing on Food Safety, edited by Jackson et al.,
Kluwer Academic / Plenum Publishers, New York, 1999.

Contamination may occur during growth, depending upon the environmental conditions in which a plant or animal is raised. Atmospheric deposition of toxic elements may contribute to the metal content of plant crops. Contamination may occur both through direct deposition on the plant itself or through deposition on soil and subsequent uptake by the plant. Use of sewage sludge as a fertilizer also contributes to the toxic metal content of foods, as does the use of contaminated water for irrigation. Another potential source of contamination is agricultural chemicals, either fertilizers or pesticides. While these products are generally used intentionally to increase crop yields, formulations often contain varying amounts of undesirable contaminants in addition to the active ingredients. Contamination may occur from fragments of harvesting equipment accidentally present in crops. Finally, animal feeds may contribute to increased toxic element levels in animal products. This may occur through the presence of trace contaminants in the feed or through the presence of elements, such as arsenic, used, or misused, as growth promoters in feed.

Post-harvest handling of food products may also lead to the contamination of food products with toxic elements. Storage at the farm after harvest, transportation between farm and processing plant, and storage at the plant all represent stages in the production of foods where additional contamination may occur.

A number of operations which occur at the processing plant itself may potentially lead to metal contamination of food products. Contact with processing equipment may lead to product contamination. Generally, high quality stainless steels, plastics and other materials approved for food contact are used. If care is taken in selecting equipment and contact surface materials, taking into account the nature of the food being processed, there is minimal chance of harmful contamination. However, misuse of equipment or use of materials incompatible with the material being processed may result in contamination. Water used at the plant in washing or rinsing operations as well as that added as an ingredient of the final food product is another potential source of undesirable metals. Water used at the plant must be metal-free to insure that food products are not contaminated. Processed foods often contain additives, used for a variety of purposes in the final product. Trace metal contamination of these additives is another potential source of undesirable toxic elements in foods. Finally, the material in which the finished product is packaged for sale may contribute to contamination of the product. Both aluminum and tin-plate cans may contribute to metal contamination of food. In the past, lead solder used to seal cans was a significant source of lead contamination. As a result, lead solder is no longer approved for food use in the United States.

Food preparation and cooking in the home, or elsewhere, is another potentially significant source of metal contamination. Foods may come in contact with contaminated surfaces such as dirty or dusty kitchen counters, pots and pans, utensils or plates. Materials used in cooking equipment and utensils may also contribute. Use of metal contaminated water in cooking or in preparation of foods and beverages such as soups and drinks, may be another significant source of dietary intake of metals. Non-ideal storage conditions in the home, such as storage of acidic foods in metal pots and pans, rather than transferring to a plastic container, may contribute to metal contamination. In fact, for some segments of the population, it is likely that contamination once the food has reached the home is the most significant source of dietary exposure to toxic metals.

The preceding paragraphs have attempted to outline some of the many potential sources of metal contamination of foods from the farm to the table. While an exhaustive discussion of each of these is beyond the scope of this chapter, several relatively recent books are either entirely devoted to this topic or contain chapters on metal contamination of foods. These reviews include Flegal et al. (1990), Gruenwedel (1990), Harrison (1993), Nriagu (1990), Nriagu and Azcue (1990), Reilly (1991), and Janssen (1997).

The remainder of this chapter will be devoted to a discussion of some examples of metal contamination of foods from the recent literature. The discussion will be confined to lead, cadmium, arsenic and mercury. These metals are all toxic to humans in that they have no known essential or beneficial effect, but exert a catastrophic effect on normal metabolic functions even at low levels. Based on considerations of usage, toxicity and environmental occurrence, these metals are amongst those given first priority by the U.S. Food and Drug Administration in its program on toxic metals in foods (Jelinek, 1985).

3. EFFECT OF PROCESSING ON TOXIC METALS

3.1. Lead

Lead exists only in small quantities in the earth's crust but has been commonly used since very early times due to the ease with which it is extracted from its ores. Current industrial uses of lead include production of batteries, lead-sheathed cables, bullets and shot gun pellets, solders, lead alloys used in printing and both organic and inorganic lead compounds with a variety of uses (Reilly, 1991). One major use of lead salts is in the glazing of ceramics. Formerly, lead was used extensively as a petroleum additive, although this use has decreased significantly throughout the world since the early 1970's.

Lead is a cumulative poison, and thus a much more potent chronic toxicant than an acute one. Chronic exposure to lead may result in brain and liver damage, tumor formation, enzyme inhibition (Gruenwedel, 1990), central and peripheral nervous system effects, anemia, disturbance of renal function and weight loss (Janssen, 1997). Acute toxicity symptoms include lassitude, vomiting, loss of appetite, poor body coordination, convulsions, stupor and coma (Gruenwedel, 1990).

The widespread use and toxicity of lead has caused a great deal of concern regarding the levels of lead in foods and beverages. It has been estimated that people in North America consume an average of 50 μg of lead per day in food, beverages and dust (Flegal et al., 1990). Lead intake due to consumption of contaminated foods has been significantly reduced since the use of lead solder in canning operations was discontinued. Nevertheless, some contamination of foods with lead still occurs, as the following examples demonstrate.

Rowarth (1990) conducted a study designed to determine lead concentrations in honey taken from different localities in New Zealand as well as from different stages of processing. Lead concentrations at different stages of processing are shown in Table 1. Av-

Table 1. Lead concentration in honey at various stages of processing

Point of sampling	Average Pb concentration (μg/g)
Comb	0.10
During Processing	0.13
Storage in soldered can	0.66
Storage in plastic	0.18

Reference: Rowarth (1990)

Table 2. Lead concentration in maple syrup during collection and processing

Sample	Pb concentration (μg/L)
Plastic tank in grove	1.5-2.5
Galvanized bucket in grove	6-8
Grove	4.3
Truck tank (thru bronze gear pump)	31.0
Diatomaceous earth filter	19.0
Stainless steel tank	20.0

Reference: Stilwell and Musante (1996)

erage lead concentration in honey samples stored in lead soldered containers was considerably higher than in raw honey, during processing or samples stored in plastic containers. In fact, the lead concentration in samples stored in lead soldered containers was more than three times that of samples stored in plastic containers. This example demonstrates the potential for contamination of a product by the material in which it is packaged and is typical of many canned foods consumed in the United States prior to removal of lead soldered cans from the market.

Stilwell and Musante (1996) conducted a survey of lead concentrations in maple syrup produced in Connecticut and identified potential sources of lead based on analysis of sap and syrup-processing samples. The contamination of maple syrup by sample handling equipment and storage containers was demonstrated. Results of this study are shown in Table 2. First, a comparison was made between lead levels in sap collected in both galvanized and plastic buckets in the grove. Lead levels were 2–5 times higher in sap collected in galvanized buckets than those collected in plastic buckets. Further contamination of the sap occurred after use of a bronze gear pump in sap transfer steps. Lead levels increased from the grove level of 4.3 μg/L to 31 μ/L in a truck tank, after pumping through the bronze gear pump. Lead was reduced to 19 μg/L after passing through a diatomaceous earth filter, but this final level remained approximately 4–5 times higher than the level in sap at the grove. This study demonstrates the need to consider chemical properties of a food and to exercise care in selection of materials which come in contact with that food in order to minimize lead contamination. Since sap is acidic and has the potential to react with many metal surfaces, contact with metals containing lead should be avoided during collection and processing.

Lead content in grapefruit juice packaged in different types of containers and uptake of lead by grapefruit juice stored in open containers has also been recently evaluated (Stilwell and Musante, 1994). Measurable lead was detected only in grapefruit juice packaged in tin-coated metal cans (Table 3). Lead levels were below detection limits in grapefruit juice packaged in glass or waxed paperboard containers. Since lead appeared only in

Table 3. Lead concentration in grapefruit juice packaged in different types of containers

Type of container	Mean Pb concentration (μg/L)
Tin-coated steel	7.7
Glass	< 1
Waxed paperboard	< 1

Reference: Stilwell and Musante (1994)

Table 4. Lead concentration in stored grapefruit juice

	Pb concentration (μg/L)				
Days of storage	Brand A	Brand B	Brand C	Brand D	Brand E
0	9	4	25	0	8
4	25	14	80	2	21
8	46	24	118	5	32
14	64	45	157	6	50

Reference: Stilwell and Musante (1994)

juices packaged in cans, it appeared likely that the source of lead was the can itself. Further investigation by these authors revealed that lead impurities in the tin-coating of the cans were the source of lead in the grapefruit juice. A leaching study designed to simulate the potential consumer practice of storing an opened can in the refrigerator for several days was also conducted. In all five brands of juice tested, lead content increased significantly during the 14 day period after opening, although there was a wide range of values for lead leached. Final lead concentrations after 14 days ranged from 6–157 μg/L (Table 4). This study again emphasizes the need to select appropriate materials for packaging and storing foods and beverages, particularly acidic ones. Lead in grapefruit juice can be minimized by selecting cans with a minimum of lead impurity in the tin-coating or using containers other than cans. Potential lead intake can further be reduced by the consumer by immediately transferring juice from cans to glass or plastic containers after opening.

The widespread use of lead salts in the glazing of ceramics is of particular concern when the ceramic is used in contact with food or beverage, such as mugs or plates. The potential for lead to leach from these materials into foods or beverages has prompted the U.S. Food and Drug Administration to establish guidelines for lead release from ceramic mugs. The current guideline is 0.5 μg/mL after 24 hours contact with acetic acid. Mindak et al. (1992) studied the leaching characteristics of lead-glazed ceramic mugs from different countries. While these authors evaluated a large sample set of mugs, results from six sets of mugs are summarized in Table 5. Detectable lead was leached into acetic acid after 30 minutes, up to 0.74 μg/mL. This level increased after 24 hours to as high as 1.49 μg/mL, and exceeding FDA's guidelines of 0.5 μg/mL in five of six samples shown. For most mugs, one fourth to one half of the lead released after 24 hours was released in the first 30 minutes. Lead was also leached into coffee after 30 minutes, up to 0.76μg/mL. Coffee and acetic acid leaching studies were not directly comparable since they were conducted at different temperatures (26°C and 85°C for acetic acid and coffee, respectively).

Table 5. Lead release from ceramic mugs with lead-containing glazes

	Pb(μg/mL) in 4% acetic acid		Pb(μg/mL) in coffee
Sample set	24 hr.	30 min.	30 min.
1	0.015	0.008	0.007
2	0.055	0.031	0.026
3	0.124	0.053	0.056
4	0.208	0.059	0.076
5	0.840	0.029	<0.001
6	1.49	0.074	0.007

Reference: Mindak et al. (1992)

Table 6. Lead In leachates from microwave heated, old ceramic dinnerware

	Pb Conc. (μg/mL)		
Sample set	Acetic acid—24 hr.	Acetic acid—micro. 2 min	Citric acid—micro. 5 min.
1	31.0	1.5	5.9
2	86.0	14.5	15.1
3	129.0	7.2	33.9
4	156.0	6.0	32.4
5	70.0	2.2	4.7
6	8.9	13.0	14.6

Reference: Sheets et al. (1996)

This study demonstrates the potential for increased lead exposure due to consumption of foods or beverages in contact with lead-containing materials. To reduce the risk of exposure, the time that the food or beverage is in contact with the lead-containing material should be minimized.

Large quantities of lead-glazed ceramic dinnerware were produced in the United States from around 1920 to the mid-1940's. While these items are no longer produced, they are considered collectibles and are often found in antique shops and flea markets. Sheets et al. (1996) investigated the effects of microwave heating on lead leaching characteristics of these items. Selected results from this study are shown in Table 6. Lead concentrations in leachates exceeded FDA guidelines, as defined for the 24 hour acetic acid leaching test. Lead values up to 156 μg/mL were measured using the 24 hour acetic acid procedure. Significant leaching of lead also occurred in both acetic acid and citric acid samples heated in the microwave for 2 minutes and 5 minutes, respectively. While the microwave heated samples had lower lead concentrations than the 24 hour acetic acid test, levels were sufficiently high to prompt the authors of this study to suggest that use of old, ceramic dinnerware to microwave common foods could result in ingestion of dangerous lead levels and thus microwave heating in ceramic ware not of recent manufacture should be avoided.

Contamination of food may also occur in hotel and restaurant operations where tinned copper pots are often used. Reilly (1991) reported lead levels in foods cooked in saucepans made of different types of materials (Table 7). These results show that lead leached into each of the four foods, fish, chicken, cabbage and potato cooked under actual kitchen conditions. The extent of leaching appeared to be dependent on the state of wear of the utensils. Lead contents were the highest in samples cooked in the previously unused tinned copper pan, up to 1.09 mg/kg in the fish samples. Lead concentrations in foods cooked in the unused tinned copper pan ranged from about 1.2 to 4 times the levels found

Table 7. Effect of cooking utensil on lead contents of foods

	Pb Concentration (mg/kg)			
Utensil	Fish	Chicken	Cabbage	Potato
Uncooked	0.31	0.14	0.15	0.19
Aluminum	0.36	0.21	0.15	0.16
Tinned copper (old)	0.42	0.25	0.29	0.16
Tinned copper (unused)	1.09	0.94	0.79	0.26

Reference: Reilly (1991)

Table 8. Lead uptake from cooking water

Food	Pb conc. (ng/g)	% Pb uptake
Potatoes	200	23
Peas	340	35
Carrots	510	48
Lima Beans	246	27
Spaghetti	282	27

Reference: Sheldon and Berry (1996)

in foods cooked in the old tinned copper pan. As expected lead concentrations in foods cooked in aluminum pans were not significantly different from levels in the uncooked foods. This study again emphasizes the need for selection of appropriate food contact materials for cooking operations to minimize potential food contamination.

The U.S. Environmental Protection Agency's dietary exposure research program has recently sponsored studies to investigate how uncontaminated foods may become contaminated by incidental contact with a polluted microenvironment. These studies have investigated interactions between foods and water, foods and surfaces and foods and air. These studies have shown that foods can become contaminated with lead through contact with both contaminated surfaces and contaminated cooking water (Sheldon and Berry, 1996). For the cooking experiments, 100 g of food were boiled for 10 minutes in 1 L water containing 10 μg/L lead. Lead uptake from the water ranged from 23% to 48% of that originally present in the water for the five foods tested (Table 8). For the surface contact studies, dust containing lead (100 ng/cm^2) was applied to plates (1 g dust/m^3 plate surface area). Foods were then placed on the plates, removed, lead measured in both the food and remaining on the plate and percent uptake calculated. A very high uptake of lead from dust contaminated surfaces was observed (Table 9). Lead uptake ranged from 80–95% for the five foods tested. This study emphasizes the potential for incidental surface contact to cause relatively high exposures from consumption of otherwise uncontaminated foods and thus the importance of insuring preparation surfaces and utensils are clean prior to contact with food.

3.2. Mercury

Mercury is not naturally widely distributed on earth. It is only the 60th most abundant element in the earth's crust and occurs in a relatively small number of areas of concentration. However, widespread use of this element has caused mercury to become ubiquitous throughout the environment. Mercury compounds have a variety of uses. Mer-

Table 9. Lead uptake from contaminated surfaces

Food	% Pb Uptake
Apple	85
Bread	85
Cheese	80
Chips	75
Hamburger	95

Reference: Sheldon and Berry (1996)

Table 10. Mercury in cooked fish

Cooking Method	Mercury (ppm - dry wt.)	
	Uncooked	Cooked
Bake	0.33	0.37
Broil	0.33	0.36
Fry	0.30	0.25
Microwave	0.42	0.44
Poach	0.27	0.28
Steam	0.37	0.38

Reference: Armbruster et al. (1988)

cury is used predominantly in electrodes, in the chlor-alkali industry, in paints and in agrochemicals. Other specialty uses include catalysts in the manufacture of plastics, slimecides in the pulp and paper industry and as germicides and pesticides (Reilly, 1991; Harrison, 1997).

The toxicity of mercury depends on its chemical form: elemental, inorganic or organic. Exposure to organic mercury compounds, such as methylmercury, is more dangerous than exposure to either elemental or inorganic mercury. Methylmercury is a neurotoxin as well as a teratogen. It damages cellular membranes and chromosomes and denatures DNA. Symptoms of acute mercury exposure include nausea, headache, abdominal pain and diarrhea. Chronic mercury exposure results in ataxia, impairment of body coordination, mental retardation and loss of taste and smell (Gruenwedel, 1990; Janssen, 1997).

Since fish is the major source of mercury in the diet, several studies have investigated the effects of processing and cooking on mercury in fish. Armbruster et al. (1988) theorized that if methylmercury were released from its association with sulfur in proteins, it would likely be volatilized by heat during cooking. However, mercury concentrations in fish cooked by baking, broiling, frying, microwaving, poaching and steaming were not significantly different from mercury concentrations in uncooked fish (Table 10). These results led the authors to conclude that volatilization losses of mercury from fish during cooking are negligible.

Hernandez-Garcia et al. (1988) reported mercury concentrations in fresh and cooked or processed tuna, anchovies and sardines. Results of this study (Table 11), in contrast to the results of Armbruster et al. (1988), suggest that heat causes loss of mercury in fish.

Table 11. Effect of cooking and processing on mercury in fish

Treatment	Hg conc. range (μg/g)
Fresh tuna	0.31–0.70
Fried tuna	0.21–0.60
Fried tuna w/ tomatoes	0.21–0.29
Fresh anchovies	0.20–0.22
Battered/Fried anchovies	0.10–0.13
Pickled anchovies	0.12–0.15
Fresh sardines	0.30–0.35
Roasted sardines	0.11

Reference: Hernandez-Garcia et al. (1988)

Table 12. Relative mercury concentration in raw and panfried walleye fillets

Cooking treatment	Hg conc. ratio[1]	Total Hg ratio[1]	Weight ratio[2]
4 min., lemon	1.12	1.01	1.11
4 min., no lemon	1.18	1.03	1.14
6 min., lemon	1.12	0.95	1.18
6 min., no lemon	1.31	1.02	1.30

[1]Hg concentration ratio and total Hg ratio expressed as cooked conc./raw conc.
[2]Weight ratio expressed as raw weight/cooked weight
Reference: Morgan et al. (1997)

This effect was most dramatic in sardines, where roasted sardines contained approximately 0.11 μg/g mercury while fresh sardines contained 0.30–0.35 μg/g mercury. Roasting caused approximately a 67% reduction in mercury content. Acetic acid also promoted a loss of mercury. Anchovies pickled in vinegar (acetic acid) for 48 hours and pressed contained 0.12–0.15 μg/g mercury as opposed to 0.20 -0.25 μg/g mercury in fresh anchovies. Fried tuna and tuna fried with tomatoes also contained slightly less mercury than fresh tuna, again suggesting that both heat and acid promote loss of mercury from fish during cooking.

Reports that treatment with acetic acid may reduce mercury concentration in fish led Morgan et al. (1997) to conduct a more extensive study of the effects of cooking on mercury in fish, taking into account commonly used cooking practices in which fish are prepared or cooked in an acidic medium, such as lemon juice. Walleye and lake trout were cooked by either pan-frying, baking, boiling or smoking. Samples were cooked for various lengths of time with and without lemon juice used in preparation or cooking. Relative mercury concentrations in raw and pan-fried walleye fillets are shown in Table 12. Mercury concentrations (wet basis) were slightly higher in pan-fried fillets than in raw fillets for all cooking treatments tested, as indicated by the Hg concentration ratios ranging from 1.12 to 1.31. However, total mercury in fillets (concentration X weight) was not affected by pan-frying at any of the study conditions. Ratios of total mercury in pan-fried and raw fillets ranged from 0.95 to 1.03. Mercury concentration ratios were very similar to weight ratios, indicating that the increased concentration of mercury resulting from pan-frying is a result of the weight loss which occurs during cooking.

Mercury concentrations in baked walleye fillets were also higher than in the raw fillets (Table 13). The ratio of Hg concentration in baked fillets to that in raw fillets ranged from 1.30 to 1.48. These ratios were somewhat higher than those for pan-fried walleye fillets, probably due to greater weight loss resulting from baking or less weight loss during

Table 13. Relative mercury concentration in raw and baked walleye fillets

Cooking treatment	Hg conc. ratio[1]	Total Hg ratio[1]	Weight ratio[2]
15 min., lemon.	1.32	1.02	1.29
15 min., no lemon	1.30	1.01	1.27
25 min., lemon	1.39	1.04	1.34
25 min., no lemon	1.48	1.07	1.40

[1] Hg concentration ratio and total Hg ratio expressed as cooked conc./raw conc.
[2] Weight ratio expressed as raw weight/cooked weight
Reference: Morgan et al. (1997)

Table 14. Relative mercury concentration in raw and boiled walleye fillets

Cooking treatment	Hg conc. ratio[1]	Total Hg ratio[1]	Weight ratio[2]
10 min., lemon.	1.27	1.04	1.23
10 min., no lemon	1.35	1.06	1.28
20 min., lemon	1.30	1.04	1.25
20 min., no lemon	1.30	1.01	1.28

[1] Hg concentration ratio and total Hg ratio expressed as cooked conc./raw conc.
[2] Weight ratio expressed as raw weight/cooked weight
Reference: Morgan et al. (1997)

frying due to uptake of cooking oil. As with pan-fried fillets, weight ratios were similar to mercury concentration ratios. The absolute amount of total mercury was unchanged by baking for 15 or 25 minutes with or without lemon juice, as evidenced by the total mercury ratios of approximately 1.

Results for boiled walleye fillets were similar to those for pan-fried and baked fillets (Table 14). Mercury concentrations increased by a factor of 1.28 to 1.35, while the absolute amount of mercury was unchanged by boiling. Weight ratios were again similar to mercury concentration ratios. Neither increasing the cooking time from 10 minutes to 20 minutes nor addition of lemon juice to the cooking water exerted any significant influence on relative mercury concentrations or absolute amounts of mercury in the cooked fillets.

Relative amounts of mercury in raw and smoked lake trout are shown in Table 15. Smoking for 3 hours increased mercury concentrations by a factor of 1.45 and 1.57 in skin-on fillets and steaks, respectively. Concentrations were further increased by increasing smoking time to 6 hours. Mercury concentrations in lake trout smoked 6 hours were almost two times the concentrations in the raw portions. As in walleye fillets, the mercury concentration ratios were similar to the weight ratios, indicating that changes in mercury concentration were related to weight lost during cooking. However, as described previously for walleye, the absolute amount of mercury in smoked lake trout fillets and steaks was not affected by the smoking process.

In general, cooking resulted in an increase in mercury concentrations in ready-to-eat fish. However, absolute amounts of mercury were not changed by cooking; no mercury was lost in the cooking process, either into the cooking media or through volatilization. Increases in mercury concentrations resulting from cooking were apparently due to the concomitant loss of weight which occurs due to moisture and fat lost during cooking. Thus, the higher mercury concentrations in fish cooked for longer periods of time is logical since moisture and fat losses would be greater in these fish. This effect was particularly noticeable in smoked lake trout where the cooking times studied were substantially

Table 15. Relative mercury concentration in raw and smoked lake trout

Cooking treatment	Hg conc. ratio[1]	Total Hg ratio[1]	Weight ratio[2]
Fillet, 3 hr.	1.45	0.98	1.49
Fillet, 6 hr.	1.98	0.96	1.98
Steak, 3 hr.	1.56	0.95	1.65
Steak, 6 hr.	1.99	0.90	2.21

[1] Hg concentration ratio and total Hg ratio expressed as cooked conc./raw conc.
[2] Weight ratio expressed as raw weight/cooked weight
Reference: Morgan et al. (1997)

Table 16. Mercury content of vegetable crops

	Total mercury (ppb - dry wt.)	
Crop	Control soil	Sludged soil
Bean	3.6	4.5
Beet	2.5	7.2
Broccoli	3.1	16.9
Cabbage	5.1	10.9
Lettuce, head	2.9	32.8
Lettuce, leaf	4.6	40.5
Tomato	1.5	7.5

Reference: Cappon (1981)

different (3 hours vs. 6 hours). The times studied in other procedures were not sufficiently different to observe these effects.

Cooking fish in an acidic media, such as lemon juice is a common practice not previously investigated with respect to its effect on mercury concentration. While a previous study had shown that pickling anchovies for 48 hours in vinegar reduced mercury (Hernandez-Garcia et. al., 1988), conditions utilized by Morgan et al. (1997) did not produce similar effects. Acid concentrations apparently were not sufficient, nor was time associated with cooking, to promote the release of mercury from its protein-bound state in fish tissue.

While the majority of research on mercury in foods has dealt with fish, other studies have shown that under certain conditions, mercury may also contaminate vegetable crops. In the early 1980's, municipalities in the United States faced with the problem of disposing of large volumes of wastewater sewage sludge in an environmentally and economically sound manner turned to land application as an alternative to other methods such as incineration, ocean dumping and landfilling. However, heavy metal content of sludge is a major drawback to land application and can pose a health hazard because of metal uptake by food crops. Cappon (1981) studied the uptake of mercury by vegetable crops grown on untreated and sludge-amended soil. On the average, mercury was four times higher in crops grown on sludge-amended soil than in crops grown on treated soil (Table 16) and in some cases up to ten times higher. Due to results of studies like this, sewage sludge is no longer used to amend soil in the United States. However, the potential still exists for metal contamination of imported foods from sludge applications. This study also demonstrates the potential for metal uptake by crops grown on contaminated soil, no matter what the source of contamination. Thus, the potential for contamination exists for crops grown near hazardous waste sites, with contaminated water used in irrigation, in areas where the potential for atmospheric deposition is high and in the vicinity of any other source of metal contamination of soil.

3.3. Arsenic

Arsenic occurs widely in the earth's crust. It is obtained commercially as a by-product of the production of copper, lead or other metals. The main commercial use of arsenic is in the chemical industry where it is used in pharmaceuticals, agricultural chemicals, preservatives and similar compounds. Agricultural chemicals containing arsenic include herbicides, fungicides, wood preservatives, insecticides, rodenticides and sheep dips. Arsenic also has many applications in the metallurgical industry (Reilly, 1991).

Acute arsenic intoxication symptoms include nausea, diarrhea, abdominal pain, skin disorders and severe irritation of mucosal tissues. Chronic symptoms include growth retardation, general weakness, muscle aching, ulceration in the gastrointestinal tract, cirrhosis

Table 17. Arsenic in manufactured seafood products

	% As			
Product	AB	MMA	DMA	Other
Fish				
Fresh	86	NEG	1.7	12
Frozen	38	NEG	0.4	>62
Canned	<23	NEG	8.7	>69
Squid				
Fresh	98	<0.25	<0.5	11
Canned	<29	<0.03	<0.4	>67
Cockles				
Fresh	52	0.15	0.8	48
Canned	28	0.01	3.7	68

AB = arsenobetaine
MMA = monomethylarsonic acid
DMA = dimethylarsinic acid
Reference: Velez et al. (1996)

of the liver, chronic hepatitis and tremors (Gruenwedel, 1990). These severe toxic effects, coupled with the widespread usage of arsenic compounds, have resulted in arsenic being considered second only to lead as a farm and household toxicant (Reilly, 1991).

Seafood products are the most significant source of dietary arsenic intake. Several arsenic compounds are found in seafood including monomethylarsonic acid (MMA), dimethylarsinic acid (DMA) and arsenobetaine (AB). Arsenic compounds differ in toxicity with organic forms such as AB being relatively nontoxic and inorganic forms such as As (III) being highly toxic. MMA and DMA fall in the middle of this range of toxicities. Due to these varying toxicities it is important to understand the forms which occur in food and the influence of processing on the chemical form of arsenic. Velez et al. (1996) studied the arsenic content of manufactured seafood products. The relatively nontoxic AB was the predominant species in fresh fish, squid and cockles (Table 17). However, when these products were canned or frozen, AB content decreased significantly with a concomitant increase in other, unidentified, arsenic compounds. MMA levels were comparatively low and essentially the same in fresh, frozen and canned seafood products. DMA increased slightly in some of the canned products. It is apparent that manufacturing processes likely cause degradation of AB, possibly to DMA, and other arsenic compounds, likely with greater toxicity than the parent AB. Thus, it would be beneficial to optimize manufacturing practices to minimize AB degradation.

Organic arsenic compounds are fed to meat-type poultry to promote growth and increase feed efficiency. These compounds also produce desirable results in egg-producing

Table 18. Arsenic in chicken eggs

	As in albumen (ppb)		As in yolk (ppb)	
Dose(ppm)	Arsanilic acid	Roxarsone	Arsanilic acid	Roxarsone
0	5	5	<50	<50
14	10	10	125	250
28	20	15	375	500
56	30	25	625	750

Reference: Donoghue et al. (1994)

Table 19. Effect of cooking on arsenic in foods

Food	Raw conc. (ppb)	Cooking method	As ratio (cook/raw)	Wt. ratio (raw/cook)
Beef steak	11	Broil	1.04	1.81
Ground beef	15	Broil	1.53	1.57
Pork	21	Roast	0.94	1.31
Veal	16	Fry	1.18	1.72
Lamb	16	Broil	0.13	1.63
Poultry	39	Roast	1.48	1.43
Marine fish	1500	Bake	1.57	1.57
Freshwater fish	1060	Bake	1.28	1.57

Reference: Dabeka et al. (1993)

poultry, but are not approved for use in them. However, it is possible that feeds containing arsenic compounds are used accidentally or illegally in egg-producing birds resulting in arsenic residues in eggs. Donoghue et al. (1994) conducted a comprehensive study utilizing multiple doses of two arsenic compounds to determine whether arsenic residues exceeded established tolerances and whether arsenic was preferentially deposited in the yolk or albumen of the egg. Results are shown in Table 18. Both arsenic compounds preferentially accumulated in the yolk, with levels exceeding the 500 ppb FDA tolerance at high doses. Relatively little arsenic accumulated in the albumen, with levels well below the 500 ppb tolerance. These investigators concluded that arsenic residues present in yolk at these levels may pose a health risk when yolks are separated from albumen and used in further processed foods.

Cooking by various methods does not have a significant effect on arsenic levels in foods. Dabeka et al. (1993) conducted an extensive survey of arsenic in Canadian foods and also evaluated the effects of cooking on arsenic levels. An increase in arsenic concentration in cooked foods, which correlated with a decrease in weight, was observed for ground beef, poultry, marine fish and freshwater fish (Table 19). These results are similar to those for mercury in fish discussed earlier.

Arsenic levels in food may be influenced by the addition of contaminated ingredients or storage in contaminated containers. Levels of several metals in various ingredients of Jordanian cheese, as well as in the final product, were determined (Ereifej and Gharaibeh, 1993). Arsenic levels in milk, cheeses, and the corresponding brines, tin and salt ranged from 0.36 to 4.54 mg/100g (Table 20). Brine solution in tin containers had the highest concentration, 1.6 mg/100g. The authors concluded that the arsenic in cheese

Table 20. Arsenic and cadmium in Jordanian cheese

Sample	As conc. (mg/100g)	Cd conc. (mg/100g)
Sheep's milk	0.36 ± 0.35	<0.01 ± 0.005
Brine in glass	0.65 ± 0.29	<0.01 ± 0.004
Brine in tin	4.54 ± 1.99	0.10 ± 0.01
Tin container	1.6 ± 1.3	0.37 ± 0.04
Salt	1.85 ± 1.15	0.22 ± 0.02
Cheese in glass	0.44 ± 0.23	<0.01 ± 0.005
Cheese in tin	0.93 ± 0.80	0.04 ± 0.009

Reference: Ereifej and Gharaibeh (1993)

Table 21. Cadmium levels in washed and cooked rice

Sample	Cd conc. (ppm-dry basis)
Polished rice	0.21 ± 0.01
Washed rice	0.13 ± 0.02
Cooked rice	0.11 ± 0.01
Total removal	48%

Reference: Lee (1990)

might have accumulated from the milk, tin and salt used in the production of the cheese. They recommend use of a purified salt for brine preparation and use of glass jars for preservation in order to minimize cheese contamination with metals from tin cans and salt.

3.4. Cadmium

Cadmium is naturally present in the environment in soils, sediments, and waters. It is obtained commercially as a by-product in the extraction and refining of other metals with which it is naturally associated. Cadmium occurs primarily with zinc, although it is also found with copper and lead. One of the primary industrial uses of cadmium is as an anti-rust coating on iron. In the United States as much as 60 percent of all cadmium is used in electroplating. Cadmium compounds are also used as stabilizers in plastics, as pigments in paints and in some solders. This widespread industrial use has led to environmental pollution with cadmium. Cadmium is emitted to air by mines, metal smelters and industries using it as described above (Reilly, 1991; Harrison, 1993).

Acute cadmium toxicity causes excessive salivation, abdominal pain, diarrhea, vertigo and loss of consciousness. Symptoms of chronic cadmium toxicity include growth retardation, impaired kidney function, hypertension and liver dysfunction. Teratogenic effects have also been observed in animals. The disease known as "Itai-Itai," a severe form of osteomalacia, is caused by cadmium (Gruenwedel, 1990).

Cadmium contamination of food may also result from addition of contaminated ingredients or storage in contaminated containers, as was described above for arsenic. Cadmium concentrations in ingredients and containers used in preparation and storage of Jordanian cheese are shown in Table 20. The milk used to prepare the cheese did not contain any detectable cadmium, nor did the brine solution in glass or the final product in glass. However, the tin container, brine solution in tin, salt and the final cheese product stored in tin contained detectable cadmium. These results suggest that cadmium contamination is derived from either the salt, which was likely naturally contaminated, or the tin container, which was likely poorly manufactured (Ereifej and Gharaibeh, 1993). Again,

Table 22. Cadmium in noodles prepared from contaminated wheat flour

Sample	Cd conc. (ppm)	% Remaining
Dough	4.89 ± 0.03	100
Cooked noodles	3.69 ± 0.04	75
Noodle broth	0.035 ± 0.004	25 (% removed)

Reference: Lee (1990)

Table 23. Cadmium in raw and cooked spanner crabs

Treatment	Cd Conc. (mg/kg)
Raw—Meat	0.03
Raw—Hepatopancreas	30.9
Microwave	0.41
Steamed	0.27
Boiled	0.26

Reference: Slattery et al. (1992)

the authors recommend use of purified salt and packaging in glass containers to minimize contamination with metals.

In some instances, cooking has been shown to reduce cadmium levels in foods such as rice (Lee, 1990). Polished rice grains were manually washed with tap water several times and cooked by adding an equal amount of water in an electric rice cooker. Cadmium concentration was reduced from 0.21 ppm in the polished rice to 0.13 ppm in washed rice and 0.11 ppm in cooked rice. In total, approximately 48 percent of cadmium was removed by washing and cooking (Table 21). Similar results were observed with noodles prepared from wheat flour (Lee, 1990). Cadmium concentrations decreased from 4.89 ppm in raw wheat flour dough to 3.69 ppm in cooked noodles (Table 22). Approximately 25 percent of total cadmium was removed and detected in the noodle broth.

Cadmium in crabs is concentrated primarily in the hepatopancreas, a digestive organ. This organ is located close to surrounding muscle tissue and any disruption of the organ, either physical or by proteolytic enzyme activity, will release the contents into the surrounding flesh causing the flesh to become mushy and possibly increasing the level of cadmium in the flesh. Crabs are typically boiled to inactivate enzymes. However, alternative heating techniques have been investigated (Slattery et al., 1992). Boiling, steaming and microwave cooking conditions which inactivated enzymes and provided acceptable shelf life were compared for effects on cadmium contents in the flesh (Table 23). Results indicate that steaming is an acceptable alternative to boiling, with cadmium concentrations in the flesh in the range of 0.26 -0.27 mg/kg. While microwave cooking resulted in only slightly higher cadmium concentrations in the flesh, 0.41 mg/kg, sensory quality was unacceptable.

The impact of amending soil with sewage-sludge on metal content of crops, previously discussed for mercury in crops grown in freshly amended soil, may also be seen many years after the last application of sludge. Crops grown on sludge-amended soils which have equilibrated for many years (12–21 years) also accumulate higher levels of cadmium and lead than crops grown on uncontaminated soil (Hooda et al., 1997). Cadmium concentrations were 2.7, 2.8 and 13.6 times higher in carrot roots, wheat grain and spinach leaves grown on sludge-amended soil, respectively, than in those crops grown in uncontaminated soil. Lead concentrations were only 1.2–1.5 times higher in crops grown on sludge-amended soil (Table 24).

4. CONCLUSIONS

The preceding examples have shown that metal contamination of foods may occur at various stages of handling and processing from the farm to the point of consumption.

Table 24. Contents of cadmium and lead in crops produced on uncontaminated and sludge-amended soils

Crop/Element	Metal concentration (mg/kg-dry weight)	
	Uncontaminated soil	Sludge-amended soil
Wheat grain		
Cadmium	0.24	0.68
Lead	0.23	0.32
Carrot roots		
Cadmium	0.63	1.71
Lead	0.33	0.48
Spinach leaves		
Cadmium	0.94	12.76
Lead	0.82	0.95

Reference: Hooda et al. (1997)

Growth of plants in contaminated soils and feeding animals toxic element containing feeds, whether intentional or accidental, contribute to increased metal content in the final product. Contact with metal used in production or processing equipment and storage or packaging containers also exert a significant influence on metal content of foods. Use of contaminated ingredients may contaminate foods. Once present in foods, traditional processing and preparation does little to remove metals, although washing in some instances decreases metal content. Cooking generally increases metal concentrations in foods due to the associated weight loss. Improper handling of foods in the home, such as preparing on contaminated surfaces, using dusty dishes or utensils or heating in lead-glazed ceramics may contribute a significant portion of dietary intake of toxic elements. Metal content of food at the point of consumption can be minimized by careful selection of growth, post-harvest handling, in-plant processing and home preparation conditions.

REFERENCES

Armbruster, G.; Gutenmann, W.H.; Lisk, D.J. The effects of six methods of cooking on residues of mercury in striped bass. *Nutr. Rep. Intl.* **1988,** 37, 123–126.

Cappon, C.J. Mercury and selenium content and chemical form in vegetable crops grown on sludge amended soil. *Arch. Environm. Contam. Toxicol.* **1981,** 10, 673–689.

Dabeka, R.W.; McKenzie, A.D.; Lacroix, M.A.; Cleroux, C.; Bowe, S.; Graham, R.A.; Conacher, H.B.S.; Verdier, P. Survey of the arsenic in total diet food composites and estimation of dietary intake of arsenic by Canadian adults and children. *J. AOAC Intl.*, **1993,** 76, 14–25.

Donoghue, D.J.; Hairston, H.; Cope, C.V.; Bartholomew, M.J.; Wagner, D.D. Incurred arsenic residues in chicken eggs. *J. Food Protection*, **1994,** 57, 218–223.

Ereifej, K.I.; Gharaibeh, S.H. The levels of cadmium, nickel, manganese, lead, zinc, iron, tin, copper and arsenic in the brined canned Jordanian cheese. *Z. Lebensm. Unters. Forsch.*, **1993,** 197, 123–126.

Flegal, A.R.; Smith, D.R.; Ellias, R.W. Lead contamination in food. In "Food Contamination from Environmental Sources," Nriagu, J.O.; Simmons, M.S. (Eds.), John Wiley and Sons, Inc., New York, NY, 1990, pp. 85–120.

Gruenwedel, D.W. Industrial and environmental chemicals in the human food chain: inorganic chemicals. In "Chemicals in the Human Food Chain," Winter, C.W.; Sieber, J.N.; Nuckton, C.F. (Eds.), Van Nostrand Reinhold, New York, NY, 1990, pp. 129–182.

Harrison, N. Metals. In "Safety of Chemicals in Food: Chemical Contaminants," Watson, D. (Ed.), Ellis Horwood Limited, West Sussex, England. 1993, pp. 109–124.

Hernandez-Garcia, M.T.; Martinez-Para, M.C.; Masoud, T.A. Changes in the content of mercury in fish samples subjected to different cooking processes. *Anales de Bromatologia*, **1988,** 40, 291–297.

Hooda, P.S.; McNulty, D.; Alloway, B.J.; Aitken, M.N. Plant availability of heavy metals in soils previously amended with heavy applications of sewage sludge. *J. Sci. Food Agric.*, **1997,** 73, 446–454.

Janssen, M.M.T. Contaminants. In "Food Safety and Toxicity," deVries, J. (Ed.), CRC Press, Boca Raton, FL. 1997, pp. 53–62.

Jelinek, C.F. Control of chemical contaminants in foods: past, present and future. *J. Assoc. Off. Anal. Chem.* **1985,** 68, 1063–1068.

Lee, S.R. Contamination and elimination of some heavy metals in Korean meals. In "Trends in Food Product Development," Ghee, A.H. (Ed.), Singapore Institute of Food Science and Technology, 1990, pp. 355–358.

Mindak, W.; Lamont, W.; Cunningham, W. Lead release from ceramic mugs with lead-containing glazes using coffee and acetic acid. Presented at the AOAC International Meeting, 1992, Cincinnati, OH.

Morgan, J.N.; Berry, M.R.; Graves, R.L. Effects of commonly used cooking practices on total mercury concentration in fish and their impact on exposure assessments. *J. Exp. Anal. Envir. Epidem.*, **1997,** 7, 119–133.

Nriagu, J. Food contamination with cadmium in the environment. In "Food Contamination from Environmental Sources," Nriagu, J.O.; Simmons, M.S. (Eds.), John Wiley and Sons, Inc., New York, NY, 1990, pp. 59–84.

Nriagu, J.O.; Azcue, J.M. Food contamination with arsenic in the environment. In "Food Contamination from Environmental Sources," Nriagu, J.O.; Simmons, M.S. (Eds.), John Wiley and Sons, Inc., New York, NY, 1990, pp. 121–144.

Reilly, C. "Metal Contamination of Food." Elsevier Science Publishers Ltd., London, England, 1991.

Rowarth, J.S. Lead concentration in some New Zealand honeys. *J. Apicultural Research*, **1990,** 29, 177–180.

Sheets, R.W.; Turpen, S.L.; Hill, P. Effect of microwave heating on leaching of lead from old ceramic dinnerware. *Sci. Total Env.*, **1996,** 182, 187–191.

Sheldon, L.S.; Berry, M.R. Evaluating food contamination scenarios for dietary exposure studies. Presented at the International Society for Exposure Analysis and Environmental Epidemiology Annual Meeting, December, 1996, New Orleans, LA.

Slattery, S.L.; Ford, A.L.; Nottingham, S.M. Cooking methods for spanner crabs *Ranina ranina (L)* and their effect on cadmium residues. *Food Australia*, **1992,** 44, 206–210.

Stilwell, D.E.; Musante, C.L. Lead content in grapefruit juice and its uptake upon storage in open containers. *J. Sci. Food Agric.*, **1994,** 66, 405–410.

Stilwell, D.E.; Musante, C.L. Lead in maple syrup produced in Connecticut. *J. Agric. Food Chem.*, **1996,** 44, 3153–3158.

Velez, D.; Ybanez, N.; Montoro, R. Monomethylarsonic acid and dimethylarsinic acid contents in seafood products. *J. Agric. Food Chem.* **1996,** 44, 859–864.

14

POLYCHLORINATED BIPHENYLS, POLYBROMINATED BIPHENYLS, AND DIOXIN REDUCTION DURING PROCESSING/COOKING FOOD

Mary E. Zabik[1] and Matthew J. Zabik[2]

[1]Food Science and Human Nutrition, College of Human Ecology
[2]National Food Safety and Toxicology Center
Michigan State University, East Lansing, Michigan 48824

1. ABSTRACT

This chapter presents information on the levels of environmental contaminants found in recent market basket surveys as well as the effect of processing and cooking on the reduction of these contaminants. Although consumers have expressed concern over the level of environmental contaminants in the food supply, market basket surveys involving over 8,000 analyses of foods ready-to-eat, found measurable amounts (ppb levels) of PCBs in only 24 foods. Processing/cooking has been shown to reduce PCBs by 20–100%. Although PBBs got into the food chain as the result of one incredible accident and thus are not expected to be found in foods today, cooking/processing was also effective in reducing PBBs. Dioxins are the result of combustion processes and chemical manufacturing processes. TCDD levels found in Great Lakes fish were in the low part per trillion level. Again, cooking and processing resulted in substantially less TCDD in fish as eaten.

2. INTRODUCTION

Industrial chemicals were not manufactured to be used in foods or in the vicinity of food production or processing but accidental contamination has led to the introduction of such compounds into soil and aquatic sediments. Climatic events or use of waterways can reintroduce these compounds into the environment in the area of food production. Biomagnification of potentially harmful chemicals in the food chain and consumer concern about unintentional chemicals in the food supply have lead to numerous studies to

Impact of Processing on Food Safety, edited by Jackson et al.,
Kluwer Academic / Plenum Publishers, New York, 1999.

quantitate the effect of processing and cooking on the possible reduction of these contaminants in food as eaten. Industrial chemicals that are halogenated are fat soluble; thus these compounds are more likely to occur in fats and oils or in meat, fish and poultry than in low fat foods. This review will concentrate on studies related to the effect of processing/cooking on polychlorinated biphenyls (PCBs), polybrominated biphenyls (PBBs) and dioxins, particularly 2,3,7,8,tetrachlorodibenzo-*p*-dioxin (TCDD). Levels of PCBs currently found in the food chain will also be reviewed.

3. POLYCHLORINATED BIPHENYLS

PCBs were synthesized by the chlorination of the biphenyl molecule to produce compounds of high thermal and chemical stability. Since there are ten possible sites for chlorine on the biphenyl ring, a total of 209 possible PCB congeners exist. PCBs manufactured in the United States had the trade name Aroclor^R followed by a four digit code; biphenyls were generally indicated by a 12 in the first two positions while the last two numbers indicated the percentage of chlorine by weight. Manufacturing of PCBs in the U.S. was terminated by 1977.

PCBs have low vapor pressure, high dielectric constants, high electric resistivity, high density, and high lipophilicity. Because of their stability and low flammability, PCBs were widely used in heat transfer fluids, hydraulic fluids and protective coatings, as well as to improve the resistance of paints, plastics and rubbers. PCB contamination of the environment resulted from accidental contamination such as migration from paint, leaky heat transfer systems, leaky hydraulic presses and the recycling of carbonless carbon paper. The first major incident of PCBs affecting humans resulted from the ingestion of highly contaminated rice oil in Japan. Thus it is not surprising that some of the earliest studies on the effects of processing on PCBs in foods were related to the effect of processing on PCBs in fats and oils.

3.1. Reduction of PCBs during the Processing of Fats and Oils

Addison and Ackman (1974) reported the levels of PCBs expressed as Aroclor^R 1254 were non-detectable (limit of detection 1 ppm) in a variety of partially hydrogenated fish and seal oils when the unprocessed oils PCB content varied from 3 to 11 ppm. Addison *et al.* (1978) further studied the hydrogenation process to establish the step in the process at which the loss of PCBs occurred. These authors reported that 100% of the PCBs quantitated as Aroclor^R 1254 were retained through the steps of alkali refining, bleaching, and hydrogenation to an Iodine Value of 79 while all the PCBs were lost when the oil was deodorized (level of detection of 0.2 ppm). A second trial by the same authors showed a slight loss of PCBs during hydrogenation but the major reduction also occurred during the deodorization step (Figure 1). The hydrogenation catalyst, which had been found to be free of PCBs before use, contained 2 ppm PCBs after use. This is about the same level as in the hydrogenated oil while the deodorized condensates had higher levels of PCBs.

Kanenatsu *et al.* (1976) found a greater loss of PCBs when the hydrogenation of soybean oil was carried out at atmospheric pressure than at high pressure (Figure 2) and the decrease in PCBs was greater if the catalyst contained copper or chromium. They also reported that the greatest loss occurred during the deodorization step. These authors attributed the loss of PCBs to chemical changes such as reduction and dechlorination rather than to evaporation out of the reaction system.

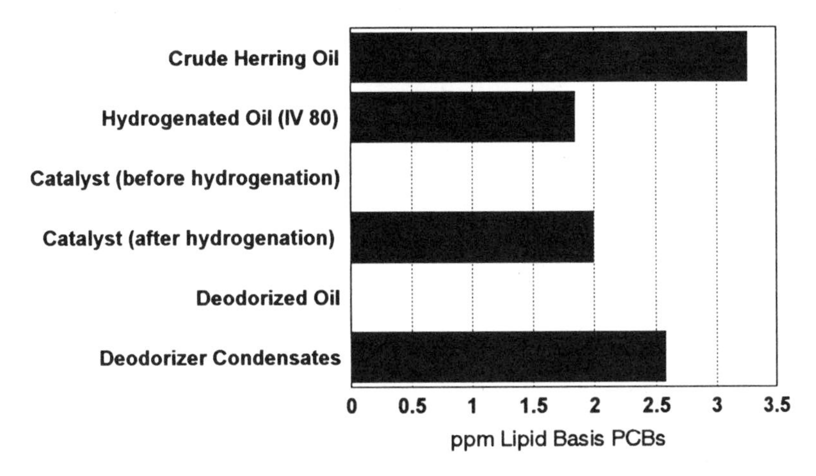

Figure 1. Residual PCB concentrations in processed herring oil and manufacture waste (Addison *et al.*, 1978).

3.2. Reduction of PCBs during the Drying of Foods

Khan (1975) reported a 100% reduction of Aroclor[R] 1254 by sun drying shrimp for 36 hours. The shrimp had been spiked with PCBs by dipping in a 5 ppm solution of 1254 prior to drying. Half the shrimp were also dipped in 1% sodium nitrate solution. The rate of reduction of PCBs for the group which was also dipped in sodium nitrate was increased and 100% reduction was reached in 30 hours. Khan *et al* (1976) studied the reduction of Aroclor[R] 1254 and 1260 during the freeze-drying of shrimp homogenate and eggs. Freeze-drying was more effective in reducing the levels of 1254 than 1260 with losses of 40.3% and 25.2%, respectively, from shrimp homogenate and of 26.8% and 22.6%, respectively, from eggs.

Recently, Santerre *et al.* (1994) investigated supercritical fluid extraction of roasted peanuts on the quality of the resulting peanut butter. Supercritical fluid extraction for four

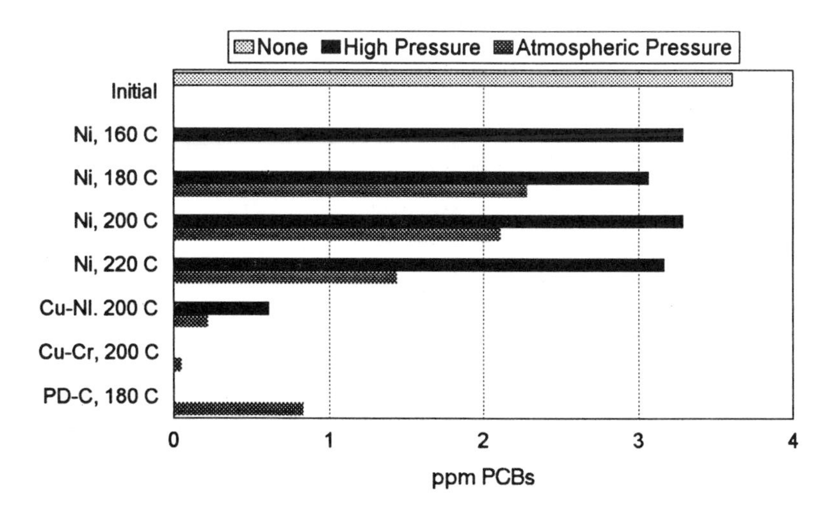

Figure 2. Effect of hydrogenation conditions on PCBs in contaminated soybean oil (Kanematsu *et al*, 1976).

hours decreased the lipid content of the roasted peanuts from 51.6% to 40.6%. The authors postulated that the supercritical fluid extraction would also remove lipophilic environmental contaminants.

3.3. Reduction of PCBs during the Processing/Cooking of Meat, Poultry, and Fish

Zabik (1974) studied the effect of cooking hens on the levels of PCBs in the cooked meat and broth. Individual drumsticks, breast pieces, thigh meat, thigh skin, and abdominal adipose tissues from hens fed Aroclor^R 1254 were stewed or pressure cooked. Raw breast, drumsticks and thigh meat had average levels of 1.5 ppm PCBs (Aroclor^R 1254) while thigh skin and adipose tissue had 7.2 and 12.3 ppm PCBs, respectively. Both cooking methods resulted in similar reductions of PCBs. Cooking significantly reduced the level of PCBs, primarily through the rendering of the fat from the chicken pieces during cooking. Percent recoveries calculated from the levels of PCBs in the cooked meat and broth as compared to that in the raw pieces ranged from 60% for the breast pieces to 95% for the drumsticks (Figure 3). Except for the adipose tissue, which had most of the recovered PCBs in the broth, the recovered PCBs were about equally divided between the meat and the broth. If one did not consume the broth, the overall reduction of PCBs from that in the raw chicken pieces was as follows: drumsticks, 56.1%; breast pieces, 69.7%; thigh meat, 55.9%; thigh skin, 60.8% and adipose tissue, 91.2%.

Zabik (1990) simulated a commercial food service operation to study the potential reduction of PCBs from light meat turkey rolls. Turkeys that were fed rations spiked with low levels of PCBs were slaughtered and the breast muscles were used to produce turkey rolls. These rolls were roasted at 105, 135 or 165°C after which half were sliced and slices were kept hot for up to 120 minutes. The remaining rolls were chilled overnight, heated at 105°C and then kept hot. Three-ounce portions from all the rolls were frozen and then heated in the microwave at either half or full power. Roasting reduced the PCBs by an average of greater than 60%. There were no significant differences in PCB residue levels due to the oven temperature, chilling, hot-holding or heating by microwave. Thus, the choice

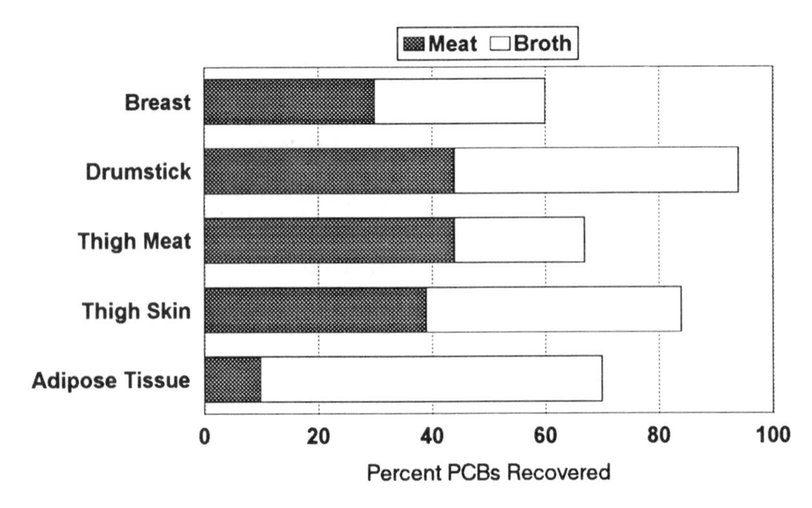

Figure 3. Percent recovery of PCBs in pressure cooked chicken meat and broth as compared to the PCBs in the raw chicken pieces (Zabik, 1974).

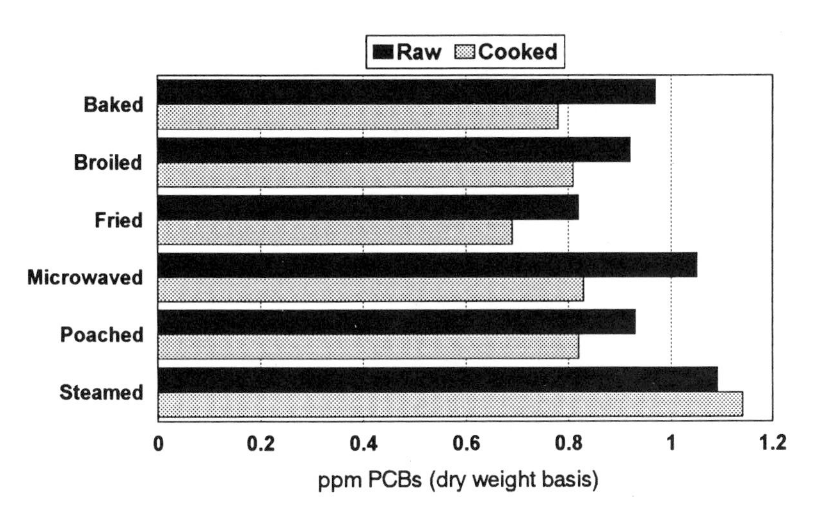

Figure 4. Comparison of PCB levels in raw and cooked striped bass (Armbruster *et al.*, 1987).

of oven-roasting temperature and whether or not to hold the turkey on a steam table or to freeze and reheat by microwave should be based on sensory, nutritional and microbial quality considerations.

Since the United States manufacture of PCBs was discontinued in 1977, PCBs deposited in the sediment of rivers and lakes have led to continued occurrences of PCB residues in fish and other aquatic organisms. Dredging, shipping, storms and marine organisms have disturbed the sediments and caused reintroduction of the PCBs into water which allows for biomagnification and results in residues in fish. Numerous studies have evaluated the effect of cooking and processing on PCB levels in fish. Armbruster and coworkers (1987) found PCB residues in striped bass were only slightly affected by a variety of cooking methods (Figure 4). Other early studies showed inconsistent or minimal losses of PCBs from fish (Smith *et al.*, 1973—chinook and coho salmon; Zabik *et al.*, 1982—carp). Nevertheless, broiling lake trout (siscowets) reduced PCBs by 53% while roasting or cooking by microwave resulted in slightly lower losses ranging from 26 to 34% (Zabik *et al.*, 1979a).

Sherer and Price (1993) used a mass basis to summarize PCB loss from a number of earlier studies. By this method, they reported an average of 22% PCB loss by baking chinook salmon, lake trout, smallmouth bass, and bluefish; 27% loss from broiling lake trout and brown trout; 56% loss from frying smallmouth bass and white croaker; and 26% loss from microwave cooking lake trout.

Zabik *et al.*, 1992 studied the effect of removing the hepatopancreas before boiling or steaming blue crab (*Callinectes sapidus* Rathbun) on the PCB residues found in the cooked crab. The hepatopancreas is a highly contaminated organ and it was feared its' presence could lead to cross contamination of the cooked muscle. Blue crab used in this study had an average of 0.22 ppm PCBs in the claw muscle and an average of 0.35 ppm PCBs in the body muscle. Losses of PCBs from the body muscle were slightly higher from crab that had the hepatopancreas removed before cooking but the losses of PCBs from the claw muscle were not affected (Figure 5). Approximately one-quarter of the PCBs were removed from the claw while one-third of the PCBs were removed from the body tissue during steaming or boiling crab.

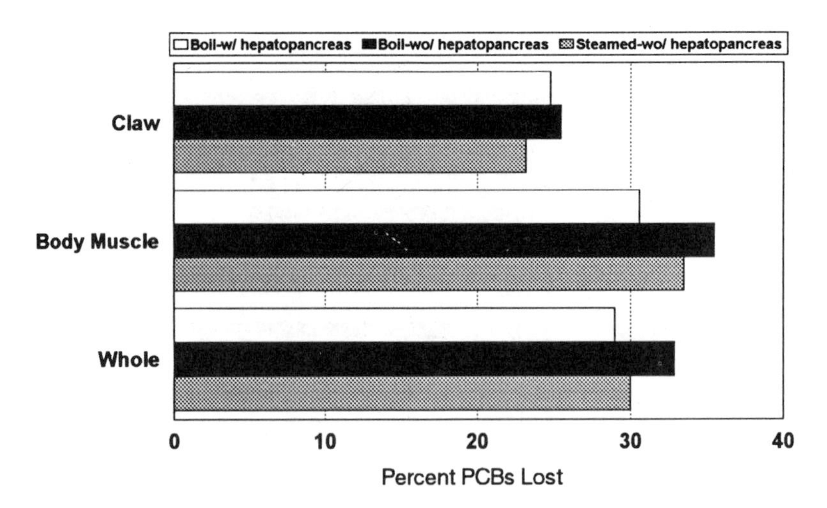

Figure 5. Effect of hepatopancreas presence on the percentage reduction of PCBs during the cooking of blue crab (Zabik *et al.*, 1994).

Higher concentrations of PCBs are found in the fatty tissue of fish so efforts have been made to reduce PCBs levels in the raw fish by trimming the belly flap and the lateral line with its associated fat. Zabik *et al.* (1978) reported that the belly flap of freshwater mullet from the upper Great Lakes had 2.6 to 5.4 times the levels of PCBs as did the muscle tissue while the lateral line of these same fish had 5.0–5.9 time the total PCBs as did the muscle tissue. Hora (1981) found 19 to 33% of the PCBs were removed from carp by trimming with the greatest loss occurring for the medium size carp. Sanders and Haynes (1988) found similar losses when they compared the level of PCBs in untrimmed to trimmed blue fish. A study by New York Sea Grant (Voiland *et al.*, 1990) found trimming the lateral line and belly flap reduced PCBs in brown trout (*Salmo trutta*) harvested from Lake Ontario by 45.6%. Standard fillets had 1.05 ppm PCBs while trimmed fillets from the same fish had 0.57 ppm PCBs. Voiland *et al.* (1990) confirmed an earlier study of PCB reduction via trimming brown trout by Skea *et al.* (1979). These authors had indicated 43.2% of the PCBs were lost when trimmed fillets (1.62 ppm PCBs) were compared to standard fillets (2.85 ppm PCBs).

Environmental contaminants in Great Lakes fish have caused consumers to be concerned with whether it is safe to consume this abundant source of high quality protein associated with low levels of saturated fats. A recently completed project provides data for public health and other government officials to quantitate the degree of exposure a human might receive from the consumption of each of five commonly sought open water game fish species prepared and cooked by commonly used methods or by a method which offers the potential for significant contaminant reduction (Zabik *et al*, 1995 a,b). The source and size of the fish were chosen on the basis of mean creel census data from sports fisherman in Michigan from the year just previous to this study. Total PCBs were determined by packed column GLC. Capillary column GLC was also used to determine selected individual congeners based on literature references of congeners found in Aroclor^{R} 1254.

Carp harvested from Lakes Erie and Huron were processed into skin-on and skin-off fillets and cooked by deep fat frying and pan frying (Zabik *et al.*, 1995a). Chinook salmon harvested from Lakes Huron and Michigan were baked, charbroiled, and scored and charbroiled as skin-on and skin-off fillets. In addition skin-off chinook salmon fillets were canned. Trimming significantly affected the total PCB levels in the current study. In this case, the skin-on fillets had the belly flap removed while the skin-off fillets had both the belly flap and the lateral line and its associated fat trimmed off. Raw skin-on carp fillets had an average of 1.9 ppm total PCBs as compared to 0.8 ppm total PCBs in the raw skin-off carp fillets. While the differences were less dramatic, raw skin-on chinook salmon fillets had significantly more total PCBs than raw skin-off chinook salmon fillets (1.4 ppm total PCBs vs 0.8 ppm total PCBs).

The cooked skin-off fillets of carp and chinook salmon also had significantly less total PCBs than the cooked skin-on fillets. Trimming fish is an important consideration to reduce the levels of PCBs ingested by consumers. With the exception of carp, which had been deep fat fried and thus the entire fish fillet normally would be covered with breading or batter, only muscle tissue was used to determine the PCB residues in the cooked sample from skin-on fillets. The percent reduction of total PCBs in the chinook salmon cooked without skin (42%) was slightly higher than that when the chinook salmon fillets were cooked skin-on (38%). Thus, not only was the level of total PCBs in the raw skin-off chinook salmon fillets less than that of skin-on fillets, the reduction during cooking of skin-off fillets was greater than the reduction in skin-on fillets resulting in lower residue levels in the skin-off chinook salmon as consumed. Cooking method, however, did not result in any significant difference in the level of residue or in the percent reduction for the chinook salmon fillets. Scoring resulted in a slightly higher, although not significantly different, loss of total PCBs in the broiled chinook salmon fillets (47% vs 42%).

Cooking method did not significantly affect the level of total PCBs in the carp nor did it affect the percentage of reduction during cooking (Zabik *et al.*, 1995a). Either pan frying or deep fat frying can be used to cook skin-off carp fillets depending on the preference of the consumer. If a consumer has to cook carp skin-on, pan frying should be recommended over deep fat frying as it is easy to separate the cooked muscle tissue from the skin and thus by discarding the skin and associated fat, reduce the amount of PCB ingested. Average losses of PCBs during the cooking of carp was 33%.

Lake trout (lean) from Lakes Huron, Michigan and Ontario and fat lake trout (siscowets) from Lake Superior were baked and charbroiled as skin-off fillets (Zabik *et al.*, 1996). In addition skin-off lake trout from Lake Michigan and siscowets from Lake Superior were salt boiled while skin-on lake trout from Lake Michigan and skin-on siscowets from Lake Superior were smoked. PCBs in the lake trout from Lake Huron averaged 0.39 ppm, from Lake Michigan 0.78 ppm, from Lake Ontario 0.82 ppm and siscowets from Lake Superior had an average of 0.89 ppm PCBs. Baking, charbroiling and salt boiling resulted in modest losses of total PCBs from the lake trout of 13%, 16%, and 12%, respectively. Smoking resulted in a 40% loss of total PCBs. This could be influenced by the long, slow processing followed by holding at a higher end temperature that resulted in significantly higher cooking losses of 40% as compared to cooking losses of approximately <20% for the other three cooking methods. Smoking did result in the formation of polynuclear aromatic hydrocarbons (PAHs) as the levels in the smoked muscle were considerably higher that those in the raw muscle. Smoked lake trout and siscowets were the only samples analyzed for PAHs.

Walleye harvested from Lakes Erie, Huron and Michigan were baked and charbroiled as skin-on fillets with additional walleye from Lake Michigan being cooked by deep fat frying (Zabik *et al.*, 1995b). Skin-on white bass fillets from Lakes Erie and Huron were pan fried. Raw walleye from Lake Erie had an average of 0.42 ppm PCBs, from Lake Huron 0.24 ppm PCBs and from Lake Michigan 0.20 ppm PCBs. Raw white bass

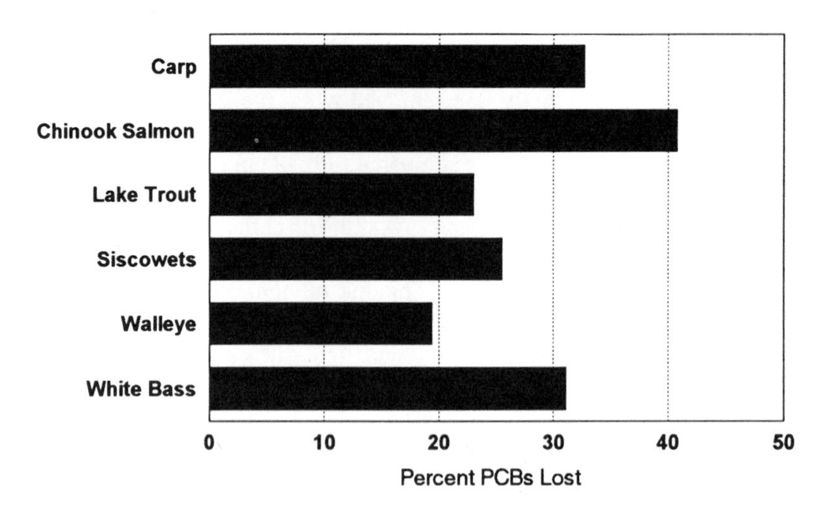

Figure 6. Average percent reduction of PCBs from Great Lakes fish.

had 0.76 ppm PCBs in Lake Erie fish and 0.50 ppm PCBs in Lake Huron fish. Cooking resulted in a 19% loss of total PCBs from the walleye and a 28% loss from the white bass.

To summarize the loss of total PCBs from the Great Lakes fish, Figure 6 shows the percent loss of PCBs by species during the cooking and processing of the Great Lakes fish. Overall losses ranged from approximately 20% for walleye to 40% for chinook salmon. Although the losses from the walleye were the lowest, this species had the lowest level of contamination ranging from 0.2 ppm total PCBs in the wet tissue of the skin-on fillets from Lakes Huron and Michigan to 0.4 ppm in the wet tissue of walleye harvested from Lake Erie.

Congener specific PCB analyses were also conducted for the congeners which have been reported in the literature to be found in Aroclor^R 1254 using capillary column GLC and using congener 30 as an internal standard to correct for losses of PCBs during the extraction and clean-up procedures (Daubenmire, 1996). Congener patterns varied slightly by lake and by species. A sample congener pattern for raw and baked lake trout is given in Figure 7.

Individual congener values were summed to calculate total PCBs based on congener specific analyses as well as grouped into the following PCB homologs: trichloro-, tetrachloro-, pentachloro-, hexachloro-, heptachloro- and octachloro-PCBs. Overall losses of total PCBs summed from the individual congener analyses during the seven cooking methods/processes used to prepare the Great Lakes fish is given in Figure 8. Losses ranged from a low of 22% for salt boiling to a high of 48% for smoking. In general, losses were about 30%.

Figure 9 shows the losses for the homologs of PCBs during baking and charbroiling lake trout and siscowets (Daubenmire, 1996). Homologs with the least and the most numbers of chlorine tended to be lost at lower percentages that did the pentachloro-, hexachloro- and heptachloro-PCBs. Pentachloro-, hexachloro- and heptachloro-PCB homologs make up the major portion of the PCBs found in these fish samples.

Irradiation also has been evaluated to reduce PCBs from fish. An early study by Cichy *et al.* (1979) used a pasteurization dosage of 1000 kilorads using a ^{60}Co source to irradiate Lake Superior lake trout (fat trout -- siscowets) before charbroiling the fish fillets. These siscowets had an average of 1.8 ppm in the raw fillets. Irradiation resulted in a 38% reduction in PCBs while irradiation and broiling resulted in a 43% reduction. The latter value was in agreement with the reduction of total PCBs by broiling these lake trout fillets

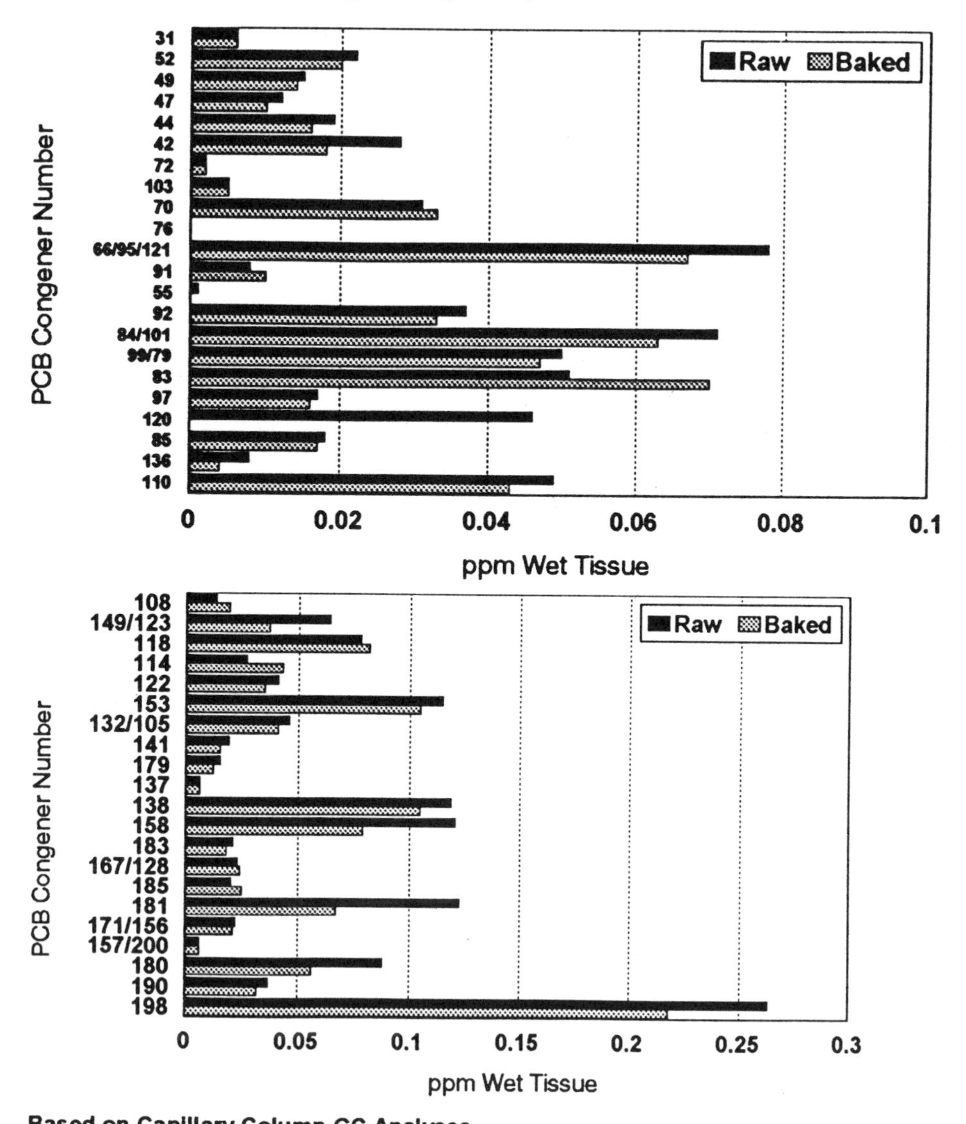

Figure 7. Congener pattern of raw and baked lake trout and siscowets.

(Zabik *et al.*, 1979a). More recently, Lépine *et al.* (1995) evaluated the effect of irradiating North Atlantic Ocean cod at 15kGy using an underwater irradiator equipped with a ^{60}Co source delivering 484 kGy/min on individual PCB congeners. These authors found that irradiation had no effect on the levels of PCB congeners found in the raw cod (Table 1).

3.4. Market Basket Survey Levels of PCBs in Foods as Eaten

The Food and Drug Administration KAN-Do Office and Pesticides Team (1995) reported data from a ten year period from 1982–1991 which analyzed 37 baskets per 230 items prepared to be eaten. This report showed that PCBs were found 27 times in a total of

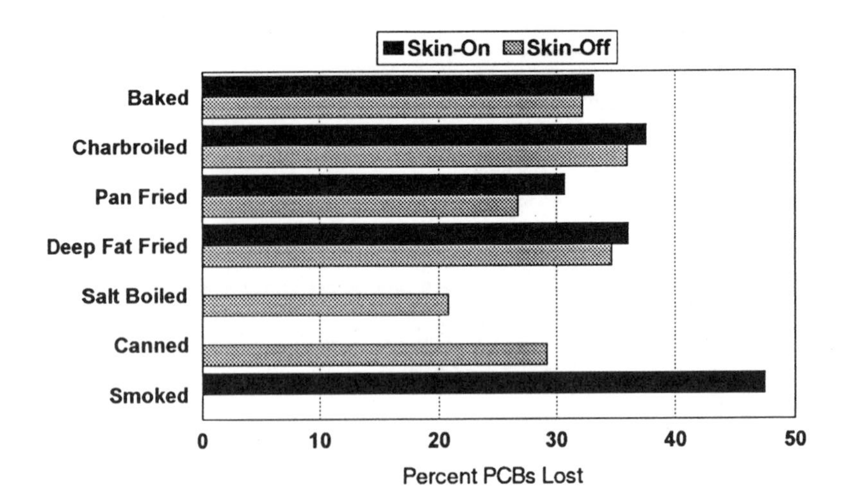

Figure 8. Effect of cooking method on the reduction of total PCBS based on the sum of individual PCB congeners from five species of Great Lakes fish (Daubenmire, 1996).

Table 1. Degradation of PCB congeners found in cod after a 15 kGy Treatment[1]

PCB congener[2]	Relative peak area before treatment	Relative peak area after treatment
80–86[3]	0.185±0.012[4]	0.200±0.025
101	0.265±0.015	0.293±0.028
99	0.417±0.037	0.398±0.07
97	0.096±0.007	0.106±0.004
87	0.344±0.05	0.389±0.016
136–112[3]	1.05±0.091	1.16±0.060
10	0.344±0.005	0.320±0.062
118	0.504±0.007	0.564±0.030
146	0.079±0.006	0.106±0.009
132	0.469±0.048	0.522±0.034
138–115[3]	0.604±0.026	0.651±0.030
187	0.144±0.004	0.151±0.01
156	0.143±0.013	0.159±0.007
180	0.510±0.008	0.551±0.04
190	0.084±0.001	0.087±0.005

[1]The peak area of each congener is expressed relative to the internal standard (dedachlorobiphenyl).
[2]PCB congeners are numbered according to International Union of Applied and Pure Chemistry nomenclature.
[3]Chromatographically unresolved congeners.
[4]n=3.

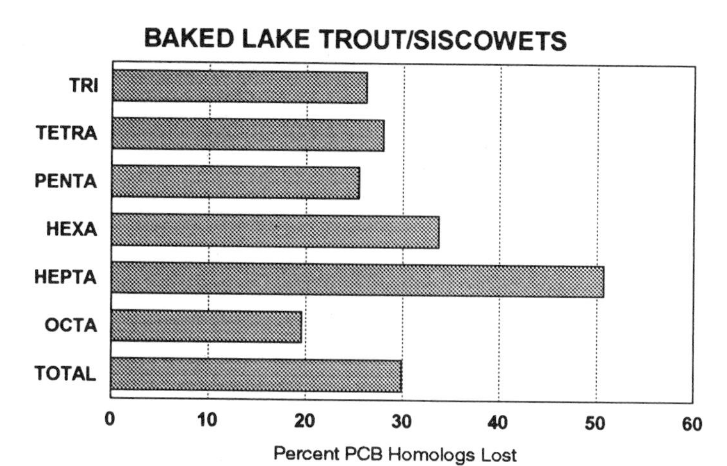

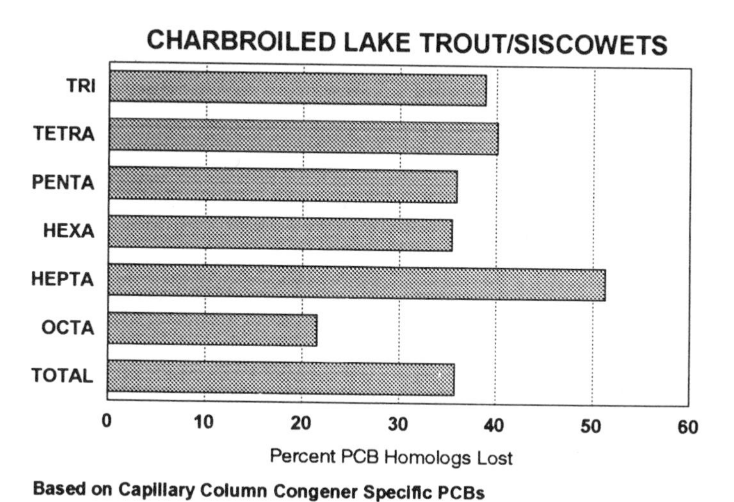

Figure 9. Comparison of loss of PCB homologs during the baking and charbroiling of lake trout/siscowets (Daubenmire, 1996).

24 foods at an average residue level of 0.0179 μg/g. Table 2 gives the specific foods in which PCBs were found. The number of each food type which had detectable residues as well as the average residue level is also given.

4. POLYBROMINATED BIPHENYLS

Polybrominated biphenyls (PBBs) are members of the halogenated hydrocarbon class of compounds with a structure, reactivity, use and toxicity similar to those attributed to PCBs of higher chlorination. Michigan Chemical Corporation manufactured a product called Firemaster[R] BP-6. This compound had an average of six bromine atoms attached to the biphenyl rings, and to meet specifications was brought to 75% bromine by weight. General properties included: solid at room temperature with a softening point of 72°C, decomposes at 300–400°C, very low water

Table 2. FDA market basket foods found to contain PCBs (FDA, 1995)

Food	Type or preparation	Residue analysis type	Number of detectable residues	Average found μg/g
Beef	Chuck roast, roasted	Fat	1	0.0100
Beef	Round steak, stewed	Fat	2	0.0110
Biscuits	Baking powder	Fat	1	0.0240
Bologna		Fat	1	0.0080
Butter	Stick type	Fat	1	0.0240
Cereal	Shredded wheat	Nonfat	1	0.0640
Fish sticks	Cooked	Fat	1	0.0090
Fish	Cod or haddock cooked	Nonfat	2	0.0115
Lamb chop	Cooked	Fat	1	0.0100
Margarine	Stick type	Fat	1	0.0200
Meatloaf	Beef	Fat	1	0.0070
Pizza	Cheese, cooked	Fat	1	0.0100
Popcorn	Popped	Fat	1	0.0090
Pork chop	Cooked	Fat	1	0.0160
Pork roast	Loin, cooked	Fat	1	0.0340
Potpie	Chicken	Fat	1	0.0250
Prunes	Dried	Nonfat	1	0.0120
Shrimp	Breaded, fried	Fat	1	0.0130
Squash	Winter, boiled	Nonfat	1	0.0260
Tomatoes	Raw	Nonfat	1	0.0200
Turkey	Breast, roasted	Fat	2	0.0165
Veal cutlet	Cooked	Fat	1	0.0090

solubility, soluble in most organic solvents, and very low volatility. PBBs were industrial compounds used primarily as fire retardants and plasticizers in such products as business machines, electrical equipment and fabricated products. PBBs were not used in food or feed or in products that would come in contact with human skin such as flame retardant fabrics. In May, 1973, an incredible error was made during the manufacture of animal feed in Michigan. Firemaster^R FF-1 was mistaken for magnesium oxide (trade name Nutrimaster) and mixed into high protein dairy pellets. Through this original contamination and subsequent cross contamination of other feeds, dairy animals, beef, poultry and swine were contaminated (Smith *et al.*, 1977). Because PBB contamination was related to one accident in Michigan, PBB residues would not be expected in be found in the general food supply today.

4.1. Effect of Processing Milk on PBB Levels

Using milk from four contaminated herds which had PBB levels of less than 0.3 ppm, Murata *et al.* (1976) followed the PBB residues during the manufacturing of a variety of dairy products. These included pasteurized milk, skim milk, cream, butter, buttermilk, and cheese. PBBs followed the fat and were not significantly reduced in most of the products when the PBBs, expressed as ppm in the fat of the finished product, were compared to the PBB levels in the fat of the raw milk. Spray drying was the only process that resulted in a significant decrease in PBB level, reducing the PBBs in whole milk by one-third and the PBBs in skim milk by more than one-half.

4.2. Effect of Cooking on PBB Levels in Beef and Poultry

Zabik *et al.* (1980) showed that roasting sirloin tip roasts, braising or broiling top or bottom round steaks and broiling ground beef and hamburger patties resulted in a minimum

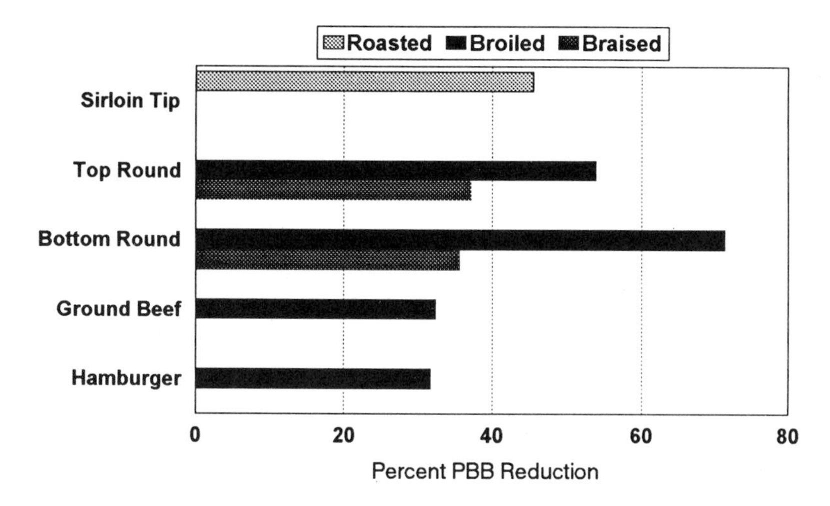

Figure 10. Percentage reduction of PBBs during the cooking of beef (Zabik *et al.*, 1980).

of 26% reduction of PBBs (Figure 10). Broiling beef round resulted in greater than a 50% reduction in PBB residues while roasting sirloin tip resulted in a 46% PBB reduction. Earlier, Smith *et al.* (1977) had studied the effect of pressure cooking on PBB residues in chicken pieces using a protocol similar to that which had been used to study the effect of stewing or pressure cooking on PCB levels in chicken pieces. These chickens had been fed 0, 30, 45, 60 and 90 ppm PBBs (Firemaster^R FF-1) which resulted in levels in the meat ranging from 0.02 to 23.17 ppm PBBs. Skin had about 5 times the levels of PBBs that were found in the muscle. Losses of PBBs were similar for all treatments. Similar overall losses of PBBs, ranging from 68 to 84%, were found for cooking chicken pieces as had been found for PCBs, but two-thirds of the recovered PBBs were found in the meat. If the broth was discarded, pressure cooking chicken pieces resulted in a 39% to 57% loss of PBBs (Figure 11).

Six of the seven peaks found in the chicken samples had been identified in the Firemaster^R FF-1 mixture (Zabik *et al.*, 1979b). 2,2',4,4',5,5'-hexabromobiphenyl accounted

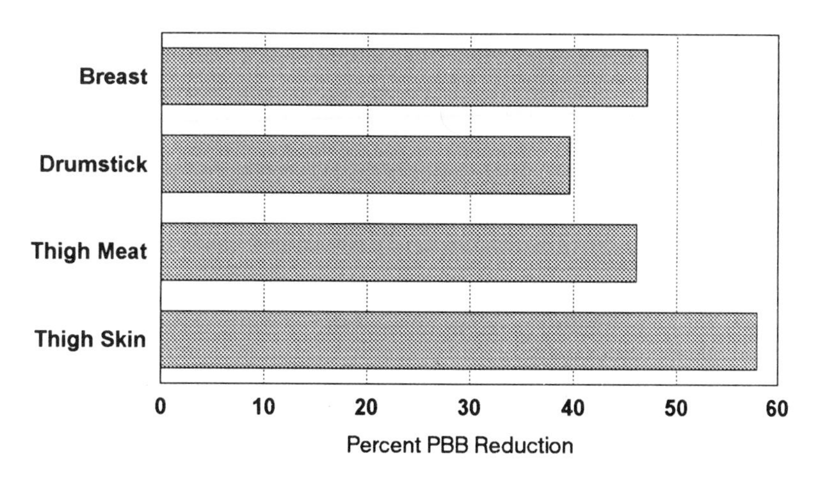

Figure 11. Percentage reduction of PBBs during pressure cooking of chicken pieces (Smith *et al.*, 1977).

for just over 60% of the PBBs found in either the raw chicken, cooked chicken or chicken broth. Two other isomers, 2,2',3,4,4',5'-hexabromobiphenyl and 2,2',3,4,4',5,5'-heptabromobiphenyl, accounted for 10–15% each of the remaining area while all other peaks were less than 5% of the total area.

5. DIOXINS

Dioxins are ubiquitous environmental contaminants produced during some combustion processes, such as waste incineration, and are also the unwanted by-products of various chemical manufacturing and bleaching processes. Dioxins were brought to public notice when the defoliant Agent Orange was used in Vietnam and the Sevesco accident in Italy in 1976. Chlorine can occur at the 1,2,3,4,6,7,8,9 positions. By for the most toxic of the dioxins is 2,3,7,8-tetrachlorodibenzo-*p*-dioxin (TCDD).

An early study involved the effect of cooking on hexa-, hepta-, and octaclorodibenzo-*p*-dioxins. Technical grade pentachlorophenol (penta) containing low levels of chlorinated dibenzodioxins had been widely used as a pesticide. Penta-treated woods had been used in livestock premises for many years. To determine whether a potential hazard to humans exists from cattle on dairy farms being exposed to substantial amounts of penta-treated wood, Zabik and Zabik (1980) studied the effect of cooking on octa-, hepta, and hexa-chlorodibenzo-*p*-dioxins. Using meat from four beef animals fed technical grade penta, liver slices were pan-fried, round steaks were braised, stew meat was pressure cooked and ground beef and hamburger patties charbroiled. Liver had 3.2 ppb hexa-, 18 ppb hepta- and 183 ppb octachlorodibenzo-*p*-dioxin. Small but significant losses of dioxins occurred during the pan frying of liver -- 20% for octa-, 11% for hepta-, and 8% for hexa-dibenzo-*p*dioxin. All other cuts had levels of about 1 ppb and the data were so variable that no significant trends were found.

All other studies being reviewed investigated the effect of cooking/processing on potential TCDD reduction. Increased precision of analyses allowed the determination of TCDD at fractions of ppt levels (Kaczmar, 1983). Using these analytical techniques, charbroiling carp fillets to 75°C resulted in 20 to 60 percent loss of TCDD.

In another study of the effect of cooking/processing on TCDD levels in fish, Stachiw *et al.* (1988) used carp surimi to form restructured carp fillets of 7.5 cm and 10.0 cm diameter by 1 cm thick. The raw surimi had about 40 ppt of TCDD. Additionally half the surimi was spiked to give levels of about 100 ppt of TCDD. Losses of TCDD were similar from spiked and unspiked restructured fillets. Increasing the surface area by increasing the diameter of the restructured carp fillets resulted in a greater TCDD loss (65% for 10.0 cm diameter fillets as compared to 55% for 7.5 cm diameter fillets) when the fillets were roasted or charbroiled to an internal temperature of 80°C (Figure 12). Increasing the internal temperature to which the carp fillets were cooked from 60 to 80°C also increased the TCDD losses (Figure 13).

The effect of cooking/processing on TCDD levels was included in the study of contaminants in the Great Lakes at the dinner table (Zabik *et al.*, 1995c). The levels of TCDD in composite samples of siscowets from Lake Superior were below the limit of detection. Of the composites which had detectable levels of TCDD, white bass were the lowest with 0.6 ppt TCDD in the composite from Lake Huron and 0.5 ppt TCDD in the composite from Lake Erie. The levels of TCDD in raw lake trout were as follows: 4.3 ppt for Lake Huron, 4.0 ppt for Lake Michigan, and 3.3 ppt for Lake Ontario. For Lake Michigan, raw skin-on chinook salmon had 7.83 ppt TCDD and raw skin-off had 7.6 ppt TCDD while for

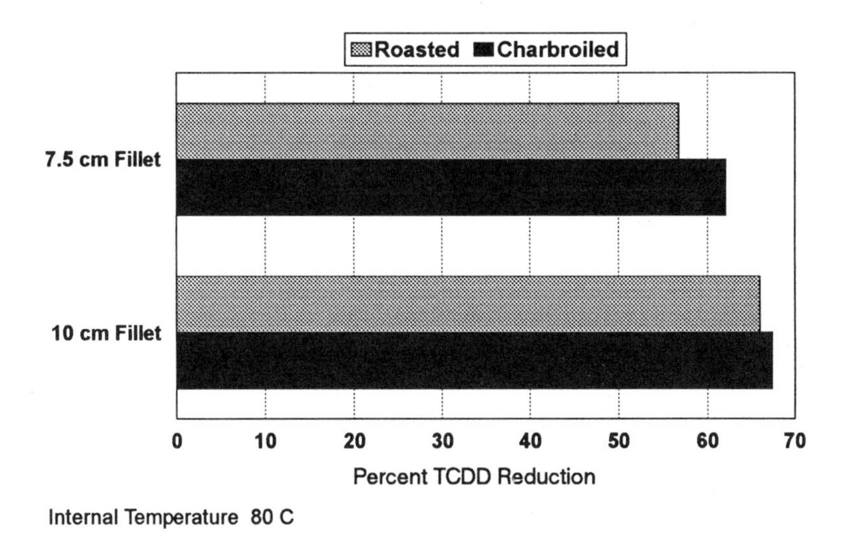

Figure 12. Effect of increased surface area on the reduction of TCDD from restructured carp fillets (Stachiw *et al.*, 1988).

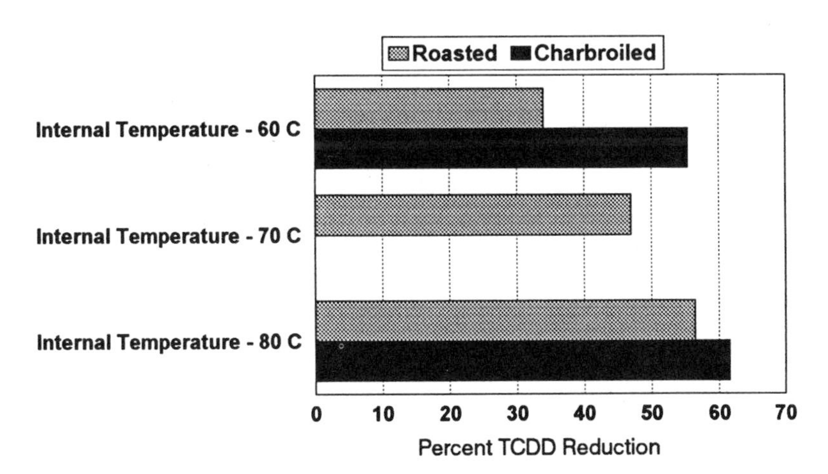

Figure 13. Effect of final internal end point temperature on the reduction of TCDD from restructured carp fillets (Stachiw *et al.*, 1988).

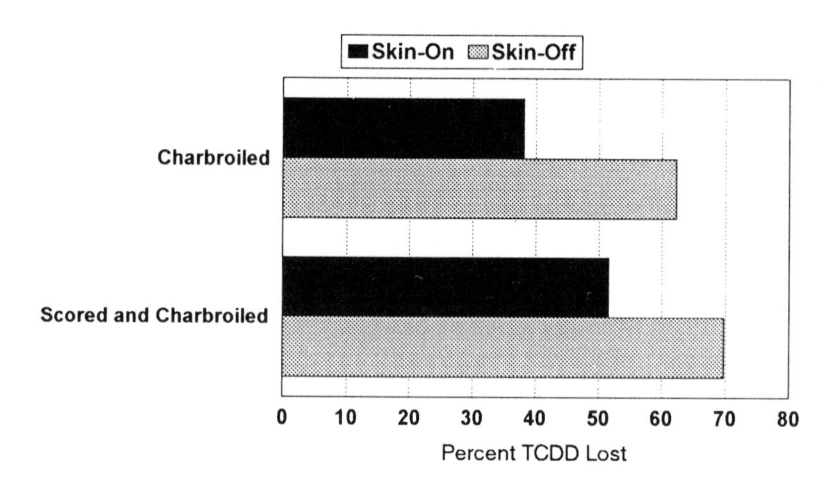

Figure 14. Influence of the use of scoring to increase the surface area of salmon fillets on the reduction of TCDD (Zabik *et al.*, 1995c).

Lake Huron, raw skin-on chinook salmon had 4.53 ppt TCDD and raw skin-off had 3.75 ppt TCDD. Walleye harvested from Lake Michigan had 2.2 ppt TCDD while walleye from Lakes Erie and Huron had 13.5 and 10.5 ppt TCDD, respectively. The bottom feeding carp from Lake Huron had the highest levels with 22.6 ppt TCDD for skin-on fillets and 23.1 ppt for skin-off. In contrast carp from Lake Erie had 5.4 ppt TCDD in skin-on fillets and 5.3 ppt in skin-off fillets.

Zabik *et al.* (1995c) also found that scoring chinook salmon to increase the surface area promoted greater losses of TCDD (Figure 14) while removing the skin before cooking resulted in at least an additional 10% TCDD loss during the preparation of the chinook salmon. As part of a comprehensive study to determine the level of environmental contaminants in five species of Great Lakes fish at the dinner table, these Great Lakes fish species were cooked/processed by seven methods. Reductions of TCDD during cooking/processing ranged from 28% for salt boiled fish to 100% for smoked fish (Figure 15). Most of the cooking methods resulted in about a 50% loss of TCDD. TCDD loss by species varied from 36% for skin-on carp to 80% for white bass.

6. SUMMARY

Although consumers have expressed concern over the level of environmental contaminants in the food supply, market basket surveys involving over 8,000 analyses of foods ready-to-eat, found measurable amounts (ppb levels) of PCBs in only 24 foods. Three of these foods had PCBs in two samples; the remaining had PCBs in only one of the samples analyzed.

Processing and cooking is responsible for PCB reductions and contributed to the levels found in the FDA market basket study. The following observations were made:

- Deodorization of edible food oils removes virtually all PCBs.
- Removal of contaminated areas reduces the level of PCBs in the final product.
  - Removing the hepatopancreas increased losses of PCBs in cooked blue crab.

  - Trimming the fatty lateral line and the belly flap resulted in 19 to 45% reductions of PCBs with most studies showing 40% or greater losses.
- Cooking/ processing also has been shown to be effective in PCB reduction.
  - Freeze-drying removes one-quarter to two-fifths of the PCBs in eggs and shrimp homogenates.
  - Cooking has been shown to reduce PCBs by 20 to 40% in a variety of studies with most studies showing at least a one-third reduction.
  - Increasing the surface area increases the percentage lost by about 5 to 10 %.
  - Smoking fish resulted in a 40%or greater loss of PCBs.
  - Canning salmon resulted in about a 30% loss of PCBs.

Although PBBs got into the food chain as the result of one incredible accident and thus are not expected to be found in foods today, cooking/processing is also effective in reducing PBBs. The following observations were made:

- Spray drying removed one-quarter of the PBBs from whole milk and more than one-half from skim milk.
- Pressure cooking chicken pieces resulted in a 39% to 57% PBB loss.
- Cooking beef resulted in a one-quarter to one-half loss of PBBs with the high heat of broiling resulting in the higher losses.

Dioxins are the result of combustion processes and chemical manufacturing processes. TCDD levels found in Great Lakes fish were in the low part per trillion level. Again, cooking and processing resulted in substantially less TCDD in fish as eaten. The following observations were made:

- Increasing surface area promoted TCDD loss.
- Increasing internal temperature promoted TCDD loss.
- Cooking/processing losses of TCDD from Great Lakes fish ranged from 28% for salt boiled fish to 100% for smoked fish with most cooking methods resulting in a 50% loss.

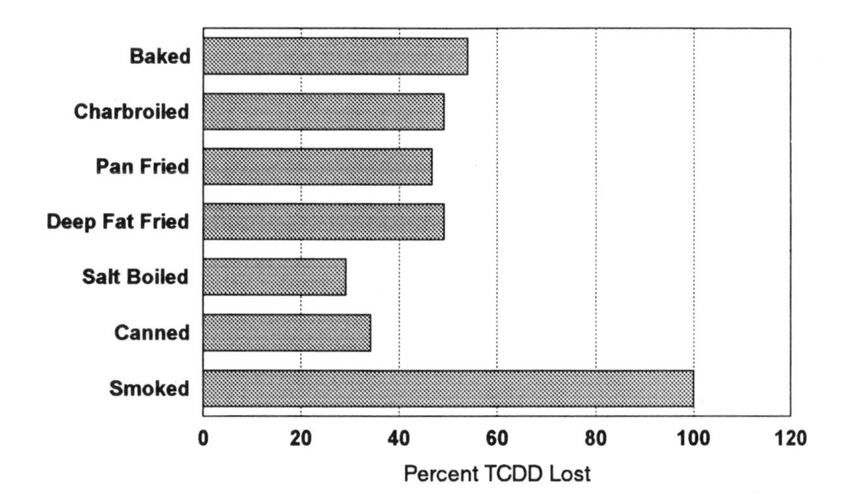

Figure 15. TCDD reduction during the cooking/processing of five species of Great Lakes fish (Zabik *et al.*, 1995c).

REFERENCES

Addison, R.F.; Ackman, R.G. Removal of organochlorine pesticides and polychlorinated biphenyls from marine oils during refining and hydrogenation for edible use. *J. Amer.Oil Chem. Soc.* **1974**, 51, 192–194.

Addison, R.F.; Zinck, R.G.; Ackman, R.G.; Sipos, J.C. Behavior of DDT, polychlorinated biphenyls (PCBs), and dieldrin at various stages of refining of marine oils for edible use. *J. Amer. Oil Chem. Soc.* **1978**, 55, 391–394.

Armbruster, G.; Gerow, K.G.; Gutenmann, W.H.; Littman, C.B.; Lisk, D.J. The effects of several methods of fish preparation on residues of polychlorinated biphenyls and sensory characteristics in striped bass. *J. Food Safety* **1987**, 8, 235–243.

Cichy, R.F.; Zabik, M.E.; Weaver, C.M. Polychlorinated biphenyl reduction in lake trout by irradiation and broiling. *Bull. Environ. Contam. Toxicol.* **1979**, 22, 807–811.

Daubenmire, S.W. Use of Great Lakes fish species as bioindicators of environmental contamination; the effect of food processing on the reduction of total PCBs and their homologs, Ph.D. Dissertation, Michigan State University Library, East Lansing, MI, 216 pp., **1996**.

Food and Drug Administration; Pesticides Team, 1995, Accumulated pesticide and industrial chemical findings from a ten-year study of ready-to-eat foods. *J. of AOAC Intern.* **1995**, 78, 614–631.

Hora, M.E. Reduction of polychlorinated biphenyl (PCB) concentrations in carp (*Cyprinus carpio*) fillets through skin removal. *Bull. Environ. Contam. Toxicol.* **1981**, 26, 364–366.

Kaczmar, S.W. Parts per trillion determination of 2,3,7,8-tetrachlorodibenzo-*p*-dioxin in Michigan Fish. Ph.D. Dissertation, Michigan State University Library, East Lansing, MI, **1983**.

Kanematsu, H.; Maruyama, T.; Niiya, I.; Imamura, M.; Suzuki, K.; Kutsuwa, Y.; Murase, I.; Matsumo, T. Studies on the behavior of trace components in oils and fats during processing for edible use. II. Variation in the amount of PCB and organochlorine pesticides during the hydrogenating Process. *J. Japan Oil Chem. Soc.* **1976**, 25, 42–46.

Khan, M.A. Radiation and processing for reducing the toxicity of polychlorinated biphenyls in foods. Ph.D. Dissertation. Louisiana State University Library, 210 pp., **1975**.

Khan, M.A.; Roa, M.R.; Novak, A.K. Reduction of polychlorinated biphenyls in shrimp and eggs by freeze-drying techniques. *J. Food Sci.* **1976**, 41, 1137–1141.

Lépine, F.L.; Brochu, F.; Milot, S.; Mamer, O.A.; Pépin, Y. γ Irradiation-induced degradation of organochlorinated pollutants in fatty acid esters and in cod. *J. Agric. Food Chem.* **1995**, 43, 491–494.

Murata, T.; Zabik, M.E.; Zabik, M.J. Polybrominated biphenyls in raw milk and processed dairy products. *J. Dairy Sci.* **1976**, 60, 516–520.

Sanders, M.; Haynes, B.L. Distribution pattern and reduction of polychlorinated biphenyls (PCB) in bluefish *Pomatomus saltatrix (Linneaus)* fillets through adipose tissue removal. *Bull. Environ. Contam. Toxicol.* **1988**, 41, 670–677.

Santerre, C.R.; Goodrum, J.W.; Kee, J.M. Roasted peanuts and peanut butter quality are affected by supercritical fluid extraction, *J. Food Sci.* **1994**, 59, 382–386.

Sherer, R.A.; Price, P.S. The effect of cooking processes on PCB levels in edible fish tissue. Qual. Assur. (San Diego) **1993**, 2, 396–407.

Skea, J.C.; Jackling, J.; Symula, H.; Simonin, H.; Harris, E.; Colquhoun, J. Summary of fish trimming and cooking techniques used to reduce levels of oil soluble contaminants. Technical Report, Division of Fisheries and Wildlife, New York Department of Environmental Conservation, Albany 36 pp., **1979**.

Smith, W.E.; Funk, K.; Zabik, M.E. Effects of cooking on concentrations of PCB and DDT compounds in chinook (*Oncorhychus tshawytscha*) and coho (*O. kisutch*) salmon from Lake Michigan. *J. Fish Res. Board Can.* **1973**, 30, 702–706.

Smith, S.K.; Zabik, M.E.; Dawson, L.E. Polybrominated biphenyl levels in raw and cooked chicken and chicken broth. *Poultry Sci.* **1977**, 56, 1289–1296.

Stachiw, N.C.; Zabik, M.E.; Booren, A.M.; Zabik, M.J. Tetrachlorodibenzo-*p*-dioxin residue reduction through cooking/processing of restructured carp fillets. *J. Agric. Food Chem.* **1988**, 36, 848–852.

Voiland, M.; Gall, K.; Lisk, D.; MacNeill, D. The effectiveness of recommended fat-trimming procedures on the reduction of PCB and mires in Lake Ontario brown trout (*Salmo trutta*). New York Sea Grant Extension Program/New York State College of Agriculture and Life Sciences Applied Research Project No. 89–002. p.16, **1990**.

Zabik, M.E. Polychlorinated biphenyl levels in raw and cooked chicken and chicken broth. *Poultry Sci.* **1974**, 53, 1785–1790.

Zabik, M.E. Effect of roasting, hot-holding or microwave heating on polychlorinated biphenyl levels in turkey. *School Food Ser. Res. Review* **1990**, 14, 98–102.

Zabik, M.E.; Olson, B.; Johnson, T.M. Dieldrin, DDT, PCBs and mercury levels in freshwater mullet from the upper Great Lakes, 1975–76, *Pesticides Monit. J.* **1978**, 12, 36–39.

Zabik, M.E.; Hoojjat, P.; Weaver, C.M. Polychlorinated biphenyls, dieldrin and DDT in lake trout cooked by broiling, roasting or microwave. *Bull. Environ. Contam. Toxicol.* **1979a**, 21, 136–143.

Zabik, M.E.; Smith, S.K.; Cala, R. Polybrominated biphenyl isomer distribution in raw and cooked chicken and chicken broth. *Poultry Sci.* **1979b**, 58, 1435–1438.

Zabik, M.E.; Zabik, M.J. Dioxin levels in raw and cooked liver, loin steaks, round and patties from beef fed technical grade pentachlorophenol. *Bull. Environ. Contam. Toxicol.* **1980**, 24, 344–349.

Zabik, M.E.; DeFouw, C.; Weaver, C.M. Polybrominated biphenyl congener levels and distribution patterns in raw and cooked beef. *Arch. Environ. Contam. Toxicol.* **1980**, 9, 651–659.

Zabik, M.E.; Merrill, C.; Zabik, M.J. PCBs and other xenobiotics in raw and cooked carp. Bull. Environ. Contam. Toxicol. **1982**, 28, 710–715.

Zabik, M.E.; Harte, J.B; Zabik, M.J.; Dickmann, G. Effect of preparation and cooking on contaminant distributions in crustaceans: PCBs in blue crab. *J. Agric. Food Chem.* **1992**, 40, 1197–1203.

Zabik, M.E.;Zabik, M.J.; Humphrey, H. Assessment of contaminants in five species of Great Lake fish at the dinner table. Final report Part I. Pesticides, total PCBs and PAHs and Part II. Congener specific PCBS and dioxins. Great Lakes Protection Fund, Chicago, IL, **1994**.

Zabik, M.E.; Zabik, M.J. Booren, A.M.; Nettles, M.; Song, J-H.; Welch, R.; Humphrey, H. Pesticides and total polychlorinated biphenyls in chinook salmon and carp harvested from the Great Lakes: Effect of skin-on and skin-off processing and selected cooking methods. *J. Agric. Food Chem.* **1995a,** 43, 993–1001.

Zabik, M.E.; Zabik, M.J.; Booren, A.M.; Daubenmire, S.; Pascall, M.A.; Welch, R.; Humphrey, H. Pesticides and total polychlorinated biphenyls residues in raw and cooked walleye and white bass harvested from the Great Lakes. *Bull. Environ. Contam. Toxicol.* **1995b**, 54, 396–402.

Zabik, M.E.; Zabik, M.J. Tetrachlorodibenzo-*p*-dioxin residue reduction by cooking/processing of fish fillets harvested from the Great Lakes. *Bull. Environ. Contam. Toxicol.* **1995c**, 55, 264–269.

Zabik, M.E.; Booren, A.; Zabik, M.J.; Welch, R.; Humphrey, H. Pesticide residues, PCBs and PAHs in baked, charbroiled, salt boiled and smoked Great Lakes lake trout. *Food Chemistry* **1996**, 55, 231–239.

15

THE EFFECT OF PROCESSING ON VETERINARY RESIDUES IN FOODS

William A. Moats

Meat Science Research Laboratory, Beltsville Agricultural Research Center
Agricultural Research Service, USDA
Beltsville, Maryland 20705-2350

1. ABSTRACT

Heat stability of antibiotics in foods to cooking has been determined by a variety of methods. These include heating in such liquid media as milk, water, buffers and meat extracts, and in solids such as buffered meat homogenates and various sausages. Inactivation of incurred residues in tissues and eggs was also studied. Time and temperature of heating were more easily controlled in liquid media, but results in actual meat products are more indicative of actual cooking processes. Ordinary cooking procedures for meat, even to "well-done", cannot be relied on to inactivate even the more heat sensitive compounds such as penicillins and tetracyclines. More severe heating as for canning or prolonged cooking with moist heat can inactivate the more heat sensitive compounds. The relevance to food safety is uncertain since the nature of the degradation products is unknown in most cases.

2. INTRODUCTION

When veterinary drugs are administered to farm animals, either therapeutically or to promote growth, residues may remain in meat, milk or eggs if proper precautions are not followed. Testing for residues is ordinarily done on raw product. However, products of animal origin are usually cooked or processed in some manner before they are consumed. It is therefore useful to determine the effect of processing in assessing actual human exposure to residues (Moats, 1988; Haagsma, 1993).

A number of approaches have been used to study the effects of cooking and other processing procedures. In studies done prior to 1988, loss of antimicrobial activity of antibiotics heated in various substrates was measured (Moats, 1988). Since then, more specific chromatographic methods of analysis have been introduced. Animal tissues and eggs

Impact of Processing on Food Safety, edited by Jackson et al.,
Kluwer Academic / Plenum Publishers, New York, 1999.

Table 1. Effect of heating antibiotics in milk (Shahani, 1957, 1958; Shahani et al., 1956)

Antibiotic	Concentration	Temp (°C)-time	% reduction	
			Milk	Water
Chlortetracycline	0.30–0.51 μg/mL	62 (30 min)	16.6	32.5
	0.20–0.62 μg/mL	71 (30 min)	27.6	51.2
	0.40–0.50 μg/mL	121 (15 min)	100	100
Oxytetracycline	0.32–3.22 μg/mL	62 (30 min)	23.6	—
	0.40–1.29 μg/mL	71 (30 min)	35.6	—
	0.50–0.55 μg/mL	71 (190 min)	100	—
Penicillin G	0.13–0.96 I.U./mL	62 (30 min)	8.2	54.7
	0.25–1.07 I.U./mL	71 (15 min)	10.1	100
	0.25–1.04 I.U./mL	121 (15 min)	59.7	100

containing incurred residues have been used as well as spiked samples. Cooking or processing of foods containing incurred residues has been studied. Incurred residues are not always distributed uniformly in tissues. However, it is difficult to simulate the distribution of incurred residues by spiking tissues. Penetration of heat is slow and uneven in solid media such as muscle and meat patties. Some investigators have studied degradation in liquid media such as milk, tissue homogenates, tissue extracts, buffers, and water. These permit better control of the time and temperature of heating, but are less representative of actual cooking conditions.

3. THERMAL PROCESSING AND VETERINARY DRUG RESIDUES

3.1. Heating in Milk

One of the earliest studies was on the effect of heating antibiotics in milk and buffers by Shahani (1957, 1958) and Shahani et al. (1956) (Table 1). The conditions ordinarily used to pasteurize milk are 62°C for 30 min. or, more commonly, 71°C for 15 sec. Pasteurization would be expected to result in only slight degradation of antibiotic residues. These studies showed that milk had a marked protective effect on penicillin G relative to heating in water. Konecny (1978) reported results of heating chloramphenicol, streptomycin, neomycin and penicillin G in milk and water (Table 2). A 30–40% reduction in antimicrobial activity was observed after heating for 30 min at 100°C. There was little

Table 2. Inactivation of some antibiotics by heating 30 min in milk and water (Konecny, 1978)

Antibiotic	Concentration	Temp (°C)	% reduction	
			Milk	Water
Chloramphenicol	1 mg/mL	70	30	11.1
		100	35	30
Streptomycin	1 mg/mL	70	8.3	25
		100	41.7	33
Neomycin	1 mg/mL	70	10	11.1
		100	35	25
Penicillin G	2.5 I.U./mL	70	30	30
		100	32.2	40

Table 3. Inactivation of some antibiotics by heating in water, milk and meat extract at 100°C (Pilet et al., 1969)

			% reduction after heating		
Antibiotic	Concentration	Substrate	30 min	60 min	90 min
Tetracycline	1–2 μg/mL	Water	80	100	100
		Bouillon	80	100	100
		Extract of chicken muscle	50	65	80
Penicillin G	0.15–0.25 μg/mL	Water	50–100	75–100	85–100
		Bouillon	35–50	65–75	88
		Milk	20–40	50–65	85–100
		Extract of chicken muscle	80–100	100	100

difference in stability between milk and water, and no protective effect of milk on penicillin G was observed. Pilet et al. (1969) reported results of heating tetracycline, oxytetracycline, penicillin G, neomycin, spiramycin, framycetin and oleandomycin in milk and water. The results for oxytetracycline and penicillin G are summarized in Table 3, and for neomycin in Table 4. Neomycin was found to be the most stable to heat, but was less stable in milk than in water. Framycetin and oleandomycin (not shown) were also less stable in milk. Penicillin G appeared to be slightly more stable in milk than in water.

3.2. Heating in Liquid Media

The studies of Pilet et al. (1969) also included heating chicken and beef muscle extracts (Tables 3 and 4). Of these, oxytetracycline was the least stable and neomycin was the most stable. Neomycin was somewhat less stable in meat extracts than in water, and spiramycin (not shown) was less stable in chicken muscle extract than in other media. Tropilo (1985) (Table 5) determined the stability of penicillin G when heated in buffers and buffered meat homogenates. Penicillin G was more stable at pH 7.0 than at pH 5.0. The presence of the meat homogenate did not seem to greatly affect degradation. Kitts et al. (1992) (Table 6) measured D-values (decimal reduction times) for degradation of oxytetracycline in buffers and ground salmon muscle. Oxytetracycline was more stable in salmon muscle homogenate than in the corresponding buffers. Cooking salmon filets 15 min at 99.4°C resulted in a 61–90% reduction which is comparable to other studies of oxytetracycline in tissues.

Table 4. Inactivation of neomycin (20–50μg/mL) heated in water, milk and meat extract (Pilet et al., 1969)

		% inactivation after heating	
Substrate	Temp (°C)	20 min	3–5 hrs
Water	100	—	0–20
	120	0–25	—
Bouillon	100	—	0–20
	120	25–100	—
Milk	100	—	75–100
	120	15–50	—
Extract of Chicken Muscle	100	—	0–10
	120	50	—

Table 5. Inactivation of penicillin G (0.2 I.U./mL) heated in buffer and meat homogenates (Tropilo, 1985)

Substrate	% inactivation after heating 15 min at: 80°C	90°C	100°C	117°C	121°C
Buffer, pH 5.0	13.5	6.5	31.0	98.0	100
Buffer, pH 7.0	15.2	10.2	18.8	68.0	81.5
Buffered meat homogenate					
pH 5.0	19.7	1.1	42.6	84.7	94.7
pH 7.0	17.8	0	25.0	62.6	87.4

3.3. Domestic Cooking Procedures—Tissues

Heating in liquid media cannot exactly duplicate actual cooking of solid tissue. However, the results from heating in liquid media may be helpful in interpreting actual cooking results. Penetration of heat during actual cooking is slow. Unless heating is prolonged, the outside reaches a higher temperature than the interior so that it is difficult to assess the actual exposure of residues to heat. It is difficult, if not impossible, to spike solid tissue in a manner simulating incurred residues from treated animals. However, residues in incurred tissues may not be evenly distributed, introducing another source of variability. Additionally, incurred tissues may contain metabolites. Some investigators have ground incurred tissues to give more uniform distribution of residues.

The earliest reported study using solid tissue was that of Escanilla et al. (1959) on the stability of chlortetracycline in ground beef patties. Considerable degradation was reported in ground beef patties fried to an internal temperature of only 42°C. The reported degradation was not greatly increased by cooking to higher temperatures. Buncic and Dakic (1981) cooked rabbit muscle and kidney containing incurred residues of penicillin G, tetracycline and streptomycin at 100°C. Penicillin G was the least stable while streptomycin was not completely degraded after heating at 100°C for 120 min. O'Brien et al. (1981) (Table 7) studied degradation of incurred residues of several antibiotics in beef muscle fried and roasted. Their data show the great variability of temperatures reached under similar cooking conditions. The maximum temperature reached after frying to "well-done" was 92°C. Little degradation was observed in steaks cooked to "rare". Steaks cooked to "well-done" showed variable degradation depending on the compound. Sulfadimidine (sulfamethazine) was stable to ordinary cooking procedures.

Ibrahim and Moats (1994) measured degradation of oxytetracycline in lamb patties fried, microwaved, and boiled in a bag (Table 8). The amount of degradation was related to the time and temperature of cooking.

Table 6. Degradation of oxytetracycline in buffers and fish muscle (Kitts et al., 1992)

Temp (°C)	D Value (min) pH 3.0 buffer	pH 6.9 buffer	Fish muscle
60	645.2	111.7	ND[a]
80	50.0	22.1	143.5
90	48.0	16.5	75.8
100	18.7	12.7	31.0

61–90% reduction after cooking 15 min at 99.4°C
[a] Not Done

Table 7. Effect of cooking on incurred antibiotic residues in beef steaks (O'Brien et al., 1981)

Antibiotic	Concentration	Reduction in zone of inhibition after cooking		
		10 min "rare" 22–56 °C	20 min "medium" 52–90 °C	30 min "well-done" 76–92 °C
Ampicillin	0.6–0.8 μg/g	3–8	2–34	25–82
Chloramphenicol	1.5–1.6 μg/g	0–7	14–50	27–61
Oxytetracycline	0.5–0.6 μg/g	4–16	12–18	22–39
Sulfadimidine	8.0 μg/g	0–5.4	0–7.6	0–6.1

Rose et al. (1996) evaluated a variety of cooking procedures on incurred oxytetracycline residues in beef. Losses were less, 35–39%, in grilled samples where final internal temperatures were only 59–70 °C, and were highest in meat roasted to "well-done" which gave both the highest internal temperature (98 °C) and the longest cooking times. Honikel et al. (1978) investigated the effect of heating on oxytetracycline and chlortetracycline in meat and bone. Degradation in meat occurred only at temperatures above 65 °C. Chlortetracycline was more stable in bone than in tissue. Some antibiotic may be extracted from bone during cooking, if the pH is below 4.0.

Hsu and Epstein (1993) (Table 9) investigated the stability of Levamisole, an anthelminthic drug, to cooking. The compound was stable to ordinary cooking, but some degradation occurred with the more severe heat treatment of canning. Curing resulted in some degradation. Rose et al. (1995b) also found that Levamisole was stable to ordinary cooking although some was lost in the drip.

Rose et al. (1995a) found that incurred clenbuterol in tissues was stable to normal cooking procedures such as frying, boiling and grilling. It did not migrate into drip or cooking water, suggesting that residues were bound to protein. This was further supported by the observation that a protease digestion step was required to free the clenbuterol prior to analysis. These results are in contrast to those of Ramos et al. (1993) who used spiked rather than incurred samples. These authors found that clenbuterol was reduced by boiling or grilling and that none remained after frying.

Steffenak et al. (1993) found that oxolinic acid, a compound used to control fish diseases, concentrated in the bones, but may migrate into muscle during cooking. Epstein et al. (1988) found that sulfamethazine was partially degraded by curing in a sausage type emulsion, but that it was stable to cooking and canning procedures. Fischer et al. (1992) did not find any degradation of sulfamethazine during curing of pork. The parent compound was stable to cooking, but metabolites such as the glucoside were partially degraded and perhaps converted to the parent compound during cooking. Rose et al. (1995c) also found that sulfamethazine was stable to cooking. Xu et al. (1996) studied stability of ormetoprim and sulfamethoxine to cooking in fish muscle. The compounds are found in a

Table 8. Degradation of oxytetracycline in ground lamb muscle during various cooking procedures (Ibrahim and Moats, 1994)

Cooking method	% reduction (temp)	
	4 min	8 min
Frying	3.6 (52 °C)	17.3 (81 °C)
Microwave cooking	12.2 (36–56 °C)	60.5 (98–102 °C)
Boiling-in-bag	64 (15 min)	95 (30 min)

Table 9. Effect of cooking/processing on incurred levamisole residues in swine muscle tissue (Hsu and Epstein, 1996)

Treatment	ppm (dry wt.)	% decrease
Uncured	1.17	—
Cured	0.78	33
Cooked		
Stir-fried	2.17	—
Smoked	1.04	0[a]
Stewed	1.01	0[a]
Grilled	1.10	0[a]
Pressure-cooked	0.98	0[a]
Microwaved	0.92	4[a]
Deep-fried	0.91	5[a]
Broiled	0.71	26
Canned	0.36	62
Frozen	0.68	29
Uncooked raw meat	0.96	—

[a]no statistically significant difference from uncooked control

commercial formulation used to treat fish diseases. Both were partially degraded. Sulfamethoxine is evidently less stable to cooking than some other sulfonamides.

Kuivinen and Slanina (1986) studied the effect of frying and boiling on residues of Ivermectin (dihydroavermectin$^{B}{}_{1a}$) in minced beef. Frying to internal temperatures of 60°C, 71°C and 77°C resulted in reduction of 38%, 37% and 32%, respectively. Boiling 9 min to an internal temperature of 70°C reduced residues 21%. Rose et al. (1996) concluded that losses of Ivermectin during cooking were a result of losses in the drip. Rose et al. (1996) observed some degradation of oxfendazole after boiling 3 hours in water. They concluded that cooking did not destroy residues in tissues. The same authors found that Lasalocid was stable at 100°C in aqueous solutions at pH 5.5 and at pH 7.0, but had a half-life of 30 min at pH 10.0. It was also stable when heated in chicken meat.

Epstein et al. (1998) found that chloramphenicol was partially degraded by curing and by cooking. More severe heating such as for canning resulted in total degradation. Rauws and Olling (1978) found that incurred residues of a tranquilizer, azaperone, in swine tissue were stable to heating.

3.4. Domestic Cooking—Eggs

Yonova (1971) found that heating for 40–60 min at 100°C was required to inactivate tetracycline or oxytetracycline in eggs. This is longer than the 15–20 min required to hard-boil eggs. Streptomycin (Inglis and Katz, 1978) and neomycin (Katz and Levine, 1978) in eggs were stable to ordinary cooking procedures such as frying, poaching, scrambling or hard boiling. Rose et al. (1996) found that Lasalocid was less stable when heated in eggs rather than in muscle, presumably because of the higher pH of eggs.

3.5. Sausage Manufacture

Escanilla et al. (1959) found that chlortetracycline was partially or completely degraded, depending on the initial concentration during processing of frankfurters. Scheibner (1972a) found that penicillin G, streptomycin and oxytetracycline were partially inactivated during scalding and smoking in sausage manufacture. More severe heating as was required for canning resulted in total degradation of all three antibiotics in the sau-

Table 10. Inactivation of antibiotics in sausages during canning (Scheibner, 1972a,b)

Antibiotic	Process	% inactivation
Penicillin G 7.2 I.U./g	Heating in glass, 90–95°C (60 min), Heating in glass and tin, 120–125°C, (65 min)	Sausage 100 Liquid 100
Oxytetracycline 40.4 μg/g	Heating in glass, 90–95°C (60 min), Heating in glass and tin, 120–125°C, (65 min)	Sausage 100 Liquid 100
Streptomycin 13.2 I.U./g	Heating in glass, 90–95°C, (60 min)	Sausage 59 Liquid 36
	Heating in glass and tin, 120–125°C,(60–65 min)	Sausage 100 Liquid 41–64

sages, although some streptomycin remained in the liquid around the sausages (Table 10)(1972b).

Ellerbrock and Steffen (1991) found that sulfamethazine and sulfapyrazine were stable during sausage manufacture except when a fermentation step was involved. Less than 40% remained after ripening for 10 days. Smit et al. (1994) studied the stability of sulfadimidine during manufacture of raw fermented sausages. Approximately 25% of the sulfadimidine was lost in the brine and some was bound or converted to metabolites.

4. SUMMARY AND CONCLUSIONS

Veterinary drug residues vary in their susceptibility to degradation by heating. Ordinary cooking procedures cause some degradation of a number of drugs, depending on the amount of heat treatment involved. The measurement of degradation in muscle or other tissues containing incurred residues is subject to large variations because of uneven heat penetration and uneven distribution. These variations reflect those which will be encountered in actual cooking. The expenditure of a great deal of effort in the attempt to obtain precise measurement under these conditions does not seem useful. More severe processing treatments such as canning may completely degrade some residues. Ordinary cooking cannot be relied on to completely degrade residues that may be present. There are only a few reports on the degradation products formed during heating in food substrates. Oxytetracycline, when heated in water, was degraded to variety of compounds, mostly unidentified and unrelated to the parent compound (Rose et al., 1996). DePaolis et al. (1978) identified the lactate ester of penicilloic acid as a major degradation product of penicillins. Penicilloates may still produce allergic reactions in sensitive individuals even though the residues have no antimicrobial activity (Sullivan et al.,1981). Schwartz and Sher (1984) reported an instance of an acute anaphylactic response to a frozen beef dinner by an individual known to be hypersensitive to penicillins. Testing showed no antimicrobial activity in the meat, but an immunoassay for the penicilloyl-moiety was positive. It cannot, therefore, be assumed that the degradation products formed by heating are always safe.

REFERENCES

Buncic, S.; Dakic, M. Influence of low and high temperatures on biological activity of antibiotic residues in meat. *Tehnol. Mesa* **1981,** 22, 66–76.

DePaolis, A.M.; Katz, S. E.; Rosen, J. D. Effect of storage and cooking on penicillin in meat. *J. Agric. Food Chem.* **1978,** 25, 1112–1115.

Ellerbrock, L.I.; Steffen, G. Effect of pasteurization and fermentation on residues of sulfonamides in sausages. *Int'l. J. Food Sci. and Technol.* **1991,** 26, 479–483.

Epstein, R.L.; Randecker, V.; Corrao, P.; Keeton, J.T.; Cross, H.R. Influence of heat and cure preservatives on residues of sulfamethazine, chloramphenicol, and cyromazine in muscle tissue. *J. Agric. Food Chem.* **1988,** 36, 1009–1012.

Escanilla, O.I.; Carlin, A.F.; Ayres, J.C. Effect of storage and of cooking on chlortetracycline residues in meat. *Food Technol.* **1959,** 13, 520–524.

Fischer, L.T.; Thulin, A.J.; Zabik, M.E.; Booren, A.M.; Poppenga, R.H.; Chapman, K.J. Sulfamethazine and its metabolites in pork: Effects of cooking and gastrointestinal absorption of residues. *J. Agric. Food Chem.* **1992,** 40, 1677–1682.

Haagsma, N. Stability of veterinary drug residues during storage, preparation and processing. Proceedings of EuroResidue II Conference on Residues of Veterinary Drugs in Food. Haagsma, N.; Ruiter, A.; Czedik-Eysenberg, P. B., Eds., Veldhoven, The Netherlands, May 3–5, 1993, pp. 41–49.

Honikel, K. O.; Schmidt, U.; Woltersdorf, W.; Liestner, L. Effect of storage and processing on tetracycline residues in meat and bones. *J. Assoc. Off. Chem.* **1978,** 61, 1222–1227.

Hsu, S.Y.; Epstein, R.L. Influence of cooking/processing conditions on Levamisole residues in swine muscle tissues. Haagsma, N.; Ruiter, A.; Czedik-Eysenberg, P. B., Eds., Proceedings of EuroResidue II Conference on Residues of Veterinary Drugs in Food, Veldhoven, The Netherlands, May 3–5, 1993, pp. 387–390.

Ibrahim, A.; Moats, W.A. Effect of cooking procedures on oxytetracycline residues in lamb muscle. *J. Agric. Food Chem.* **1994,** 42, 2561–2563.

Inglis, J.M.; Katz, S. E. Determination of streptomycin residues in eggs and stability of residues after cooking. *J. Assoc. Off. Anal. Chem.* **1978,** 61, 1098–1102.

Katz, S.E.; Levine, P.R. Determination of neomycin residues in eggs and stability of residues after cooking. *J. Assoc. Off. Anal. Chem.* **1978,** 61, 1103–1106.

Kitts, D.D.; Yu, C.W.Y.; Burt, R.G.; McErlane, K. Oxytetracycline degradation in thermally processed farm salmon. *J. Agric. Food Chem.* **1992**, 140, 1977–1981.

Konecny, S. Effect of temperature and time on reduction of the biological activity of some kinds of antibiotics in milk. *Veternarstvi.* **1978,** 28, 409–410.

Kuivinen, J.; Slanina, P. Effect of cooking on Ivermectin residues in meat. *Vaar Foeda* **1986,** 38, 280–284.

Moats, W.A. Inactivation of antibiotics by heating in foods and other substrates - A Review. *J. Food Prot.* **1988,** 51, 491–497.

O'Brien, J.J.; Campbell, N.; Conaghan, T. The effect of cooking and cold storage on biologically active antibiotic residues in meat. *J. Hyg., Camb.* **1981,** 87, 511–523.

Pilet, C.; Toma, B.; Muzet, J.; Renard, F. Investigation of the thermostability of several antibiotics. *Cahier Med. Vet.* **1969,** 6, 227–234.

Ramos, F.; Castillo, M.C.; DeSilvera, M.I.N. The effect of domestic cooking on clenbuterol residues in meat. Haagsma, N.; Ruiter, A.; Czedik-Eysenberg, P. B., Eds., Proceedings of EuroResidue II Conference on Residues of Veterinary Drugs in Food, May 3–5, 1993, pp. 563–566.

Rauws, A.G.; Olling, M. Residues of azaperone and azaperol in slaughter pigs. *J. Vet. Pharm. Therap.* **1978,** 1, 57–62.

Rose, M.D.; Shearer, G.; Farrington, W.H.H. The effect of cooking on veterinary drug residues in food: 1. Clenbuterol. *Food Addit. Contam.* **1995a,** 12, 67–76.

Rose, M.D.; Argent, L.; Shearer, C.G.; Farrington, W.H.H. The effect of cooking on veterinary drug residues in food: 2. Levamisole. *Food Addit. Contam.* **1995b,** 12, 185–194.

Rose, M.D.; Shearer, G.; Farrington, W. H. H. The effect of cooking on veterinary drug residues in food: 3. Sulfamethazine. *Food Addit. Contam.* **1995c,** 12, 739–750.

Rose, M.D.; Bygrave, J.; Farrington, W.H.H.; Shearer, G. The effect of cooking on veterinary drug residues in food: 4. Oxytetracycline. *Food Addit. Contam.* **1996,** 13, 275–286.

Rose, M.D.; Shearer, G.; Farrington, W.H.H. The thermal stability and effect of cooking on veterinary drug residues in food. Haagsma, N.; Ruiter, A., Eds., Proceedings of EuroResidue III Conference on Veterinary Drug Residues in Food, Veldhoven, The Netherlands, May 6–8, 1996, pp. 829–834.

Scheibner, G. Studies into the effect of scalded sausage technology on certain antibiotics. *Monatsch. Veternaermed.* **1972a,** 27, 161–164.

Scheibner, G. Inactivation of several antibiotics in meat tinning. *Monatsch. Veternaermed.* **1972b,** 27, 745–747.

Schwartz, H.J.; Sher, T.H. Anaphylaxis to penicillin in a frozen dinner. *Ann. Allergy* **1984,** 52, 342–343.

Shahani, K.M. The effect of heat and storage on the stability of Aureomycin in milk, buffer, and water. *J. Dairy Sci.* **1957,** 40, 289–296.

Shahani, K.M. Factors affecting Terramycin activity in milk, broth, buffer, and water. *J. Dairy Sci.* **1958,** 41, 382–391.

Shahani, K.M.; Gould, I.A.; Weiser, H.H.; Slatter, W.L. Stability of small concentrations of penicillin in milk as affected by heat treatment and storage. *J. Dairy Sci.* **1956,** 39, 971–977.

Smit, L.A.; Hoogenboom, L.A.P.; Berghmans, M.C.J.; Haagsma, N. Stability of sulfadimidine during raw fermented sausage preparation. *Z. Lebensm.-Unters. Forsch.* **1994,** 198, 480–485.

Steffenak, I.; Hormazabel, V.; Yndestad, M. Residues of Quinolones in fish and the effect of cooking on the residues in the fish. Haagsma, N.; Ruiter, A.; Czedik-Eysenberg, P. B., Eds., Proceedings of the EuroResidue II Conference on Residues of Veterinary Drugs in Food, Veldhoven, The Netherlands, May 3–5, 1993, pp. 646–649.

Sullivan, T.J.; Wedner, J.; Shatz, G.S.; Yecies, L.D.; Parker, C.W. Skin testing to detect penicillin allergy. *J. Allergy Clin. Immunol.* **1981,** 68, 171–180.

Tropilo, J. Effect of heating on the inactivation of penicillin G. *Med. Weter.* **1985,** 41, 276–279.

Xu, D.; Grizzle, J.M.; Rogers, W.A.; Santerre, C.R. Effect of cooking on residues of ormetoprim and sulfadimethoxine in the muscle of channel catfish. *Food Res. Int'l.* **1996,** 29, 339–334.

Yonova, I. Studies on the thermal resistance of tetracycline and oxytetracycline residues in eggs and poultry meat. *Veterinarnomed. Nauki* **1971,** 8(10), 75–82.

16

EFFECT OF PROCESSING ON *FUSARIUM* MYCOTOXINS

Lauren S. Jackson[1] and Lloyd B. Bullerman[2]

[1]National Center for Food Safety and Technology
Food and Drug Administration
6502 S. Archer Rd., Summit, Argo, Illinois 60501
[2]Department of Food Science and Technology, University of Nebraska-Lincoln
Lincoln, Nebraska 68583

1. ABSTRACT

Mycotoxins are secondary metabolites produced by a wide variety of fungal species that contaminate food or feed. Fumonisins (FUM), deoxynivalenol (DON) and zearalenone (ZEN) are examples of common mycotoxins in grains that have been shown to affect human and/or animal health. Physical, chemical and biological methods have been used for decontaminating grains containing these toxins. Some treatments reduce the concentration of mycotoxins while others are ineffective. For example, removal of damaged grain by density segregation can reduce DON and ZEN concentrations in corn and wheat. In contrast, thermal processing is usually ineffective for reducing the FUM and ZEN content of foods. More work is needed to identify effective methods for detoxifying mycotoxin contaminated food.

2. INTRODUCTION

Mycotoxins are a chemically diverse group of toxic secondary metabolites produced by fungi. The United Nations Food and Agricultural Organization (FAO) has estimated that over 25% of the world's food crops are lost due to mycotoxin contamination (Mannon et al., 1985). They are responsible for significant financial losses for the food industry, particularly any aspect of the industry that harvests, stores, processes or uses raw agricultural products. Economic losses from contaminated foods and feed are estimated to be annually in the billions of dollars worldwide (Pohland, 1993). Fungal species in the genera

Impact of Processing on Food Safety, edited by Jackson et al.,
Kluwer Academic / Plenum Publishers, New York, 1999.

Aspergillus, *Penicillium* and *Fusarium* are the most important mycotoxin-producing fungi in food and feed. Examples of mycotoxins produced by these fungi include aflatoxins, trichothecenes, zearalenone, fumonisins, moniliformin, ochratoxins, patulin and citrinin.

The major route of exposure to mycotoxins is the consumption of contaminated agricultural products such as peanuts, corn, wheat, barley, tree nuts, cassava, sorghum, fruits, milk and meat (Pestka and Casale, 1990). The severity of mycotoxin contamination of agricultural products varies yearly (Coulombe, 1993). Factors that affect mycotoxin formation include moisture levels and pH of the food, temperature extremes, harvesting practices and stresses such as drought and insect damage. Mycotoxin production can occur in the field and during harvest, processing, transport and storage of food or feed.

Mycotoxins elicit a variety of acute and chronic toxic effects in domestic animals, including reduced growth efficiency, vomiting, reproductive problems, liver cancer and immunosuppression (Pestka and Casale, 1990; Coulombe, 1993). In humans, many mycotoxins have been implicated in disease outbreaks and some are believed to be carcinogens (Coulombe, 1993). For this reason, mycotoxins pose a threat to human and animal health and the determination of methods for reducing the mycotoxin content of food is desirable. Efforts to control mycotoxin levels in food and feed include prevention of contamination, regulatory limits or guidelines and decontamination procedures.

Prevention of mycotoxin contamination, although desirable, is not always possible. Under certain environmental conditions, mold infestation and mycotoxin contamination is inevitable (Trenholm et al., 1992). However, advances in molecular biology have provided the means for developing crops that resist fungal infection and/or mycotoxin contamination. Another preharvest control currently under investigation is biocompetitive exclusion, a technique by which nontoxigenic strains of fungi are added to the soil to compete with toxin-producing strains. Methods for preventing fungal growth in food during storage include use of fungistatic agents, modified atmosphere storage and γ-irradiation (Paster and Bullerman, 1988; Hooshmand and Klopfenstein, 1995).

Since the discovery of aflatoxins in the 1960's, many countries have developed legislation or guidelines to reduce exposure to mycotoxins in food and feed. The guidelines are based on known toxicological data and take into account reductions that take place during cleaning, milling, and processing operations that usually precede consumption (Patey and Gilbert, 1989). Mycotoxins considered important enough for tolerance levels include patulin, ochratoxin A, trichothecenes and zearalenone. In the U.S., corn containing more than 20 μg/kg total aflatoxins can neither be used for human food or fed to dairy cows. Milk must contain less than 0.5 μg/kg aflatoxin M_1 (Van Egmond, 1989). Currently, the U.S. Food and Drug Administration (FDA) has set an advisory level for DON in finished products at 1 μg/g for humans and is considering whether advisory levels are needed for fumonisins and other toxins.

Decontamination treatments for mycotoxin contaminated products include physical removal of the affected food or portion of food; treatment of the food with chemicals, heat or radiation to decompose or change the toxin into chemically innocuous compounds; and biological removal of the toxin. A decontamination treatment must be economically feasible and meet the following criteria. An effective process must 1) inactivate, destroy or remove the toxin; 2) not produce or leave toxic residues in foods; and 3) not alter the food physically, organoleptically, or nutritionally (Beaver, 1991). Several excellent reviews exist on the effects of processing on mycotoxins in food (Scott, 1984; Patey and Gilbert, 1989; Charmley and Prelusky, 1993; Bennett and Richard, 1996). This chapter focuses on the effects of processing on *Fusarium* mycotoxins and includes a section on the fumonisins, a recently discovered mycotoxin found in corn-based foods.

3. EFFECT OF PROCESSING ON MYCOTOXINS

3.1. Trichothecenes

Fusarium and other mold species produce a diverse group of mycotoxins known as the trichothecenes. More than 80 different trichothecenes have been isolated and characterized and all possess similar antibiotic, antifungal and cytostatic activities (Prelusky et al., 1994). The trichothecenes are sesquiterpenoid compounds with a C12, C13 epoxy group (Figure 1). The trichothecenes include T-2 toxin, HT-2 toxin, diacetoxyscirpenol (DAS), neosolaniol, fusarenon-X, nivalenol (NIV) and deoxynivalenol (DON).

Types of agricultural products found to be contaminated with trichothecenes include grains and some fruits. Cool temperatures, high moisture and high humidity are believed to favor fungal colonization and trichothecene formation in food (Pestka and Casale,

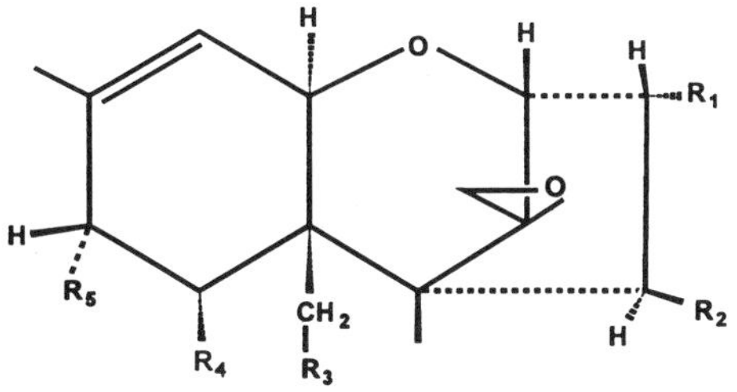

TYPE A

NAME	R_1	R_2	R_3	R_4	R_5
T-2 toxin	OH	OAc	OAc	H	$OCOCH_2CH(CH_3)_2$
HT-2 toxin	OH	OH	OAc	H	$OCOCH_2CH(CH_3)_2$
Neosolaniol	OH	OAc	OAc	H	OH
Diacetoxyscipenol	OH	OAc	OAc	H	H
T-2 tetraol	OH	OH	OH	H	OH
Acetyl T-2 toxin	OAc	OAc	OAc	H	$OCOCH_2CH(CH_3)_2$

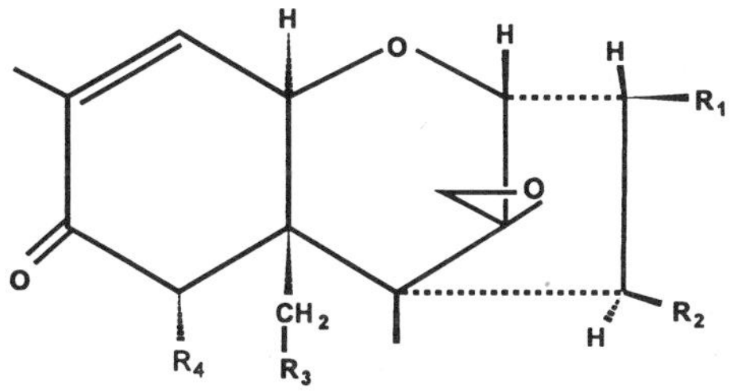

TYPE B

NAME	R_1	R_2	R_3	R_4
Nivalenol	OH	OH	OH	OH
Fusarenon-X	OH	OAc	OH	OH
Neosolaniol	OH	OAc	OAc	OH
Diacetylnivalenol	OH	OAc	OAc	OH
Deoxynivalenol	OH	H	OH	OH

Figure 1. Structures of trichothecenes.

1990). In the U.S. and Canada, the most common trichothecene contaminants in food are DON, otherwise known as vomitoxin, and NIV (Prelusky et al., 1994). Both toxins are produced by *Fusarium graminearum*, a fungal species that most commonly infects wheat, corn, rye and barley.

Biochemically, the trichothecenes are among the most potent inhibitors of protein synthesis in eukaryotic cells and have been shown to damage DNA both *in vitro* and *in vivo* (Sharma and Kim, 1991). The acute symptoms of trichothecene poisoning in humans and animals include skin irritation, feed refusal, vomiting, diarrhea, hemorrhages, neural disturbance, abortion and death (Prelusky et al., 1994; Coulombe, 1993). Given in sublethal doses, the trichothecenes are highly immunosuppresive in mammals (Pestka and Casale, 1990), and have been implicated in human mycotoxicoses in India (Bhat et al., 1989) and in China (Wang et al., 1993).

There have been surveys of trichothecene levels in grain products from the U.S. (Trucksess et al., 1995; Trigo-Stockli et al., 1995), Canada (Scott, 1997), Europe (Jelinek et al., 1989; Perkowski et al., 1990; Hietaniemi and Kumpulainen, 1991), South America (Pacin et al., 1997), and Asia (Luo et al., 1990). Advisory levels for DON exist for foods in the U.S. and Canada. The U.S. FDA has set an advisory level for DON in finished wheat products (e.g. flour, bran and germ) used for human consumption at 1μg/g (Trucksess et al., 1995). In Canada, the maximum level of DON permitted in uncleaned soft wheat destined for nonstaple foods is 2.0 μg/g. The maximum level of DON in wheat used as an ingredient in baby foods is 1.0 μg/g (Scott, 1997).

3.1.1. Physical Processing. Research on physical methods for removing trichothecenes in grain has focused on cleaning, dry and wet milling, and thermal processing (Table 1). Some methods for cleaning or removing contaminated kernels from untainted grain have been moderately successful. Tkachuk et al. (1991) used specific gravity to separate and remove shrunken, broken and severely sprouted wheat kernels from intact, undamaged kernels. They found that DON was highly concentrated in the least dense fractions (shrunken and broken kernels) and that the most dense fractions contained considerably less DON than unfractionated wheat. Using sieves to fractionate ground grain, Trenholm et al. (1991) found that removing fractions containing small particles (>+9 mesh for barley and wheat and >+16 mesh for corn) resulted in a 67–83% reduction of DON levels. Removing corn and wheat buoyant in water and in 30% sucrose decreased the DON present by 53–96% (Huff and Hagler, 1985). In contrast to these studies, Seitz et al. (1985) found that using screens and air flow was not an effective cleaning treatment, lowering DON levels in contaminated wheat by only 16%.

Trenholm et al. (1992) studied the use of washing steps to remove DON from contaminated grain. Washing barley and corn kernels contaminated with 16–24 μg DON/g three times in distilled water reduced DON levels by 65–69%. Stirring the kernels in 1 M sodium carbonate solution and then washing with water reduced DON by 72–74%. This method may be useful for decontaminating grain used in manufacturing processes that require the grain to be wetted or tempered before processing (Trenholm et al., 1992).

Microscopic analysis of wheat kernels infected with *Fusarium graminearum* has shown that although the fungus concentrates mainly in the tissues near the exterior of the kernel, hyphae can be found in the endosperm (Bechtel et al., 1985; Seitz and Bechtel, 1985). Consequently, although higher concentrations of DON and NIV are found in low-grade flour streams, they are still present in most refined flours (Scott et al, 1984; Young et al., 1984; Seitz et al., 1985; Seitz et al., 1986). Hart and Braselton (1983), Tanaka et al. (1986), Lee et al. (1987), Nowicki et al. (1988), and Trigo-Stockli et al. (1996) determined

Table 1. Physical methods for reducing the trichothecene content of food

Processing Method	Effect	Reference
Cleaning (specific gravity tables)	Reduced DON levels in naturally contaminated wheat (1.89–7.96 μg DON/g) by > 66%.	Tkachuk et al. (1991)
Cleaning (sieving)	Removal of small particles from sound grain (corn, wheat and barley) containing 5–23 μg DON/g reduced DON levels by 67–83%	Trenholm et al. (1991)
Cleaning (screening + air flow)	Reduced DON levels in naturally contaminated wheat (0.03–2.89 μg DON/g) by 16%.	Seitz et al. (1985)
Cleaning (density floatation)	Reduced DON levels in naturally contaminated wheat (0.60–2.4 μg DON/g) by 53–96%.	Huff and Hagler (1985)
Cleaning (water)	Reduced DON levels in barley and corn (16.1–23.9 μg DON/g) by 65–69%.	Trenholm et al. (1992)
Cleaning (sodium carbonate + water)	Reduced DON levels in barley and corn (16.1–23.9 μg DON/g) by 72–74%.	Trenholm et al. (1992)
Dry milling	Flour made from contaminated wheat contained 0–46% less DON than whole wheat; DON concentrated in bran and shorts fractions.	Hart and Braselton (1983); Young et al. (1984); Scott et al. (1984); Lee et al. (1987); Trigo-Stockli et al. (1996)
Dry milling	Wheat flour contained 20–69% less NIV than whole wheat; NIV concentrated in the bran fraction.	Lee et al. (1987)
Wet milling	Corn starch made from contaminated corn (20μg T-2 toxin/g) contained 92% less T-2 than corn from which it was derived.	Collins and Rosen (1981)
	High levels of NIV and DON were found in steep water while low levels were found in the corn solids (starch, germ, gluten and fiber).	Lauren and Ringrose (1997)
Baking	No appreciable losses of DON in bread baked (205°C/30 min or 350°C/2 min) from naturally contaminated wheat (1.4–7.5μg DON/g).	Scott et al. (1984); El-Banna et al. (1983)
	0-35% reduction in DON in cookies, bread and cake baked with DON contaminated flour	Tanaka et al. (1986); Young et al. (1984); Seitz et al. (1986); Boyacioglu et al. (1993)
Heating (dry)	No decomposition of pure DON, NIV, fusarenon-X, DAS, neosolaniol and T-2 toxin at 120°C for 45 min; Complete decomposition of these toxins at 210°C for 30 min	Kamimura et al. (1979)
Heating (1 h, 100°C)	No decomposition of fusarenon-X, DAS or T-2 toxin in aqueous solution	Kamimura et al. (1979)
Heating (100, 120 and 170°C; 0–60 min; pH 4, 7 and 10 buffer)	Stability of DON was greatest at pH 4 and least at pH 10. At pH 10, total loss of DON at 100°C for 60 min, 120°C for 30 min and 170°C for 15 min.	Wolf-Hall and Bullerman (1998)
Heating (microwave and convection)	50–90% loss of DON in corn contaminated with 1000 µg DON/g.	Young (1986a)
Cooking (boiling in water)	50–60% loss of DON in spaghetti and noodles during cooking	Nowicki et al. (1988)
Extrusion cooking	27–40% loss of DON in spiked corn grits; No loss of DON when spiked dog food (22% moisture) was extruded.	Wolf-Hall et al. (1998)
γ-irradiation	3–41% reduction in DON and T-2 toxin levels in soy and wheat irradiated at 5–20 kGy	Hooshmand and Klopfenstein (1995)

that 50–80% of DON and 30% of nivalenol in wheat carried over into the milled flour. The bran or shorts, which are used for animal feed, contained 2–3 times more DON and NIV than the original wheat.

Several researchers traced the trichothecene mycotoxins during a wet milling operation. Using a laboratory simulated process, Collins and Rosen (1981) found that 66% of T-2 toxin in corn was removed by the steep and process water, 4% was found in the starch, and approximately 30% was in the germ. Analyzing fractions from a commercial wet milling operation, Lauren and Ringrose (1997) found high concentrations of NIV and DON in steep water and low concentrations in the solid fractions of corn. Both studies suggest that contaminated corn may be converted to toxin-free starch.

Work has been done to determine the thermal stability of mycotoxins during food processing operations involving heat. Patey and Gilbert (1989) and Kamimura et al. (1979) found that DON, NIV, fusarenon-X, DAS, neosolaniol and T-2 toxin in crystalline form have high thermal stability. Kamimura et al. (1979) heated a mixture of trichothecenes (fusarenon-X, DAS, T-2 toxin) in water for 2 h at 100°C and in aqueous alkaline solutions. They found little decomposition of toxins when boiled in water for 1 h. However, the toxins were found to be relatively unstable in alkaline solutions (sodium hydroxide, sodium carbonate, sodium hydrogen carbonate, ammonia) even at room temperature. Wolf-Hall and Bullerman (1998) studied the effect of heat (100, 120 and 170°C) and pH (4.0, 7.0 and 10.0) on the stability of DON in aqueous buffer solutions over different time periods (15, 30 and 60 min). At pH 4.0, they found that DON was very stable with no loss at 100 or 120°C and only partial loss at 170°C after 60 min. At pH 7.0, they found that DON was still quite stable but that there was greater loss at 170°C after 15 min. At pH 10.0, it was found that DON was partially lost at 100°C after 60 min and totally lost at 120°C after 30 min and at 170°C after 15 min.

Although heating studies using purified toxins are useful for predicting potential decomposition, it is essential to study the effects of heat on toxins in food, since the physical environment can lead to enhanced or decreased thermal stability. Young et al. (1984) and Tanaka et al. (1986) found 0–35% reduction in DON and NIV levels in baked products not containing yeast (cookies and cakes). An unexpected result was the increase in DON levels during the preparation of yeast doughnuts (Young et al., 1984). The increase was explained by a biological conversion of precursors into DON. In contrast, El-Banna et al. (1983), Scott et al. (1983;1984), Seitz et al. (1986) and Boyacioglu et al. (1993) found no change in DON levels when naturally contaminated wheat was baked into a yeast-containing bread. In contrast to these studies, Young (1986a) reported that microwave and convection heating of naturally contaminated corn resulted in 50–90% reduction of DON levels. It is not known whether the reduction was due to true losses since percent recovery of DON was not measured. Wolf-Hall et al. (1998b) reported that up to 40% of DON was lost in a non-mixing extrusion process and up to 27% was lost in a mixing extrusion process using spiked corn grits. When a dog food extrusion mixture was spiked with DON and extruded at 22% moisture, no loss of DON was observed. Likewise no loss of DON was observed in canning processes for a mixed cereal infant food and a dog food that were spiked with DON. However, the canning of spiked cream style corn resulted in a 12% loss of DON. Nowicki et al. (1988) studied the retention of DON during the cooking of wheat spaghetti and Japanese and Chinese-style wheat noodles. Retention of DON in spaghetti and noodles ranged from 40–50%, with the remainder leaching into the cooking water. Few reports have been found on the effects of thermal processing of DON in corn or other food matrices or on other trichothecenes. In addition, little is known about the identity and the toxicity of decomposition products of the trichothecenes.

Hooshmand and Klopfenstein (1995) studied the effects of ionizing radiation on mycotoxin contaminated foods. At 5 and 7.5 kGy doses, DON and T-2 concentrations in soybeans and wheat, respectively decreased slightly (3–7%). Irradiation doses of 10 kGy, the maximum allowable dose for food products, destroyed 16% of T-2 toxin in wheat and 33% of DON in soybeans.

3.1.2 Chemical Processing. Chemical treatments that have been tested for their effectiveness in destroying trichothecene toxins in foods include sodium bisulfite, hydrogen peroxide, ascorbic acid, ammonium hydroxide, cysteine, hydrochloric acid, sodium hypochlorite, sulfur dioxide, ozone, chlorine, ammonia, and calcium hydroxide (Table 2). Studies by Young (1986a,b) and Young et al. (1986) have shown that levels of DON in contaminated grains can be reduced by at least 95% through treatment with sodium bisulfite. DON reacts with sodium bisulfite to form the 10-sulfonate adduct which is stable in acid but hydrolyzed to DON under alkaline conditions (Young, 1986b). In one feeding trial, a corn-based diet containing 7.2 mg DON/kg caused reductions in feed consumption and weight gain by pigs (Young et al., 1987). When the corn was autoclaved with sodium bisulfite, mixed with basal diet and fed to pigs, feed intake and body weight gain were improved compared with pigs fed untreated corn. Treatment with sodium bisulfite may not be suitable for direct application to human foods because it adversely affects the rheological properties of doughs made from the treated flour. In addition, DON-sulfonate is unstable in the presence of alkali and thereby hydrolyzed to the parent DON during some processing conditions. Young et al. (1987) suggests that bisulfite treatment may be useful for decontaminating DON tainted animal feeds.

Young et al. (1986) reported complete destruction of DON when corn containing 1000 μg/g DON was treated with 30% chlorine (v/v) for 30 min. However, bleaching wheat flour with chlorine in a commercial mill resulted in only a small (10%) reduction in DON levels (Young et al., 1984). Presumably the lack of destruction was due to the low levels of chlorine and relatively short contact times (Young, 1986a). Treatment of naturally contaminated field corn with moist and dry ozone achieved a 90% and 70% reduction of DON levels, respectively (Young, 1986a). Exposing corn to ammonia (100%) for at least 18 h resulted in substantial reductions (85%) in DON levels. Boiling DON contaminated corn in lime water (2%$Ca[OH]_2$) removed 72–82% of DON and 100% of 15-acetyl-DON (Abbas et al., 1988). Ascorbic acid, hydrochloric acid and ammonium hydroxide were moderately effective in reducing the DON levels (53–65%) in wheat.

3.1.3 Biological Processing. Little information exists on the effects of biological treatments on trichothecenes. Boswald et al. (1995) found that none of the tested strains of yeast *(Brettanomyces* spp., *Candida* Spp., *Hansunula anomala*, *Pichia* spp., *Kloeckera apiculata*, *Saccharomyces* spp., *Schizosaccaromyces* spp. and *Zygosaccharomyces rouxii*) metabolized DON.

3.2. Zearalenone

Zearalenone (ZEN; F-2 toxin) and related metabolites (Figure 2) are resorcylic lactones produced by several *Fusarium* species in corn, wheat, sorghum, barley, sesame meal, oats and hay grown throughout the world (Bennett et al., 1980). ZEN is often found in the U.S. and Canada in corn-based products such as breakfast cereals and cornmeal (CAST, 1989). ZEN is produced primarily by *F. graminearum* and occurs most notably in

Table 2. Chemical methods for reducing the trichothecene content of food

Reagent	Concentration	Food	Trichothecene	% loss of trichothecene	Reference
Ammonia	100%, 18 h	Corn (1000 μg DON/g)	DON	85	Young (1986a)
Ammonium hydroxide	5%	Wheat (1 μg DON/g)	DON	65	Young et al. (1986)
Ammonium phosphate, monobasic	1000 μg/g bread	Wheat bread (from wheat flour containing 3.13 μg DON/g)	DON	38	Boyacioglu et al. (1993)
Ascorbic acid	2%	Wheat (1 μg DON/g)	DON	53	Young et al. (1986)
	50 μg/g bread	Wheat bread (from wheat flour containing 3.13 μg DON/g)	DON	14	Boyacioglu et al. (1993)
	100 μg/g bread	Wheat bread (from wheat flour containing 3.13 μg DON/g)	DON	26	Boyacioglu et al. (1993)
Calcium hydroxide	2%	Corn (3.28–12.26 μg DON/g; 1.49–9.83 μg 15-acetyl-DON/g)	DON	72–82	Abbas et al. (1988)
			15-acetyl-DON	100	
Chlorine	30% v/v; 30 min	Corn (1000 μg DON/g)	DON	100	Young (1986a)
	0.1–0.5% w/w	Wheat flour (0.33 μg DON/g)	DON	0	Young et al. (1984)
Cysteine	10, 40, 90 μg/g	Wheat bread (from wheat flour containing 3.13 μg DON/g)	DON	40–44	Boyacioglu et al. (1993)
Hydrochloric acid	0.1 M	Wheat (1 μg DON/g)	DON	65	Young et al. (1986)
Hydrogen peroxide	5%	Wheat (1 μg DON/g)	DON	8	Young et al. (1986)
Ozone (moist)	1.1 mol%	Corn (1000 μg DON/g)	DON	90	Young (1986a)
Ozone (dry)	1.1 mol%	Corn (1000 μg DON/g)	DON	70	Young (1986a)
Potassium bromate	25 and 75 μg/g bread	Wheat bread (from wheat flour containing 3.13 μg DON/g)	DON	0	Boyacioglu et al. (1993)
Sodium bisulfite	10% SO_2	Wheat (1 μg DON/g)	DON	> 98%	Young et al. (1986)
	25 and 50 (μg/g bread)	Wheat bread (from wheat flour containing 3.13 μg DON/g)	DON	37–45%	Boyacioglu et al. (1993)
Sodium hydroxide	0.01 N	–	DAS and T-2 toxin	95%	Kamimura et al. (1979)
Sodium hypochlorite	1%	Wheat (1 μg DON/g)	DON	0	Young et al. (1986)

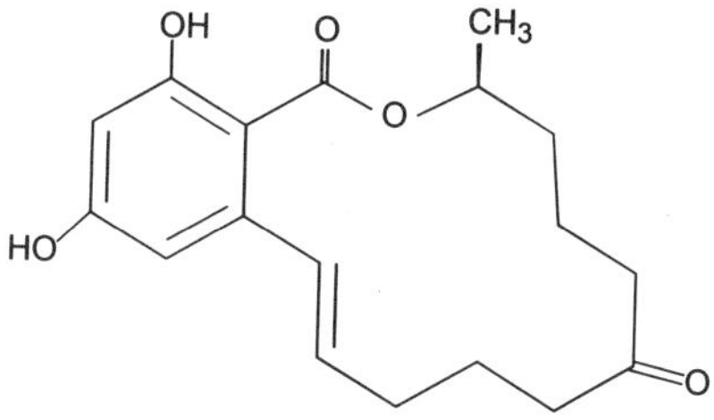

Figure 2. Structure of zearalenone.

high moisture grain at low temperatures. Frequently, ZEN contaminated grain also contains DON (Luo et al., 1990).

ZEN and related metabolites have been shown to have strong estrogenic effects in experimental animals and in humans (Kuiper-Goodman, 1994; Verdeal and Ryan, 1979). Field cases of ZEN-induced disorders in cattle, sheep and swine have been well documented (Allen et al., 1981; Meronuck et al., 1970; Miller et al., 1973). Responses in swine, one of the most sensitive species to ZEN, occurred when the ZEN levels in corn used for feeds exceeded 1 μg/g (Coulombe, 1993). Results of carcinogenicity assays in rats and mice were considered by the U.S. Department of Health and Human Services National Toxicology Program to demonstrate "positive evidence of carcinogenicity" (National Toxicity Program, 1982). It has been speculated that the high incidence of esophageal cancer in certain parts of the world may be due to ZEN in conjunction with other mycotoxins (e.g. trichothecenes, fumonisins) (Marasas et al., 1979).

Several investigations have been made on the ZEN content of agricultural products. In U.S. surveys, ZEN has been found to contaminate about 6% of corn; in Canada 9–29% of samples surveyed contained levels up to 141 μg/g (Pohland, 1993). In the U.S. or Canada, there are no regulations or guidelines with regard to ZEN levels in food or feed. Physical, chemical and biological treatments have been studied for removing ZEN in contaminated grains.

3.2.1. Physical Processing. Physical processes had varying success at removing ZEN from contaminated grain (Table 3). Using a commercial dehuller, Trenholm et al. (1991) reduced ZEN levels in barley, wheat and rye by 40–100%. Trenholm et al. (1991) also found that sieving out grain (barley, wheat or corn particles > +16 mesh) decreased the ZEN content by 67–83%. Density segregation has been effective at reducing ZEN levels in wheat. Huff and Hagler (1985) reported that removing wheat kernels buoyant in 30% sucrose solution produced wheat free of ZEN. Washing barley and corn kernels with distilled water reduced ZEN levels by 2–61% (Trenholm et al., 1992). Soaking barley and corn kernels in sodium carbonate (0.1–1.0 M) for 2–72 h resulted in 46–100% removal of ZEN in the contaminated grain (Trenholm et al. 1992).

Bennett et al. (1976), Lee et al. (1987), and Trigo-Stockli et al. (1996) determined that in the dry-milling process, ZEN concentrates in the germ and feed fractions of wheat and corn. Dry milling was not effective in removing all ZEN in grains, and the concentration of ZEN remaining in wheat flour was 30–90% (Lee et al., 1987; Tanaka et al., 1986). Bennett et al., (1976) found that wet milling was an effective method for salvaging ZEN contaminated corn. The starch fraction, the largest and most important for food purposes, was essentially free of ZEN. However, the germ and bran fractions, which are used as ani-

Table 3. Physical methods for reducing the ZEN content of food

Processing method	Effect	Reference
Dehulling	Reduced ZEN levels in barley and wheat (0.5–1.21 μg ZEN/g) by 40–100%	Trenholm et al. (1991)
Dry milling	Reduced ZEN levels in barley and wheat (0.5–1.21 μg ZEN/g) by 40–100%	Trenholm et al. (1991)
	Flour contained < 10% of the ZEN found in wheat (8 ng ZEN/g)	Tanaka et al. (1986)
	ZEN levels were highest in bran and lowest in flour	Trigo-Stockli et al. (1996)
	Reduced ZEN levels in wheat (2.05 μg ZEN/g) by 48–66%	Lee et al. (1987)
Wet milling	Produced ZEN-free starch; ZEN levels in the fractions were in the order of gluten> solubles> fiber> germ	Bennett et al. (1978)
Cleaning (density segregation)	Removing kernels buoyant in 30% sucrose produced ZEN-free wheat	Huff and Hagler (1985)
Cleaning (sieving)	Sieving out small particles from intact wheat, barley and corn kernels (0.5–1.21 μg ZEN/g) reduced ZEN levels by 67–83%	Trenholm et al. (1991)
Washing (water)	Reduced ZEN levels in corn (0.89–1.58 μg ZEN/g) by 2–61%	Trenholm et al. (1992)
Washing (sodium carbonate)	Reduced ZEN levels in corn (0.89–1.58 μg ZEN/g) by 80–87%	Trenholm et al. (1992)
Wet milling	Wet milling produced ZEN-free starch	Bennett et al. (1980)
Baking, (150°C/44h), (170°C/30 min)	No loss of purified ZEN or ZEN in corn	Bennett et al. (1980), Tanaka et al. (1986)
Extrusion cooking	65–83% loss of ZEN during extrusion cooking of spiked corn grits	Ryu et al. (1998)

mal feed contained much higher ZEN concentrations than the original corn. The distribution of ZEN in products from wet milling was in the order of gluten> solubles> fiber> germ (Bennett et al., 1978).

ZEN is a fairly heat resistant mycotoxin. Exposure to 150°C heat for 44 h did not cause degradation of pure ZEN or ZEN in ground corn (Bennett et al., 1980). In cake naturally contaminated with ZEN, no significant toxin reduction was observed after baking at 170°C for 30 min (Tanaka et al., 1986). However, Ryu et al. (1998) reported 65–83% losses of ZEN during extrusion cooking of spiked corn grits.

3.2.2. Chemical Processing. Several chemical treatments were studied for decreasing ZEN levels in contaminated corn (Table 4). Ammoniation had no effect on ZEN levels in yellow corn (Bennett et al., 1980) however, use of formaldehyde vapors, 3% ammonium hydroxide and ozone destroyed significant quantities of ZEN in naturally contaminated and spiked corn grits. Other chemical treatments such as use of propionic acid, acetic acid, hydrochloric acid, sodium bicarbonate and hydrogen peroxide were not effective treatments (Bennett et al., 1980). Abbas et al. (1988) studied the effects of the tortilla-making process on the stability of ZEN in naturally contaminated and spiked corn. The process involved boiling corn in lime ($Ca[OH]_2$) water, preparing a dough from the alkali treated corn, forming the dough into tortillas, and baking the tortillas at 110–120°C for 14–16 min. Losses ranged from 59–100% with the majority of ZEN removed with the lime water.

Table 4. Chemical methods for reducing ZEN levels in food

Reagent	Conditions	Food	% loss of ZEN	Reference
Propionic acid	3%; 3 days at room temperature	Corn grits (3–5 μg ZEN/g)	0	Bennett et al. (1980)
Acetic acid	3%; 3 days at room temperature	Corn grits (3–5 μg ZEN/g)	0	Bennett et al. (1980)
Hydrochloric acid	1.85%; 3 days at room temperature	Corn grits (3–5 μg ZEN/g)	0	Bennett et al. (1980)
Sodium bicarbonate	10%; 16 h at 50°C	Corn grits (3–5 μg ZEN/g)	0	Bennett et al. (1980)
Hydrogen peroxide	3%; 3 days at room temperature	Corn grits (3–5 μg ZEN/g)	0	Bennett et al. (1980)
Hydrogen peroxide	3%; 16 h at 50°C	Corn grits (3–5 μg ZEN/g)	0	Bennett et al. (1980)
Formaldehyde, solution	3.7%, 16 h at 50°C	Corn grits (3–5 μg ZEN/g)	100	Bennett et al. (1980)
Formaldehyde, vapor	10 days at room temperature	Corn grits (3–5 μg ZEN/g)	96	Bennett et al. (1980)
Ammonium hydroxide	3%, 16 h at 50°C	Corn grits (3–5 μg ZEN/g)	80	Bennett et al. (1980)
Calcium hydroxide	2%	Corn (0.23–4.23 μg ZEN/g)	59–100	Abbas et al. (1988)
Ozone	10%, 15 sec	—	100	McKenzie et al. (1997)

3.2.3. Biological Processing. The possible metabolism of ZEN by yeasts in beer and wine, or by yeasts responsible for contamination or spoilage of fermented foods and feeds was investigated by Boswald et al. (1995). They found that all of the yeasts tested (*Brettanomyces* spp., *Candida* spp., *Hansenula anomala*, *Pichia* spp., *Kloeckera apiculata*, *Saccharomyces* spp., *Schizosaccharomyces* spp. and *Zygosaccharomyces rouxii*) reduced ZEN to both α- and β-zearalenol, less toxic forms of the compound.

Okoye (1987) studied the effects of beer making on the ZEN levels in beer brewed with naturally contaminated corn. ZEN carryover into the finished product was 51%; 12% was removed with the discarded solid residue and the remainder was completely destroyed or not detected by the analytical method used. Bennett et al. (1981) reported that fermentation of ZEN contaminated corn by *Saccharomyces uvarum* resulted in toxin-free ethanol. However, the ZEN concentrated in the residual solids which made them unsuitable for animal feed.

3.3. Fumonisin

Fumonisins are mycotoxins that are produced primarily by *Fusarium moniliforme* and *F. proliferatum*, two common fungal contaminants of corn and other grains. Fumonisins are ubiquitous contaminants of corn and corn-based foods (Sydenham et al., 1991). Of the over eight different forms of fumonisin that have been characterized (Bezuidenhout et al., 1988; Branham and Plattner, 1993; Cawood et al., 1991; Plattner et al., 1992), fumonisin B_1 (FB_1), fumonisin B_2 (FB_2) and fumonisin B_3 (FB_3) are the major forms found in food (Figure 3). FB_1 is the diester of propane-1,2,3-tricarboxylic acid and 2-amino-12,16-dimethyl-3,5,10,14,15-pentahydroxyeicosane (Bezuidenhout et al., 1988). FB_2 and FB_3 contain one less hydroxyl group than FB_1 at the C-10 and C-5 positions, respectively. FB_1 also known as macrofusin, is the most abundant of the fumonisin family and usually accounts for about 60–70% of the total fumonisin content of *F. moniliforme* cultures and naturally contaminated foods (Ross et al., 1991). FB_2 and FB_3 represent between 30–40% and 1–5% of the fumonisins in food, respectively.

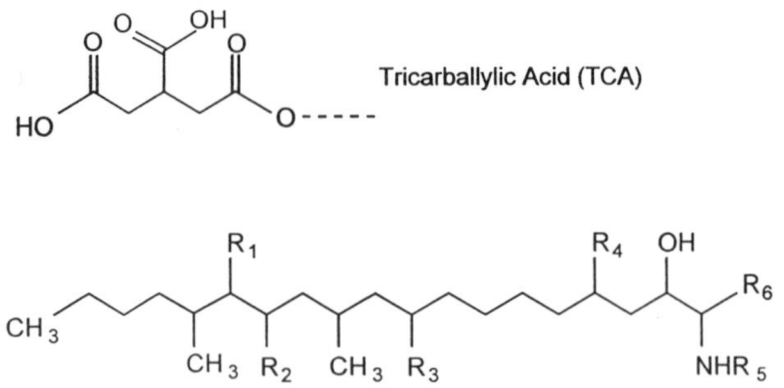

Tricarballylic Acid (TCA)

	R_1	R_2	R_3	R_4	R_5	R_6
FB_1	TCA	TCA	OH	OH	H	CH_3
FB_2	TCA	TCA	H	OH	H	CH_3
FB_3	TCA	TCA	OH	H	H	CH_3
FB_4	TCA	TCA	H	H	H	CH_3
FA_1	TCA	TCA	OH	OH	$COCH_3$	CH_3
FA_2	TCA	TCA	H	OH	$COCH_3$	CH_3
FA_3	TCA	TCA	OH	H	$COCH_3$	CH_3
FC_1	TCA	TCA	OH	OH	H	H

Figure 3. Structures of fumonisins.

Laboratory studies have shown that fumonisins can cause equine leukoencephalomalacia (Marasas et al., 1988; Wilson et al., 1992), porcine pulmonary edema (Harrison et al., 1990; Colvin et al., 1993), and liver cancer and toxicity in rats (Gelderblom et al., 1991). In humans, consumption of food containing *F. moniliforme* has been linked epidemiologically to the high incidence of esophageal cancer in some areas of the world (Sydenham et al., 1991; Rheeder et al., 1992). Because of their toxicity and widespread natural occurrence, the fumonisins are of public health concern. At present, no guidelines or regulations exist in the U.S. or Canada for fumonisin levels in corn.

3.3.1. Physical Processing. Table 5 lists the physical processes that have been studied for reducing fumonisin levels in food. Treatments such as sieving 'fines' from bulk shipments of corn have reduced fumonisin levels by 26–69% (Sydenham et al., 1994). Katta et al. (1997) reported that dry milling of fumonisin contaminated corn tended to concentrate the fumonisins in the bran and germ fractions and produced grits relatively free of contamination. Since many processed foods are made from flaking grits, this would explain the relatively low levels of fumonisins in these products. Preliminary work by Canela et al. (1996) has shown that steeping in water may reduce the fumonisin content of naturally contaminated corn.

The fumonisins are fairly heat stable compounds. Jackson et al. (1996a,b) and Alberts et al. (1990) found minor losses when aqueous solutions of FB_1 and FB_2 were heated at temperatures < 150°C. Similarly, Dupuy et al. (1993) found minimal losses of FB_1 in

Table 5. Physical methods for reducing the fumonisin content of food

Processing method	Effect	Reference
Dry milling	Fumonisins were found in the germ, bran and fines of corn; Flaking grits contained low levels of fumonisins.	Katta et al. (1997)
Wet milling	Wet milling produced fumonisin-free starch; Fumonisin levels in fractions were in the order of gluten>fiber>germ.	Bennett et al. (1996)
Cleaning (sieving)	Sieving out 'fines' from intact corn kernels (0.53–1.89 μg fumonisin/g) reduced fumonisin levels by 26–29%.	Sydenham et al. (1994)
Steeping (water; 0.3% sodium bisulfite)	Steeping corn kernels (0.53–2.32 μg fumonisin/g) in water or a solution of sodium bisulfite resulted in fumonisin in the steep solution.	Canela et al. (1996)
Heating (100–235°C; 0–60 min; pH 4, 7 and 10 buffer)	Overall, FB_1 and FB_2 were least stable at pH 4 followed by pH 10 and 7; Decomposition began at temperatures ≥ 150°C; Hydrolysis products of fumonisin were major decomposition products.	Jackson et al. (1996a,b)
Heating (50–150°C; 0–960 min)	Decomposition of FB_1 in dry corn (1530 μg FB_1/g) heated at 100–150°C followed first order kinetics.	Dupuy et al. (1993)
Heating (pasteurization)	Pasteurization at 62°C for 30 min had no effect on loss of FB_1 or FB_2 spiked into milk (50 ng/ml).	Maragos and Richard (1994)
Heating (190 and 220°C)	Heating moist corn meal at 190 (60 min) and 220°C (25 min) resulted in 40–100% loss of FB_1 and FB_2.	Scott and Lawrence (1994)
Extrusion cooking	Extruding corn grits spiked with 5 μg FB_1/g resulted in 34–95% loss of FB_1.	Katta et al. (1998)
Baking (175 and 200°C; 20 min)	Baking corn muffins (spiked with 5 μg FB_1/g) resulted in 16–28% loss of FB_1.	Jackson et al. (1997)
Baking (204 and 232°C; 20 min)	No significant loss of FB_1 at 204°C; 48% loss of FB_1 at 232°C.	Castelo et al. (1998)
Canning (121°C; 60 min)	9% loss of FB_1 during canning of spiked cream-style corn.	Castelo et al. (1998)
Roasting (dry heat; 218°C; 15 min)	Complete loss of FB_1 in corn meal (5 μg FB_1/g).	Castelo et al. (1998)
Frying (140–190°C; 0–15 min)	FB_1 began to degrade when corn chips were fried at temperatures ≥ 180°C and times ≥ 8 min.	Jackson et al. (1997)

naturally contaminated dry corn meal heated at temperatures < 125°C. Maragos and Richard (1994) found that heating whole milk spiked with FB_1 and FB_2 for 30 min at 62°C did not reduce levels of these toxins. Jackson et al. (1996 a,b) found that temperatures ≥ 150°C were required to observe decomposition of fumonisins in aqueous solutions. Decomposition products found in the thermally processed solutions were mainly hydrolysis products of FB_1. Scott and Lawrence (1994) found that heating moist corn meal at 190°C for 60 min resulted in approximately 80% reduction in FB_1 and FB_2 levels. Heating dry corn meal spiked with FB_1 and FB_2, at 190 (60 min) and 220°C (25 min) resulted in 60 and 100% loss of both toxins, respectively (Scott and Lawrence, 1994). Jackson et al. (1997) reported baking corn muffins at 175 and 200°C for 20 min resulted in 16% and 27% loss of FB_1, respectively. Castelo et al. (1998) round that baking corn muffins at 204°C for 20 min resulted in no significant loss of FB_1 whereas baking corn bread at 232°C for 20 min gave a 48% loss of FB_1. In contrast, Scott and Lawrence (1994) observed >70% reduction in FB_1 levels in corn muffins that were baked at 220°C for 25 min. Greater losses reported by Scott and Lawrence (1994) may be due to the higher baking temperatures, longer baking times and/or analytical problems that prevented accurate quantitation of fumonisins. Castelo et al. (1998) also found that canning spiked cream style corn resulted in a 9% loss of FB_1 and roasting (dry heating) spiked and naturally contaminated corn meal at 218°C for 15 min resulted in almost complete losses of FB_1. Jackson et al. (1997) reported that no significant losses of FB_1 were found when spiked corn masa was fried at 140–170°C for 0 to 6 min. However, FB_1 began to degrade at frying temperatures ≥ 180°C and times ≥ 8 min. Extrusion appears to be an effective method for reducing fumonisin levels in corn. Katta et al. (1998) found that losses of FB_1 spiked into corn grits increased as extrusion temperature (140–200°C) increased and screw speed (40–160 rpm) decreased. Losses of FB_1 ranged from 46–76% depending on extrusion conditions.

3.3.2. Chemical Processing. Very little is known about the effect of chemical treatments on fumonisins (Table 6). Norred et al. (1991) found that atmospheric pressure/ambient temperature ammoniation reduced the fumonisin content of *F. moniliforme* culture material but did not reduce the toxicity of the material when fed to rats. In contrast, Park et al. (1992) reported 79% reduction in fumonisin levels of corn after high-pressure/ambient temperature ammoniation followed by a low-pressure/high-temperature treatment. However, they did not measure the toxicity of the treated corn.

Survey by Sydenham et al. (1991) and Scott and Lawrence (1996) showed that corn products (masa, tortillas) from South America and the U.S. that were treated with lime water and heat had very low levels of fumonisins. Hendrich et al. (1993) and Sydenham et al. (1995a,b) reported that treating corn or culture material with lime water and heat, resulted in hydrolysis of FB_1 into the aminopentol backbone and tricarballylic acid. However, the treated corn and culture material were still toxic to rats (Hendrich et al., 1993; Voss et al., 1996).

McKenzie et al. (1997) found that treating an aqueous solution of FB_1 with 10% (w/w) ozone (O_3) gas for 15 sec resulted in the conversion of the parent compound to the 3-keto FB_1 (3k-FB_1) derivative. In two separate toxicity tests, 3k-FB_1 was found to retain most of the toxicity present in the parent compound. Consequently, O_3 treatment is not an effective method for detoxifying FB_1.

Reports by Murphy et al. (1996) and Lu et al. (1997) suggest that a combination of chemical and thermal treatment may reduce fumonisin levels in food. Murphy et al. (1996) reported that in a model system, fumonisins participated in a non-enzymatic browning reaction that appeared to detoxify these compounds. Murphy et al. (1996) found that heating (80°C; 48 h) 100 mM fructose or glucose with 5 μg/ml (6.93 μM) FB_1 in pH 7.0 buffer resulted in an first-order rate loss of FB_1. At present, the FB_1-sugar product(s) have not been identified and it is not known if the FB_1-sugar reaction occurs in thermally processed food or if the reaction can be enhanced through the addition of reducing sugars to fumonisin contaminated food. Work done by Jackson et al. (unpublished data) suggests the browning reaction involving FB_1 does occur in food. Adding glucose to corn masa dough before frying at 180°C for 8 min resulted in reduction of fumonisin levels by several fold.

3.3.3. Biological Processing. Very little is known about the effects of biological processing on fumonisins. Scott et al. (1995) determined the stability of FB_1 and FB_2 dur-

Table 6. Chemical methods for reducing fumonisin levels in food

Treatment	Conditions	Food	% loss of fumonisins	Reference
Ammoniation	2% ammonia, 15% moisture, 20°C, 60 psi, 60 min	Ground corn	79%	Park et al. (1992)
	2% ammonia, 50°C, 4 days	Ground corn	45%	Norred et al. (1991)
Nixtamalization	1.2% $Ca[OH]_2$; 80–100°C; 1 h	Ground corn	100%[1]	Hendrich et al. (1993)
	0.1 M $Ca[OH]_2$; ambient temperature	Ground corn	>80%[1]	Sydenham et al. (1995)
Ozone	10%, 15 sec	—[2]	100%[3]	McKenzie et al. (1997)
Sugar + heat	fructose; 80°C; 48 h	—	>95%	Murphy et al. (1996) Lu et al. (1997)

[1]Formed amino pentol backbone of FB_1
[2]Aqueous model system
[3]Degradation products of FB_1 remained toxic

ing the beer making process. Both toxins, which were spiked into the wort, were fairly stable in the fermentation process. Similarly, little degradation of FB_1 was found in a 3-day yeast fermentation of corn (Bothast et al., 1992).

4. CONCLUSIONS

Mycotoxin contamination of food will remain a global problem in the foreseeable future. Consequently, continued efforts will be made to reduce mycotoxin levels in food through processing. Although a number of effective processes have been developed, no single method can remove all toxins from food. More work is needed to develop a method for eliminating a variety of mycotoxins simultaneously. In addition, more research is needed to determine the effects of processing on other *Fusarium* mycotoxins, especially moniliformin. Finally, more work is needed to identify and determine toxicological effects of products resulting from physical decomposition or chemical modification of mycotoxins.

ACKNOWLEDGMENTS

This publication was partially supported by a cooperative agreement no. FD-000431 from the U.S. Food and Drug Administration and the National Center for Food Safety and Technology. Its contents are solely the opinions of the authors, and do not necessarily represent official views of the U.S. Food and Drug Administration.

REFERENCES

Abbas, H.K.; Mirocha, C.J.; Rosiles, R.; Carvajal, M. Decomposition of zearalenone and deoxynivalenol in the process of making tortillas from corn. *Cereal Chem.* **1988**, *65*, 15–19.

Alberts, J.F.; Gelderblom, W.C.A.; Thiel, P.G.; Marasas, W.F.O.; van Schalwyk, D.J.;

Behrend, Y. Effects of temperature and incubation period on production of fumonisin B_1 by *Fusarium moniliforme. Appl. Environ. Microbiol.* **1990**, 56, 1729–1733.

Allen, N.K.; Mirocha, C.J.; Aakus-Allen, S.; Bitgood, J.J.; Weaver, G.; Bates, F. Effect of dietary zearalenone on reproduction of chickens. *Poult. Sci.* **1981**, *60*, 1165–1174.

Beaver, R.W. Decontamination of mycotoxin-containing foods and feedstuffs. *Trends in Food Sci. and Technol.* **1991**, 170–173.

Bechtel, D.B.; Kaleikau, L.A.; Gaines, R.L.; Seitz, L.M. The effects of *Fusarium graminearum* infection on wheat kernels. *Cereal Chem.* **1985**, 62, 191–197.

Bennett, G.A.; Richard, J.L. Influence of processing on *Fusarium* mycotoxins in contaminated grains. *Food Technol.* **1996**, 50, 235–238.

Bennett, G.A.; Peplinski, A.J.; Brekke, O.L.; Jackson, L.K. Zearalenone: Distribution in dry-milled fractions of contaminated corn. *Cereal Chem.* **1976**, 53, 299–307.

Bennett, G.A.; Vandegraft, E.E.; Shotwell, O.L.; Watson, S.A.; Bocan, B.J. Zearalenone distribution in wet-milling fractions from contaminated corn. *Cereal Chem.* **1978**, 55, 455–461.

Bennett, G.A.; Shotwell, O.L.; Hesseltine, C.W. Destruction of zearalenone in contaminated corn. *J. AOAC Int.* **1980**, 57, 245–247.

Bennett, G.A.; Lagoda, A.A.; Shotwell, O.L.; Hesseltine, C.W. Utilization of zearalenone-contaminated corn for ethanol production. *J. Am. Oil Chem. Soc.* **1981**, 58, 974–976.

Bezuidenhout, S.C.; Gelderblom, W.C.A.; Spiteller, G.; Vleggaar, R. Structure elucidation of the fumonisins, mycotoxins from *Fusarium moniliforme. J. Chem. Soc. Chem. Commun.* **1988**, 743–745.

Bhat, R.V.; Beedu, S.R.; Ramakrishna, Y.; Munshi, K.L. Outbreak of trichothecene mycotoxicosis associated with consumption of mould-damaged wheat products in Kashmir valley, India. *The Lancet*, **1989**, 1, 35–37.

Boswald, C.; Engelhardt, G.; Vogel, H.; Wallnofer, P.R. Metabolism of the Fusarium mycotoxins zearalenone and deoxynivalenol by yeast strains of technological relevance. *Natural Toxins* **1995**, 3, 138–144.

Bothast, R.J.; Bennett, G.A.; Vancauwenberge, J.E.; Richard, J.L. Fate of fumonisin B_1 in naturally contaminated corn during ethanol fermentation. *Appl. Environ. Microbiol.* **1992**, 58, 233–236.

Boyacioglu, D.; Hettiarachchy, N.S.; D'appolonia, B.L. Additives affect deoxynivalenol (vomitoxin) flour during breadmaking. *J. Food Sci.* **1993**, 58, 416–418.

Branham, B.E.; Plattner, R.D. Isolation and characterization of a new fumonisin from liquid cultures of *Fusarium moniliforme. J. Nat. Prod.* **1993**, *56*, 1630–1633.

Canela, R.; Pujol, R.; Sala, N.; Sanchis, V. Fate of fumonisins B_1 and B_2 in steeped corn kernels. *Food Add. Contamin.*, **1996**, *13*, 511–517.

CAST. Mycotoxins: Economic and Health Risks. Council for Agricultural Science and Technology, Report 116, 1989.

Castelo, M.M.; Sumner, S.S.; Bullerman, L.B. Stability of fumonisins in thermally processed corn products. *J. Food Prot.* **1998**, In Press

Cawood, M.E.; Gelderblom, W.C.A.; Veggaar, R.; Behrend, Y.; Thiel, P.G.; Marasas, W.F.O. Isolation of the fumonisin mycotoxins: A quantitative approach. *J. Agric. Food Chem.* **1991**, *39*, 1958–1962.

Charmley, L.L.; Prelusky, D.B. Decontamination of *Fusarium* mycotoxins. In "Mycotoxins in Grain," Miller, J.D.; Trenholm, H.L. (Eds.), Eagan Press, St. Paul, MN 1994, pp. 421–435.

Collins, G.J. and Rosen, J.D. Distribution of T-2 toxin in wet-milled corn products. *J. Food Sci.* **1981**, 46, 877–879.

Colvin, B.M.; Cooley, A.J.; Beaver, R.W. Fumonisin toxicosis in swine: clinical and pathologic findings. *J. Vet. Diagn. Invest.* **1993**, 5, 232–241.

Coulombe, R.A. Biological action of mycotoxins. *J. Dairy Sci.* **1993**, 76, 880–891.

Dupuy, J.; Le Bars, P.; Boudra, H.; Le Bars, J. Thermostability of fumonisin B_1, a mycotoxin from *Fusarium moniliforme*, in corn. *Appl. Environ. Microbiol.* **1993**, *59*, 2864–2867.

El-Banna, A.; Lau, P.-Y.; Scott, P.M. Fate of mycotoxins during processing of food stuffs. II Deoxynivalenol (vomitoxin) during making of Egyptian bread. *J. Food Protect.* **1983**, 46, 484–484.

Gelderblom, W.C.A.; Kriek, N.P.J.; Marasas, W.F.O.; Thiel, P.G. Toxicity and carcinogenicity of the *F. moniliforme* metabolite, FB_1, in rats. *Appl. Environ. Microbiol.* **1991**, *12*, 1247–1251.

Harrison, L.R.; Colvin, B.M.; Greene, T.J.; Newman, L.E.; Cole, R.J. Pulmonary edema and hydrothorax in swine produced by fumonisin B_1, a toxic metabolite of *Fusarium moniliforme. J. Vet. Diag. Invest.* **1990**, *2*, 217–221.

Hart, L.P.; Braselton, W.E. Distribution of vomitoxin in dry milled fractions of wheat infected with *Gibberella zeae. J. Agric. Food Chem.* **1983**, 31, 657–659.

Hendrich, S; Miller, K.A.; Wilson, T.M.; Murphy, P.A. Toxicity of *Fusarium proliferatum*-fermented nixtamilized corn-based diets fed to rats: effect of nutritional status. *J. Agric. Food Chem.* **1993**, *41*, 1649–1654.

Hietaniemi, V.; Kumpulainen, J. Contents of *Fusarium* toxins in Finnish and imported grains and feeds. *Food Add. Contamin.* **1991**, 8, 171–182.

Hooshmand, H.; Klopfenstein, C.F. Effects of gamma irradiation on mycotoxin disappearance and amino acid contents f corn, wheat, and soybeans with different moisture contents. *Plant Foods for Human Nutrition* **1995**, 47, 227–238.

Huff, W.E.; Hagler, W.M. Density segregation of corn and wheat naturally contaminated with aflatoxin, deoxynivalenol and zearalenone. *J. Food Protection* **1985**, 48, 416–420.

Jackson, L. S.; Hlywka, J. J.; Senthil, K. R.; Bullerman, L. B.; Musser, S.M. Effects of time, temperature, and pH on the stability of fumonisin B_1 in an aqueous model system. *J. Agric. Food Chem.* **1996a**, *44*, 906–912.

Jackson, L.S.; Hlywka, J.J.; Senthil, K.R.; Bullerman, L.B. Effects of thermal processing on the stability of fumonisin B_2 in an aqueous system. *J. Agric. Food Chem.* **1996b**, *44*, 1984–1987.

Jackson, L.S.; Katta, S.K.; Fingerhut, D.D.; DeVries, J.W.; L.B. Bullerman. Effects of baking and frying the fumonisin B_1 content of corn-based foods. *J. Agric. Food Chem.* **1997**, 45, 4800–4805.

Jelinek, C.E.; Pohland, A.E.; Wood, G.E. Worldwide occurrence of mycotoxins in foods and feeds. *J. Assoc. Off. Anal. Chem.* **1989**, 72, 223–230.

Kamimura, H.; Nishijima, M.; Sait, K.; Yasuda, K.; Ibe, A.; Nagayama, T.; Ushiyama, T.; Naoi, Y. The decomposition of trichothecene mycotoxins during food processing. *J. Fd. Hyg. Soc., Japan* **1979**, 20, 352–357.

Katta, S.K.; Cagampang, A.E.; Jackson, L.S; L.B. Bullerman. Distribution of Fusarium molds and fumonisins in dry-milled corn fractions. *Cereal Chem.* **1997**, 74, 858–863.

Katta, S.K.; Jackson, L.S.; Hanna, M.A.; Bullerman., L.B. Screw speed and temperature effects on the stability of fumonisin B_1 (FB_1) in extrusion cooked corn grits. *Cereal Chem.* **1998**, Submitted for publication.

Kuiper-Goodman, T. Prevention of human mycotoxicosis through risk assessment and risk management. In "Mycotoxins in Grain," Miller, J.D.; Trenholm, H.L. (Eds.), Eagan Press, St. Paul, MN 1994, pp. 439–469.

Lauren, D.R.; Ringrose, M.A. Determination of the fate of three *Fusarium* mycotoxins through wet-milling of maize using an improved HPLC analytical technique. *Food Add. Contamin.* **1997**, 14, 435–443.

Lee, U.-S.; Jang, H.-S.; Tanaka, T.; Oh, Y.-J.; Cho, C.-M.; Ueno, Y. Effect of milling on decontamination of Fusarium mycotoxins nivalenol, deoxynivalenol, and zearalenone in Korean wheat. *J. Agric. Food Chem.* **1987**, 35, 126–129.

Lu, Z.; Dantzer, W.R.; Hopmans, E.C.; Prisk, V.; Cunnick, J.E.; Murphy, P.A.; Hendrich, S. Reaction with fructose detoxifies fumonisin B_1 while stimulating liver-associated natural killer cell activity in rats. *J. Agric. Food Chem.* **1997**, 45, 803–809.

Luo, Y.; Yoshizawa, T.; Yatayama, T. Comparative study on the natural occurrence of *Fusarium* mycotoxins (trichothecenes and zearalenone) in corn and wheat from high-and low-risk areas for human esophageal cancer in China. *Environ. Microbiol.* **1990**, 56, 3723.

Mannon, J.; Johnson, E. Fungi on the farm. *New Sci.* **1985**, 105, 12–16.

Maragos, C.M.; Richard, J.L. Quantitation and stability of fumonisins B_1 and B_2 in milk. *J. AOAC Int.* **1994**, *77*, 1162–1167.

Marasas, W.F.O., Van Rensburg, S.; Mirocha, C. Incidence of *Fusarium* species and mycotoxins deoxynivalenol and zearalenone in corn produced in esophageal cancer areas in the Transkei. *J. Agric. Food Chem.* **1979**, 27, 1108–1112.

Marasas, W.F.O.; Kellerman, T.S.; Gelderblom, W.C.A.;Coetzer, J.A.W.; Thiel, P.T.; van der Lugt, J.J. Leukoencephalomalacia in a horse induced by fumonisin B_1 isolated from *Fusarium moniliforme*. *Onderstepoort J. Vet. Res.* **1988**, 55, 197–203.

McKenzie, K.S.; Sarr, A.B.; Mayura, K.; Bailey, R.H.; Miller, D.R.; Rogers, T.D.; Norred, W.P.; Voss, K.A.; Plattner, R.D.; Kubena, L.F.; Phillips, T.D. Oxidative degradation and detoxification of mycotoxins using a novel source of ozone. *Food Chem. Toxicol.* **1997**, 35, 807–820.

Meronuck, R.A.; Garren, K.H.; Christensen, C.M.; Nelson, G.H.; Bates, F. Effects of turkey poults and chicks of rations containing corn invaded by *Penicillium* and *Fusarium* species. *Am. J. Vet. Res.* **1970**, 31, 551–555.

Miller, J.K.; Hacking, A.; Harrison, J. Gross, V.J. Stillbirths, neonatal mortality, and small litters in pigs associated with the ingestion of *Fusarium* toxin by pregnant sows. *Vet. Rec.* **1973**, 93, 555–559.

Murphy, P.A.; Hendrich, S.; Hopmans, E.C.; Hauck, C.C.; Lu, Z.; Buseman, G.; Munkvold, G. Effect of processing on fumonisin content of food. In "*Fumonisins in Food*," Jackson, L.S.; DeVries, J.W.; Bullerman, L.B. (Eds.), Plenum Press, NY, NY, 1996, pp. 323–334.

Nowicki, T.W.; Gaba, D.G.; Dexter, J.E.; Matsuo, R.R.; Clear, R.M. Retention of the *Fusarium* mycotoxin deoxynivalenol in hweat during processing and cooking of spaghetti and noodles. *J. Cereal Sci.* **1988**, 8, 189–202.

Norred, W.P.; Voss, K.A.; Bacon, C.W.; Riley, R.T. Effectiveness of ammonia treatment in detoxification of fumonisin-contaminated corn. *Food Chem. Toxicol.* **1991**, *29*, 815–819.

NTP (National Toxicology Program) Carcinogenesis Bioassay of Zearalenone in F344/N Rats and B6C3F1 Mice. NTP, Technical Report Series No. 235, Department of Health and Human Services, Research Park, NC 1982.

Okoye, Z.S.C. Stability of zearalenone in naturally contaminated corn during Nigerian traditional brewing. *Food Add. and Contamin.* **1987**, 4, 57–59.

Pacin, A.M.; Resnik, S.L.; Neira, M.S.; Molto, G.; Martinez, E. Natural occurrence of deoxynivalenol in wheat, wheat flour and bakery products in Argentina. *Food Add.Contamin.* **1997**, 14, 327–331.

Park, D.L.; Rua, S.M., Jr.; Mirocha, C.J.; Abd-Alla, E.S.A.M.; Weng, C.Y. Mutagenic potentials of fumonisin contaminated corn following ammonia decontamination procedure. *Mycopathologia* **1992**, *117*, 105–108.

Paster, N.; Bullerman, L.B. Mould spoilage and mycotoxin formation in grains as controlled by physical means. *Int. J. Food Micr.* **1988**, 7, 257–265.

Patey, A.L.; Gilbert, J. Fate of Fusarium mycotoxins in cereals during food processing and methods for their detoxification. In "Fusarium: Mycotoxins, Taxonomy and Pathogenicity," Chelkowski, J. (Ed.), Elsevier, Amsterdam 1989, pp. 299–420.

Perkowski, J.; Plattner, R.D.; Golinski, P.; Vesonder, R.F.; Chelkowski, J. Natural occurrence of deoxynivalenol, 3-acetyldeoxynivalenol, 15-acetyl deoxynivalenol, nivalenol, 4,7-dideoxynivalenol and zearalenone in Polish wheat. *Mycotoxin Res.* **1990**, 6, 7–12.

Pestka, J.J.; Casale, W.L. Naturally occurring fungal toxins. In "Food Contamination from Environmental Sources," J.O. Nriagu and M.S. Simmons (Eds), J Wiley, NY, NY 1990, pp 613–638.

Plattner, R.D.; Weisleder, D.; Shackelford, D.D.; Peterson, R.; Powell, R.G. A new fumonisin from solid cultures of *Fusarium moniliforme*. *Mycopathologia*, **1992**, *117*, 23–28.

Pohland, A.E. Mycotoxins in review. *Food Add Contamin.* **1993**, 10, 17–28.

Prelusky, D.B.; Rotter, B.A.; Rotter, R.G. Toxicology of mycotoxins. In "Mycotoxins in Grain," Miller, J.D.; Trenholm, H.L. (Eds.), Eagan Press, St. Paul, MN 1994, pp. 359–403.

Rheeder, J.P.; Marasas, W.F.O.; Thiel, P.G.; Sydenham, E.W.; Shephard, G.S.; Van Schalkwyk, D.J. *Fusarium moniliforme* and fumonisins in corn in relation to human esophageal cancer in Transkei. *Phytopath.* **1992**, *82*, 353–357.

Ross, P.F.; Rice, L.G.; Plattner, R.D.; Osweiller, G.D.; Wilson, T.M.; Owens, D.L.; Nelson, H.A.; Richard, J.L. Concentrations of fumonisin B_1 in feeds associated with animal health problems. *Mycologia* **1991**, *114*, 129–135.

Ryu, D.; Hanna, M.A.; Bullerman, L.B. The effect of extrusion on the stability of zearalenone. *J. Food Prot.* **1998**, In Press

Scott, P.M. Effects of food processing on mycotoxins. *J. Food Protect.* **1984**, 47, 489–499.

Scott, P.M. Multi-year monitoring of Canadian grains and grain-based foods for trichothecenes and zearalenone. *Food Add. Contamin.*, **1997**, 14, 333–339.

Scott, P.M.; Lawrence, G.A. Stability and problems in recovery of fumonisins added to corn-based foods. *J. AOAC Int.* **1994**, *77*, 541–545.

Scott, P.M.; Lawrence, G.A. Determination of hydrolyzed fumonisin B_1 in alkali-processed corn foods. *Food Add. Contamin.* **1996**, 13, 823–832.

Scott, P.M.; Kanhere, S.R.; Lau, P.-Y.; Dexter, J.E.; Greenhalgh, R. Effects of experimental flour milling and breadbaking n retention of deoxynivalenol (vomitoxin) in hard red spring wheat. *Cereal Chem.* **1983**, 60, 421–424.

Scott, P.M.; Kanhere, S.R.; Dexter, J.E.; Brennan, P.W.; Trenholm, H.L. Distribution of the trichothecene mycotoxin deoxynivalenol (vomitoxin) during the milling of naturally contaminated hard red spring wheat and its fate in baked products. *Food Add. Contam.* **1984**, 1, 313–323.

Scott, P.M.; Kanhere, S.R.; Lawrence, G.A.; Daley, E.F.; Farber, J.M. Fermentation of wort containing added ochratoxin A and fumonisins B_1 and B_2. *Food Addit. Contamin.* **1995**, 12, 31–40.

Seitz L.M.; Eustace, W.D.; Mohr, H.E.; Shogren, M.D.; Yamazaki, W.T. Cleaning, milling and baking tests with hard red winter wheat containing deoxynivalenol. *Cereal Chem.* **1986**, 63, 146–160.

Seitz, L.M; Bechtel, D.B. Chemical, physical and microscopical studies of scab-infected hard red winter wheat. *J. Agric. Food Chem.* **1985**, 33, 373–377.

Seitz, L.M.; Yamazaki, W.T.; Clements, R.L.; Mohr, H.E.; Andrews, L. Distribution of deoxynivalenol in soft wheat mill streams. *Cereal Chem.* **1985**, 62, 467–469.

Sharma, R.P.; Kim, Y.-W. Trichothecenes. In "Mycotoxins and Phytoalexins," Sharma, R.P.; Salunkhe, D.K., (Eds.), CRC Press, Boca Raton, FL 1991, pp. 339–359.

Sydenham, E.W.; Thiel, P.G.; Shephard, G.S.; Koch, K.R.; Hutton, T. Preparation and isolation of the partially hydrolyzed moiety of fumonisin B_1. *J. Agric. Food Chem.* **1995**, 43, 2400–2405.

Sydenham, E.W.; Stockenstrom, S.; Thiel, P.G.; Shephard G.S.; Koch, K.R.; Marasas, W.F.O. Potential of alkaline hydrolysis for the removal of fumonisins from contaminated corn. *J. Agric. Food Chem.* **1995**, 43, 1198–1201.

Sydenham, E.W.; Van der Westhuizen, L.; Stockenstrom, S.; Shephard, G.S.; Thiel, P.G. Fumonisin-contaminated maise: physical treatment for the partial decontamination of bulk shipments. *Food Addit. Contam.* **1994**, *11*, 25–32.

Sydenham, E.W.; Shephard, G.S.; Thiel, P.G.; Marasas, W.F.O.; Stockenstrom, S. Fumonisin contamination of commercial corn-based human foodstuffs. *J. Agric. Food Chem.* **1991**, 39, 2014–2018.

Tanaka, T.; Hasegawa, A.; Yamamoto, S.; Matsuki, Y.; Ueno, Y. Residues of Fusarium mycotoxins, nivalenol, deoxynivalenol and zearalenone, in wheat and processed food after milling and baking. *J. Food Hyg. Soc. Japan* **1986**, 27, 653–655.

Tkachuk, R.; Dexter, J.E.; Tipples, K.H.; Nowicki, T.W. Removal by specific gravity table of tombstone kernels and associated trichothecenes from wheat infected with *Fusarium* head blight. *Cereal Chem.* **1991**, 68, 428–431.

Trenholm, H.L.; Charmley, L.L.; Prelusky, D.B.; Warner, R.M. Two physical methods for the decontamination of four cereals contaminated with deoxynivalenol and zearalenone. *J. Agric. Food Chem.* **1991**, 39, 356–360.

Trenholm, H.L.; Charmley, L.L.; Prelusky, D.B.; Warner, R.M. Washing procedures using water or sodium carbonate solutions for the decontamination of three cereals contaminated with deoxynivalenol and zearalenone. *J. Agric. Food Chem.* **1992**, 40, 2147–2151.

Trigo-Stockli, D.M.; Curran, S.P.; Pedersen, J.R. Distribution and occurrence of mycotoxins in 1993 Kansas wheat. *Cereal Chem.* **1995**, 72, 470–474.

Trigo-Stockli, D.M.; Keyoe, C.W.; Satumbaga, R.F.; Pedersen, J.R. Distribution of deoxynivalenol and zearalenone in milled fractions of wheat. *Cereal Chem.* **1996**, 73, 388–391.

Trucksess, M.A.; Thomas, F.; Young, K., Stack, M.E.; Fulgueras, W.J.; Page, S.W. Survey of deoxynivalenol in US 1993 wheat and barley crops by enzyme-linked immunosorbent assay. *J. AOAC Int*, **1995**, 78, 631–636.

Van Egmond, H.P. Current situation on regulations for mycotoxins. Overview of tolerances and status of standard methods of sampling and analysis. *Food Add.Contamin.* **1989**, 139–188.

Verdeal, K.; Ryan, D.S. Naturally-occurring estrogens in plant foodstuffs- A review. *J. Food Protect.* **1979**, 42:577–583.

Voss, K.A.; Bacon, C.W.; Meredith, F.I.; Norred, W.P. Comparative subchronic toxicity studies of nixtamalized and water-extracted *Fusarium moniliforme* culture material. *Food Chem. Toxicol.* **1996**, *34*, 623–632.

Wang, Z.-G.,; Feng, J.-N.; Tong, Z. Human toxicosis caused by mouldy rice contaminated with *Fusarium* and T-2 toxin. *Biomedical and Environmental Sciences.* **1993**, 6, 65–70.

Wilson, T.M.; Ross, P.R.; Owens, D.L.; Rice, L.G.; Green, S.A.; Jenkins, S.J.; Nelson, H.A. Experimental reproduction of ELEM. *Mycopathologia* **1992**, *117*, 115–120.

Wolf-Hall, C.E.; Bullerman, L.B. Heat and pH alter the concentration of deoxynivalenol in an aqueous environment. *J. Food Prot.* **1998a**, In Press.

Wolf-Hall, C.E.; Hanna, M.A.; Bullerman, L.B. Stability of deoxynivalenol during extrusion cooking. J. Food Prot. **1998b**, In Press.

Young, J.C. Reduction in levels of deoxynivalenol in contaminated corn by chemical and physical treatment. *J. Agric. Food Chem.* **1986a**, 34, 465–467.

Young, J.C. Formation of sodium bisulfite addition products with trichothecenes and alkaline hydrolysis of deoxynivalenol and its sulfonate. *J. Agric. Food Chem.* **1986b**, 34, 919–923.

Young, J.C.; Fulcher, R.G.; Hayhoe, J.H.; Scott, P.M.; Dexter, J.E. Effect of milling and baking on deoxynivalenol (vomitoxin) content of Eastern Canadian wheats. *J. Agric. Food Chem.* **1984**, 32,659–664.

Young, J.C.; Subrayan, L.M; Potts, D.; McLaren, M.E.; Gobran, F.H. Reduction in levels of deoxynivalenol in contaminated wheat by chemical and physical treatment. *J. Agric. Food Chem.* **1986**, 34, 461–465.

Young, J.C.; Trenholm, H.L.,; Friend, D.W.; Prelusky, D.B. Detoxification of deoxynivalenol with sodium bisulfite and evaluation of the effects when pure mycotoxin or contaminated corn was treated and given to pigs. *J. Agric. Food Chem.* **1987**, 35, 259–261.

INDEX